Molecular Biology of Colorectal Cancers

Molecular Biology of Colorectal Cancers

Editors

María Jesús Fernández Aceñero
Rodrigo Barderas Manchado
Javier Martínez Useros
Cristina Díaz del Arco

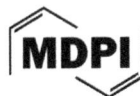

Basel • Beijing • Wuhan • Barcelona • Belgrade • Novi Sad • Cluj • Manchester

Editors

María Jesús Fernández Aceñero
Universidad Complutense de Madrid
Madrid
Spain

Rodrigo Barderas Manchado
Instituto de Salud Carlos III
Madrid
Spain

Javier Martínez Useros
Rey Juan Carlos University
Madrid
Spain

Cristina Díaz del Arco
Hospital Clínico Universitario San Carlos
Madrid
Spain

Editorial Office
MDPI
St. Alban-Anlage 66
4052 Basel, Switzerland

This is a reprint of articles from the Special Issue published online in the open access journal *Cancers* (ISSN 2072-6694) (available at: https://www.mdpi.com/journal/cancers/special_issues/Cancer_Molecular_Biology).

For citation purposes, cite each article independently as indicated on the article page online and as indicated below:

Lastname, A.A.; Lastname, B.B. Article Title. *Journal Name* **Year**, *Volume Number*, Page Range.

ISBN 978-3-7258-0427-6 (Hbk)
ISBN 978-3-7258-0428-3 (PDF)
doi.org/10.3390/books978-3-7258-0428-3

© 2024 by the authors. Articles in this book are Open Access and distributed under the Creative Commons Attribution (CC BY) license. The book as a whole is distributed by MDPI under the terms and conditions of the Creative Commons Attribution-NonCommercial-NoDerivs (CC BY-NC-ND) license.

Contents

Olfat Khannous-Lleiffe, Jesse R. Willis, Ester Saus, Victor Moreno, Sergi Castellví-Bel,
Toni Gabaldón and on behalf of the CRIPREV Consortium
Microbiome Profiling from Fecal Immunochemical Test Reveals Microbial Signatures with
Potential for Colorectal Cancer Screening
Reprinted from: *Cancers* 2023, *15*, 120, doi:10.3390/cancers15010120 1

Can Lu, Josefine Schardey, Ulrich Wirth, Viktor von Ehrlich-Treuenstätt, Jens Neumann,
Clemens Gießen-Jung, et al.
Analysis of Circulating Immune Subsets in Primary Colorectal Cancer
Reprinted from: *Cancers* 2022, *14*, 6105, doi:10.3390/cancers14246105 23

Ferran Moratalla-Navarro, Anna Díez-Villanueva, Ainhoa Serrano, Adrià Closa,
David Cordero, Xavier Solé, et al.
Identification of a Twelve-microRNA Signature with Prognostic Value in Stage II Microsatellite
Stable Colon Cancer
Reprinted from: *Cancers* 2023, *15*, 3301, doi:10.3390/cancers15133301 41

Lina Lambis-Anaya, Mashiel Fernández-Ruiz, Yamil Liscano and Amileth Suarez-Causado
High OCT4 Expression Might Be Associated with an Aggressive Phenotype in Rectal Cancer
Reprinted from: *Cancers* 2023, *15*, 3740, doi:10.3390/cancers15143740 54

Arne Rotermund, Martin S. Staege, Sarah Brandt, Jana Luetzkendorf, Henrike Lucas,
Lutz P. Mueller and Thomas Mueller
Luciferase Expressing Preclinical Model Systems Representing the Different Molecular
Subtypes of Colorectal Cancer
Reprinted from: *Cancers* 2023, *15*, 4122, doi:10.3390/cancers15164122 65

Mateo Paz-Cabezas, Tania Calvo-López, Alejandro Romera-Lopez, Daniel Tabas-Madrid,
Jesus Ogando, María-Jesús Fernández-Aceñero, et al.
Molecular Classification of Colorectal Cancer by microRNA Profiling: Correlation with the
Consensus Molecular Subtypes (CMS) and Validation of miR-30b Targets
Reprinted from: *Cancers* 2022, *14*, 5175, doi:10.3390/cancers14215175 86

Jakub Kryczka and Joanna Boncela
Characteristics of ABCC4 and ABCG2 High Expression Subpopulations in CRC—A New
Opportunity to Predict Therapy Response
Reprinted from: *Cancers* 2023, *15*, 5623, doi:10.3390/cancers15235623 99

Anna Citarella, Giuseppina Catanzaro, Zein Mersini Besharat, Sofia Trocchianesi,
Federica Barbagallo, Giorgio Gosti, et al.
Hedgehog-GLI and Notch Pathways Sustain Chemoresistance and Invasiveness in Colorectal
Cancer and Their Inhibition Restores Chemotherapy Efficacy
Reprinted from: *Cancers* 2023, *15*, 1471, doi:10.3390/cancers15051471 121

Ruoxuan Ni, Jianwei Jiang, Mei Zhao, Shengkai Huang and Changzhi Huang
Knockdown of UBQLN1 Functions as a Strategy to Inhibit CRC Progression through the
ERK-c-Myc Pathway
Reprinted from: *Cancers* 2023, *15*, 3088, doi:10.3390/cancers15123088 137

Aldona Kasprzak
Prognostic Biomarkers of Cell Proliferation in Colorectal Cancer (CRC): From
Immunohistochemistry to Molecular Biology Techniques
Reprinted from: *Cancers* 2023, *15*, 4570, doi:10.3390/cancers15184570 149

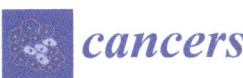

Article

Microbiome Profiling from Fecal Immunochemical Test Reveals Microbial Signatures with Potential for Colorectal Cancer Screening

Olfat Khannous-Lleiffe [1,2], Jesse R. Willis [1,2], Ester Saus [1,2], Victor Moreno [3,4,5,6], Sergi Castellví-Bel [6,7], Toni Gabaldón [1,2,8,9,*] and on behalf of the CRIPREV Consortium [†]

1. Barcelona Supercomputing Center (BSC-CNS), Carrer de Jordi Girona, 29, 31, 08034 Barcelona, Spain
2. Institute for Research in Biomedicine (IRB), Carrer de Baldiri Reixac, 10, 08028 Barcelona, Spain
3. Catalan Institute of Oncology (ICO), L'Hospitalet de Llobregat, 08908 Barcelona, Spain
4. Bellvitge Biomedical Research Institute (IDIBELL), L'Hospitalet de Llobregat, 08908 Barcelona, Spain
5. Consortium for Biomedical Research in Epidemiology and Public Health (CIBERESP), Av. de Monforte de Lemos, 3–5, 28029 Madrid, Spain
6. Gastroenterology Department, University of Barcelona, 08036 Barcelona, Spain
7. Gastroenterology Department, Institut d'Investigacions Biomèdiques August Pi i Sunyer (IDIBAPS), Centro de Investigación Biomédica en Red de Enfermedades Hepáticas y Digestivas (CIBERehd), Hospital Clínic, 08036 Barcelona, Spain
8. Institució Catalana de Recerca i Estudis Avançats (ICREA), Pg. Lluís Companys 23, 08010 Barcelona, Spain
9. Centro Investigación Biomédica En Red de Enfermedades Infecciosas (CIBERINFEC), 08028 Barcelona, Spain
* Correspondence: toni.gabaldon@bsc.es
† Authorship Appendix—CRIPREV Consortium: See Appendix A for the full list.

Simple Summary: Colorectal cancer (CRC) is a global healthcare challenge that involves both genetic and environmental factors. Several pieces of evidence suggest that alterations of the gut microbiome can influence CRC development. In the present study we analyzed 16S rRNA sequencing data from fecal immunochemical test (FIT) samples from a large cohort, observing a predictive potential of the microbiome, revealing changes along the path from healthy tissue to carcinoma. Our work has implications in the understanding of the roles of microbes on the adenoma to carcinoma progression and opens the door to an improvement of the current CRC screening programmes.

Abstract: Colorectal cancer (CRC) is the third most common cancer and the second leading cause of cancer deaths worldwide. Early diagnosis of CRC, which saves lives and enables better outcomes, is generally implemented through a two-step population screening approach based on the use of Fecal Immunochemical Test (FIT) followed by colonoscopy if the test is positive. However, the FIT step has a high false positive rate, and there is a need for new predictive biomarkers to better prioritize cases for colonoscopy. Here we used 16S rRNA metabarcoding from FIT positive samples to uncover microbial taxa, taxon co-occurrence and metabolic features significantly associated with different colonoscopy outcomes, underscoring a predictive potential and revealing changes along the path from healthy tissue to carcinoma. Finally, we used machine learning to develop a two-phase classifier which reduces the current false positive rate while maximizing the inclusion of CRC and clinically relevant samples.

Keywords: colorectal cancer; microbiome; 16S rRNA sequencing; screening; diagnosis

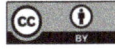

1. Introduction

Colorectal cancer (CRC) is the third most common cancer type and the second leading cause of cancer-related deaths worldwide [1], accounting for nearly 900,000 deaths each year. This malignant disease develops from the pathological transformation of normal colonic epithelium to adenomatous polyps, which ultimately leads to invasive cancer.

This process is gradual and involves the accumulation of genetic and/or epigenetic alterations [2]. CRC incidence increases with economic development and Westernization of dietary and lifestyle habits, hinting at a significant effect of environmental and lifestyle factors, likely in combination with genetic predisposition [3]. In this regard, a growing body of evidence has linked alterations of the gastrointestinal tract microbiota with CRC development [4]. Earlier research has shown that alterations in the gut microbiota may influence colon tumorigenesis [5] through chronic inflammation or the production of carcinogenic compounds [6]. Differences in the relative abundances of some microbial species or genera have been found when comparing paired tumor and normal tissues, or fecal samples from CRC patients and healthy subjects [7,8].

Diagnosis of CRC is challenging and involves a complex process that usually starts with the detection of the first symptoms by the patient, and is followed by clinical diagnostic procedures, mainly based on colonoscopy. The implementation of preventive measures and early diagnosis of CRC can save many lives [9,10] and routine screening of asymptomatic populations following an age-selected criteria has been implemented in many countries. Current CRC screening in the vast majority of Western countries consists of a two-step procedure with a non-invasive test (most commonly a fecal immunochemical test (FIT) for quantification of occult hemoglobin in the stool) followed by colonoscopy if the test is positive (FIT-positive, or more accurately, above a given threshold of hemoglobin concentration) [11,12]. This approach is effective but results in a high rate of false positives (around 65% FIT-positive samples reveal no clinically relevant feature at colonoscopy) at the first step and many unnecessary colonoscopies, with a FIT sensitivity of around 35% [13]. Colonoscopy is an invasive, expensive and time-consuming procedure, and hence additional biomarkers that could better stratify individuals with higher risk for CRC or premalignant lesions to undergo a colonic examination would significantly reduce healthcare costs. Much current research is directed towards finding additional criteria, such as risk factors and alternative biomarkers to be considered by the decision algorithms used to personalize positive FIT testing to colonoscopy. To search for potential predictive biomarkers present in FIT samples and to shed light on the potential roles of the gut microbiome in CRC development, we performed microbiome profiling using targeted sequencing of the 16S V3-V4 region from DNA extracted directly from FIT containers collected within the population-based organized screening program implemented in Catalonia, Spain [14]. We analyzed a total of 2889 FIT-positive samples and assessed their microbial composition and metabolic potential, and how they varied across samples with different colonoscopy results (i.e., different diagnostic outcome after colonoscopy exploration, including, among others, the absence of any clinical feature, the presence of lesions and their risk, the presence of colorectal cancer, and the presence of polyps).

2. Materials and Methods

Our study followed the Strengthening the Organization and Reporting of Microbiome Studies (STORMS) checklist (Data S1).

2.1. Sample Collection and Subjects

A total of 2889 FIT-positive (>20 µg hemoglobin/g feces) samples recruited in two rounds (2009 and 2017–2019) from asymptomatic participants from the Catalan CRC screening program were analysed. Individuals were selected within the age criteria implemented by the screening programme (50 to 69 years old) and the diagnosis and sex selection were based on an ideal balanced dataset (aimed to obtain equal numbers within each class). Collected metadata comprised six different clinical variables for each sample, including the diagnosis after colonoscopy evaluation (Data S2), the number of polyps, the FIT value (µg of hemoglobin/g of feces), the hospital at which the sample was collected, and the donor's sex and age. The considered colonoscopy diagnoses were negative (N), colorectal cancer (CRC) and different lesions that can be relevant in CRC development: carcinoma in situ (CIS), high risk lesion (HRL), intermediate risk lesion (IRL), low risk lesion (LRL) and lesion not associated to risk (LNAR) [15] (Table S1). Additionally, we classified the samples into two groups according to the clinical relevance of the colonoscopy-based diagnosis [16]: CRC, CIS, HRL and IRL were considered clinically relevant (CR) lesions (indeed, they are the goal of CRC screening programs), and N, LNAR and LRL as non-clinically relevant (non-CR) lesions (Table S1). Individuals with inflammatory bowel disease or polyposis were excluded from the study. Our study was approved by the institutional ethical committees of the involved institutions and informed consent was obtained from the participants.

2.2. DNA Extraction and 16S Sequencing

Aliquots of 500 µL of buffer contained in FIT collection devices (OC-Sensor, Eiken Chemical Co., Tokyo, Japan) were prepared in a test tube and stored at −80 °C until further processing. DNA was extracted from FIT samples using the DNeasy PowerLyzer PowerSoil Kit (Qiagen, ref. QIA12855) following manufacturer's instructions. The extraction tubes were agitated twice in a 96-well plate using the TissueLyser II (Qiagen) at 30 Hz/s for 5 min.

Four µL of each DNA sample were used to amplify the V3–V4 regions of the bacterial 16S ribosomal RNA gene, using the following universal primers in a limited cycle PCR: V3-V4-Forward (5′-TCGTCGGCAGCGTCAGATGTGTATAAGAGACAGCCTACGGGNGGCWG-CAG-3′) and V3-V4-Reverse (5′-GTCTCGTGGGCTCGGAGATGTGTATAAGAGACAGGA-CTACHVGGGTATCTAATCC-3′). To prevent unbalanced base composition in further MiSeq sequencing, we shifted sequencing phases by adding a variable number of bases (from 0 to 3) as spacers to both forward and reverse primers (we used a total of 4 forward and 4 reverse primers). The PCR was performed in 10 µL volume reactions with 0.2 µM primer concentration and using the Kapa HiFi HotStart Ready Mix (Roche, ref. KK2602). Cycling conditions were initial denaturation of 3 min at 95 °C followed by 25 cycles of 95 °C for 30 s, 55 °C for 30 s, and 72 °C for 30 s, ending with a final elongation step of 5 min at 72 °C.

After the first PCR step, water was added to a total volume of 50 µL and reactions were purified using AMPure XP beads (Beckman Coulter) with a 0.9X ratio according to manufacturer's instructions. PCR products were eluted from the magnetic beads with 32 µL of Buffer EB (Qiagen) and 30 µL of the eluate were transferred to a fresh 96-well plate. The primers used in the first PCR contained overhangs allowing the addition of full-length Nextera adapters with barcodes for multiplex sequencing in a second PCR step, resulting in sequencing ready libraries. To do so, 5 µL of the first amplification was used as template for the second PCR with Nextera XT v2 adaptor primers in a final volume of 50 µL using the same PCR mix and thermal profile as for the first PCR but for only 8 cycles. After the second PCR, 25 µL of the final product was used for purification and normalization with the SequalPrep normalization kit (Invitrogen), according to the manufacturer's protocol. Libraries were eluted in 20 µL and pooled for sequencing.

Final pools were quantified by qPCR using the Kapa library quantification kit for Illumina Platforms (Kapa Biosystems) on an ABI 7900HT real-time cycler (Applied Biosystems). Sequencing was performed in the Illumina MiSeq with 2 × 300 bp reads using v3 chemistry with a loading concentration of 18 pM. To increase the diversity of the sequences, 10% of PhIX control libraries were spiked in.

Two bacterial mock communities were obtained from the BEI Resources of the Human Microbiome Project (HM-276D and HM-277D), each containing genomic DNA of ribosomal operons from 20 bacterial species [17]. Mock DNAs were amplified and sequenced in the same manner as all other FIT samples. Negative controls of the DNA extraction and PCR amplification steps were also included in parallel, using the same conditions and reagents. These negative controls provided no visible band or quantifiable DNA amounts by Bioanalyzer, whereas all our samples provided clearly visible bands after 25 cycles.

2.3. Microbiome Analysis

We used the dada2 (v. 1.10.1) pipeline [18] to obtain an amplicon sequence variants (ASV) table for each of the sequencing runs separately. The quality profiles of forward and reverse sequencing reads were examined using the plotQualityProfile function of dada2 and, according to these plots, low-quality sequencing reads were filtered and trimmed using the filterAndTrim function. We obtained a matrix with learned error rates with the learnErrors dada2 function. We performed dereplication (combining identical sequencing reads into unique sequences), sample inference (from the matrix of estimated learning error rates) and merged paired reads to obtain full denoised sequences. From these, chimeric sequences were removed. Taxonomy was assigned to ASVs by mapping to the SILVA 16s rRNA database (v. 132) [19]. Negative controls (non-template samples) and positive controls (mock microbial communities comprising a mixture of 20 strains with known proportions) were sequenced and analyzed in each of the runs to assess the possible contamination background and evaluate the accuracy of the pipeline. We obtained ASV and taxonomy tables for each run separately, and then merged the results. Samples without metadata information and the controls were discarded in further analyses.

We reconstructed a phylogenetic tree by using the phangorn (v. 2.5.5) [20] and Decipher R packages (v 2.10.2) [21] and integrated it with the merged ASV and Taxonomy tables and their assigned metadata creating a phyloseq (v. 1.26.1) object [22]. We characterized alpha diversity metrics including Observed index, Shannon, Simpson, InvSimpson, PD Chao1, ACE and standard error measures such as se.Chao1 and se.ACE using the estimate_richness function of the phyloseq package. Using the picante package (v. 1.8.1) we computed Faith's phylogenetic diversity, an alpha diversity metric that incorporates branch lengths of the phylogenetic tree. Additionally, we calculated different distance metrics based on the differences in taxonomic composition between samples using the Phyloseq and Vegan (v. 2.5–6) [23] packages. These metrics include Jensen-Shannon Divergence (JSD), Weighted-Unifrac, Unweighted-unifrac, Bray-Curtis dissimilarity, Jaccard and Canberra. We also computed Aitchison distances between samples using the cmultRepl and codaSeq.clr functions from the CodaSeq (v. 0.99.6) [24] and zCompositions (v. 1.3.4) [25] packages. Normalization was performed by transforming counts to centered log-ratios (clr) [26]. We performed multiplicative simple zero replacement as implemented in the cmultRepl function of the zCompositions package (v. 1.3.4) (indicating method = "CZM"). Samples with fewer than 1000 reads and taxa that appeared in fewer than 10 samples and at low abundances (fewer than 100 reads) were filtered out. Finally, we agglomerated taxa at each taxonomic rank to study trends at different taxonomic depths.

We made a comparison of our overall microbiome profiles with samples studied in a previous study [27]. We treated the samples from their 2×300 pb cycle run by applying the same procedure state in the present section.

2.4. Statistical Analysis

We assessed associations between clinical variables and the overall microbial composition of the samples by performing permutational multivariate analysis of variance (PERMANOVA) using the adonis function from the Vegan R package (v. 2.5–6) with the seven distance metrics mentioned above. Diagnosis, sex and age variables were considered as covariates. Additionally, we performed an analysis of similarities (ANOSIM) test using the anosim function from the Vegan R package to assess differences between and within groups.

We performed a differential abundance analysis using clr data for the different taxonomic ranks across various clinical variables using linear models implemented in the R package lme4 (v. 1.1–21) [28]. We built a linear model including diagnosis (Dx), hospital, sex, age, number of polyps and FIT value as fixed effects, and the sequencing run as a random effect to account for possible batch effects: tax_element~Dx + hospital + sex + age + number_polyps + FIT_value + (1 | run). This linear model was evaluated considering all the diagnoses, but also made a comparison of CRC versus non-CRC samples by changing all other diagnoses to "others". A second linear model was applied that considered as fixed effect a variable called risk instead of the diagnosis in order to assess the differences between samples with CR or non-CR colonoscopy, as defined above (Table S1).

We applied analysis of variance (ANOVA) to assess the significance for each of the fixed effects included in the models using the Car R package (v. 3.0–6) [29]. To assess differences between groups, we performed multiple comparisons to the results obtained in the linear models using the Tukey test in the function glht from the multcomp R package (v. 1.4–12) [30]. We applied Bonferroni as a multiple testing correction as implemented in the summary.glht function of the multcomp package, and statistical significance was defined at p values lower than 0.05. In addition, we used the selbal package (v. 0.1.0) [31] to study groups of taxa (balances) with potential predictive power for CRC status.

2.5. Co-Occurrence and Networks

Co-occurrence networks for microbial species were inferred and represented for each of the diagnostic groups, considering the top 50 taxa and using the SpiecEasi R package (v. 1.1.0) [32]. We used neighborhood selection based on penalized regression as the graphical model inference. The resulting networks, following the path transition from healthy colon (N) to cancer (CRC), were compared by computing hamming distances with the netdist function from the R package nettools (v. 1.1.0). We represented the weights of the correlations of the co-occurrence networks by using the chordDiagram function from the circlize package (v. 0.4.12).

We also calculated taxa correlation matrices for each diagnosis group by using the function corr.test from the R psych package (v. 2.0.12) and using the Spearman method, adjusting for multiple comparisons with the Holm-Bonferroni method. The significance threshold was set at p.adjust < 0.05.

2.6. Genome Content Inference

Given the ASV and taxonomy tables in the phyloseq object, we applied the t4f function from the themetagenomics package (v. 1.0.0) [33] to predict the functional content in terms of functional genes (kegg orthologous groups (OGs), which are families of genes that descent from a common ancestral gene and that generally perform similar functions). Then, we applied a linear model (ortholog~Dx + hospital + sex + age + number_polyps + FIT_value + (1 | run)) to determine OGs that were significantly differentially abundant according to the diagnosis, and a multiple comparison test (Tukey) correcting by Bonferroni. From these differentially abundant OGs, we extracted all the functional pathways in which they were involved and performed a test for pathway enrichment only considering pathways with 10 or more predicted OGs and having at least 10% of their OGs being differentially abundant. Using custom scripts and text mining tools implemented in the easyPubMed R package (v.2.13) [34], we retrieved pubmed articles in which these pathways appeared related to CRC.

2.7. Machine Learning Classification

We developed a predictive model based on a two-phase classification using a neural network (NN) algorithm implemented in the caret package (v. 6.0–85) [35]. For each phase we trained a random 75% of the data with a 10-fold cross validation and tested with the remaining samples. The process was repeated 100 times to avoid "lucky" splits and to evaluate the variability in predictive performance. We performed a feature selection based on the differential abundance results including taxa found as having significantly different abundances in our study and incorporating FIT-value, age and sex variables. Samples with missing values for the considered metadata were removed. Taxa abundances were included as clr. The two-phase classifier proceeds as follows: in the first phase the method classifies CRC vs. non-CRC samples. Samples that are classified as non-CRC in the first phase are subjected to a second model that classifies CR vs. non-CR samples. At the end of the two-phase classification, the mean percentage of misclassified CRC and CR samples was calculated, and the performance of the model was evaluated.

To validate our strategy we built a model training with all the CRIPREV samples and tested it in two independent datasets: a cohort from the USA [36,37] and 100 extra samples from the same Catalan screening. For the USA cohort, we applied the Catalan hemoglobin threshold (>20 µg of hemoglobin/g of feces) to select the FIT-positive samples to include in the validation. We processed their raw data following the same methodology as in our study (see Microbiome analysis, Materials and Methods). We unfortunately could not assign *Bacteroides fragilis*, likely because that study only used the V4 region of the 16S rRNA gene as compared to V3-V4 in our study.

We assessed possible subsets of taxa with classification potential by using the 100 extra samples from the same local screening. We identified a total of 27 taxa, found as differentially abundant in both the CRC vs. others and CR vs. non-CR comparisons, intersecting between the CRIPREV project and these extra samples, that are those included in the results presented here. We assessed different combinations of the taxa, considering the effect size observed in our statistical test. We defined top and down taxa from the list, per each phase, and made an assessment of subsets of taxa as follows: 4 taxa from the top of the list (50 random combinations), 4 taxa from the bottom of the list (50 random combinations), 4 random taxa (50 random combinations), 2 taxa from the top of the list (all the possible combinations), 2 taxa from the bottom of the list (all the possible combinations), 1 taxa from the top of the list (all the possible combinations) and 1 taxa from the bottom of the list (all the possible combinations).

We tested a total of 948 models using our validation set. We filtered the models based on some classification metrics: AUC1 >= 0.55, specificity1 > 0.2, AUC2 > 0.5 and specificity2 > 0.

ROC curves were represented using the package pROC (v 1.16.1) [38].

3. Results

3.1. 16S Metabarcoding from FIT Samples Is a Valid Proxy for Gut Microbiome

To assess the diagnostic and research potential of microbiome analyses performed on FIT samples collected within currently ongoing CRC screening programs, we enrolled asymptomatic participants of the Catalan CRC screening program that had a FIT-positive test. We froze their FIT cartridges until the results from the colonoscopy examination were obtained. These outcomes were categorized into clinically relevant (CR) lesions -including CRC, carcinoma in situ (CIS), high risk lesion (HRL) and intermediate risk lesion (IRL)-, and non-CR lesions—including negative (N), lesion not associated to risk (LNAR) and low risk lesion (LRL). Using the colonoscopy information, we selected a representative set of samples for microbiome characterization, aiming for a balanced representation of clinically relevant colonoscopy outcomes. We performed DNA extraction and 16S metabarcoding analysis of the V3-V4 region on the selected samples (see Materials and Methods, Section 2.2). A total of 2889 FIT-positive samples passed all quality filters and were included in the study (see Materials and Methods, Section 2.3). A summary of the distribution of these samples across several characteristics is shown in Table S2. We obtained a mean value of 56,219.03 filtered reads per sample, which comprised a total of 376 assigned taxa. Bacteroidetes and Firmicutes were the most represented phyla, and the ten most abundant genera were, in this order: *Bacteroides*, *Faecalibacterium*, *Prevotella*, *Blautia*, F.Lachnospiraceae.UCG, *Ruminococcus*, *Agathobacter*, *Bifidobacterium*, *Alistipes* and *Akkermansia* (Figure S1). These results are consistent with previous studies using stool samples [39–43], and with earlier analyses showing a high correspondence between stool and FIT samples from the same individuals [36,37]. We compared our data with that of a recent Spanish population gut microbiome study [27]. The two cohorts differ in several features such as the age range, but most notably our cohort was entirely formed by individuals with blood in stool, a factor shown to impact the gut microbiome [44], and hence differences are expected. Nevertheless, the two sample sets were largely similar in terms of dominating phyla and genera, reinforcing the validity of FIT sampling as a proxy of the gut microbiome (Figure S2).

3.2. Changes in Microbiome Composition along the Path from Healthy Colon to Colorectal Cancer

We quantified the overall microbiome diversity by computing alpha and beta diversity metrics. We only observed significant differences (Kruskal-Wallis, $p < 0.05$) in the observed index alpha diversity metric (which measures the number of species per sample), and in the Simpson index (which considers taxa abundances) when considering all diagnoses, but not when specifically comparing clinically relevant (CR) vs. non-CR samples (Figure S3). For the Shannon and Simpson indices, which consider differences in taxa abundances, we only observed significant differences with the Simpson index (which assigns more weight to dominant species) when considering all diagnoses. We produced multidimensional scaling (MDS) plots using distances between the microbial profiles of samples (beta diversity) such as the Aitchison distance (Figure S4). We did not observe a clear clustering of samples with the same diagnosis or risk (CR vs. non-CR). However, with the adonis test and Aitchison distance, we detected a significant effect of the diagnosis ($p = 0.001$) considering sex and age as covariates, and the sequencing run as a possible source of batch effect. The ANOSIM test also supported significant differences between the diagnostic groups and a higher similarity within groups (R: 0.07463, p-value: 0.001). Altogether, these results suggest the existence of significant but subtle differences in the overall microbiome composition between FIT-positive samples with different colonoscopy outcomes.

We next used comparative analysis to detect significant differences in the relative abundance of taxa according to the variables considered (Table S3). These analyses identified 34 species whose abundance varied significantly across colonoscopy diagnosis (Data S3 and Figure 1).

Based on the observation that CRC was the diagnosis with the most distinct microbiome (Figure 1), we specifically compared CRC to non-CRC samples, which revealed 41 differentially abundant species (Figure 2a and Data S4). These included overrepresentation of *Akkermansia muciniphila* and *Akkermansia* spp., as well as underrepresentation of *Bacteroides plebeius* and *Bacteroides fragilis* in CRC compared to non-CRC samples. In addition, we found that the ratio between species abundance (balance) most associated with CRC-status was given by a decrease (as compared to non-CRC samples) in a group of taxa comprising *B. fragilis* (G1: *Bifidobacterium* spp., *Bacteroides fragilis*, *Sutterella wadsworthensis*, and *Eggerthella* spp.), with respect to a second group of taxa including *Akkermansia* spp. (G2: *Akkermansia* spp., *Gemella* spp., *Peptostreptococcus stomatis*, *Adlercreutzia* spp. and *Butyrivibrio* spp.). We explored the progression of the levels of *Akkermansia* genus along the path from normal colon to CRC, observing an increase from HRL to carcinoma in situ and from carcinoma in situ to CRC. (Figure S5).

Finally, we applied the same linear model to the comparison of CR vs. non-CR samples, which identified 34 differentially abundant species, of which six were shared with the comparison above (Figure 2b and Data S5).

We next explored whether changes in the microbiome correlated with other variables collected in the study such as the number of polyps observed in the colonoscopy examination and lifestyle parameters collected by a questionnaire. Colorectal polyps, which are benign tumors that project onto the colon mucus and protrude into intestinal lumen [45], have long been identified as potential precursors of CRC. Polyp size, localization and histology, among other factors, may influence their role in CRC development. Our study includes the information of the presence or absence of polyps, wherein colonoscopy detected the presence of polyps in 66.82% of samples, with the numbers of polyps ranging from one to 22. We observed that some CRC (32/134, 23.88%) samples had no polyps, whereas some negative samples had from 1 to 3 polyps (21/925, 2.27%), and some lesions that were not associated with a clinically relevant colonoscopy had a considerable amount of polyps (from 1 to 11 polyps, e.g., two individuals diagnosed by LNAR and LRL had 11 polyps). We searched for species whose abundance correlated significantly with the number of polyps and found 33 such cases (Data S6), including *B. vulgatus*, which was associated with systemic inflammation and CRC progression [46]. Finally, we found no significant effect of the CRC tumor stage on the microbiome composition, although this may relate to limited sample size (n = 101, Adonis test, R2: 0.03104 *p* value: 0.386). A subset of the included individuals (n = 2016) responded to a lifestyle questionnaire. We assessed the impact of different variables on microbiome composition, and found a significant impact of weight, height, regular exercise, smoking, alcohol, vegetables and processed meat intake and anti-inflammatory drug use, as observed in previous studies. When this impact was considered in conjunction with the diagnosis, we observed only a significant effect of the vegetable's intake (Figure S6).

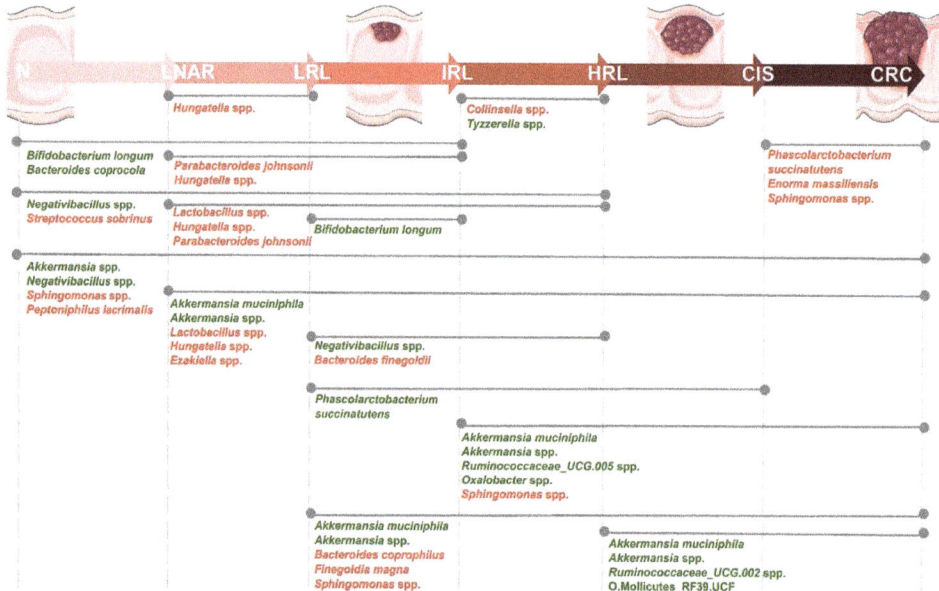

Figure 1. Representation of the 34 bacterial species found as significantly differentially abundant in pairwise comparisons of diagnoses following the path from healthy colon to colorectal cancer (Tukey test, p.adjusted < 0.05, n = 2565). Different colonoscopy diagnoses are depicted from left to right following this path, with healthier states at the left and in the following order: N, negative; LNAR, lesion not associated to risk; LRL, low risk lesion; IRL, intermediate risk lesion; HRL, high risk lesion; CIS, carcinoma in situ; CRC, colorectal cancer. Lines connecting different diagnoses indicate comparisons, with differentially abundant species names indicated. Colors in the species names indicate the direction of the change with red indicating decrease and green increased relative abundance with respect to the healthier state.

3.3. Diagnosis-Specific Co-Occurrence and Functional Profiles

To gain further insights into the changes of microbial composition along the path from healthy tissue to CRC, we used proxies for community interactions (co-occurrence networks), and functional potential (functional inference from taxonomic assignment). We first built species networks showing patterns of correlated abundances for samples with each specific diagnosis and compared them (see Materials and Methods, Section 2.5). By constructing and representing co-occurrence networks based on the 50 most abundant taxa, we qualitatively observed differences across the diagnoses along the path from healthy colon to CRC (Figure 3). These differences were confirmed by computing hamming distances between co-occurrence networks of successive pairs of diagnoses along this path: 0.024 (N vs. LNAR), 0.023 (LNAR vs. LRL), 0.014 (LRL vs. IRL), 0.016 (IRL vs. HRL),

0.030 (HRL vs. CIS) and 0.028 (CIS vs. CRC). According to this, the last two steps in the progression from healthy tissue towards CRC (HRL to CIS and CIS to CRC) display the largest dissimilarities. Similar results were obtained using an alternative approach based on Spearman correlations: 66% (N vs. LNAR), 65% (LNAR vs. LRL), 53% (LRL vs. IRL), 53% (IRL vs. HRL), 79% (HRL vs. CIS) and 73% (CIS vs. CRC).

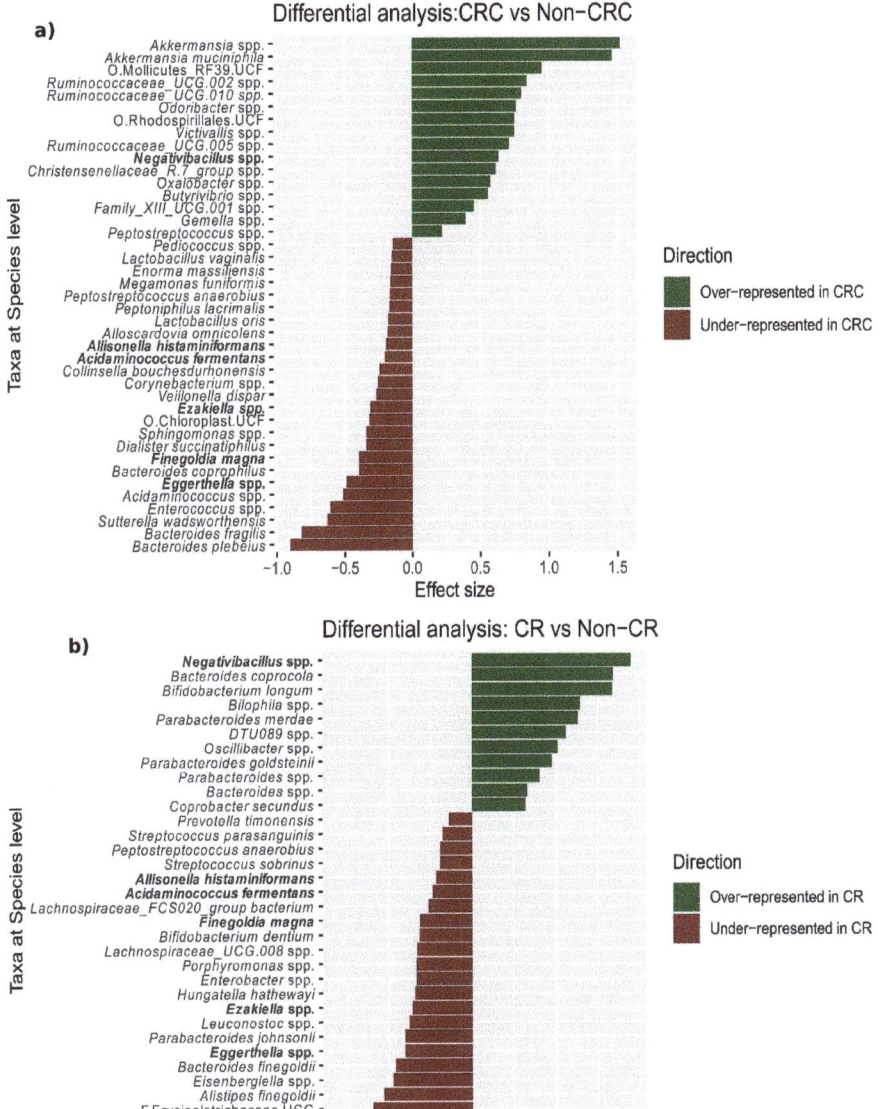

Figure 2. The effect size of species found as significantly differentially abundant when comparing CRC vs. non-CRC samples (n = 2565) (**a**) and CR vs. non-CR samples (**b**). Bars are green for overrepresentation and red for underrepresentation. The bars are sorted according to the effect size. In bold are the highlighted taxa that appeared as differentially abundant in both comparisons.

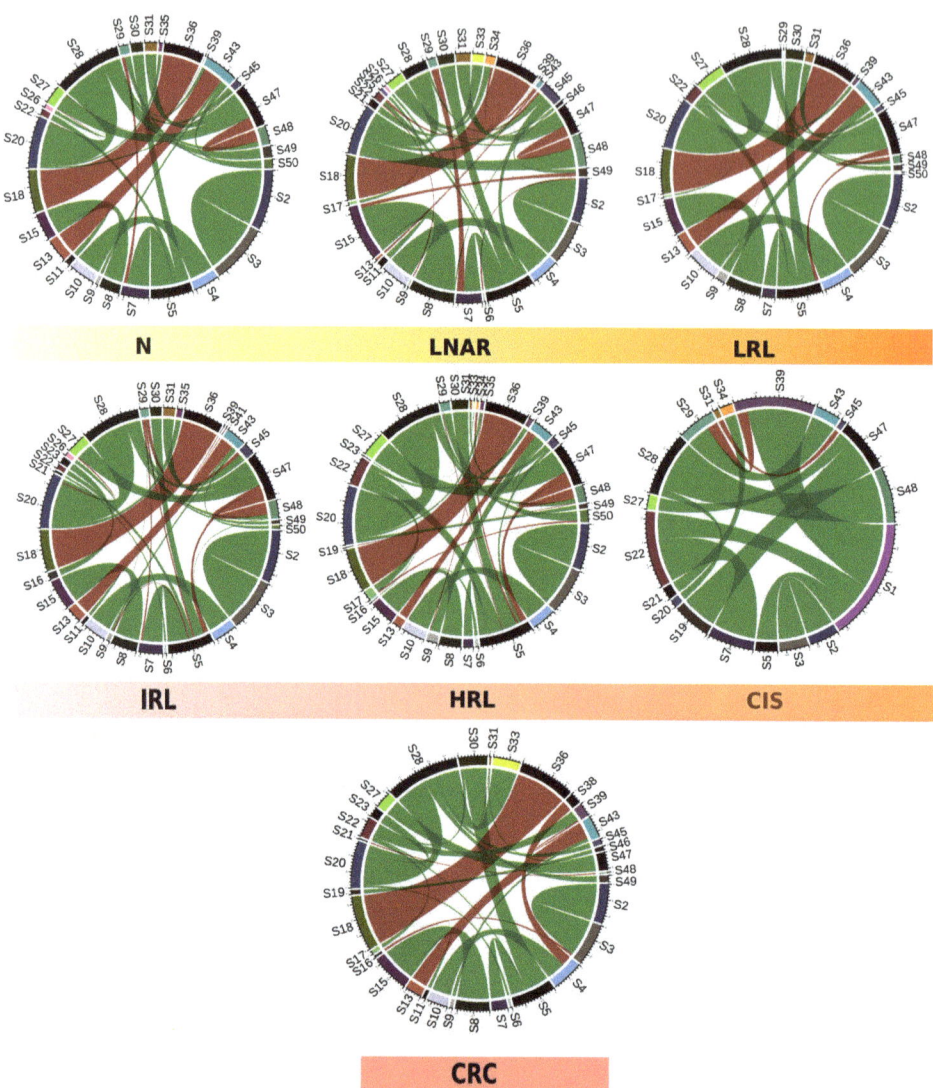

Figure 3. Circos plots representing the correlation weight matrices obtained from the computed networks of co-occurrence according to the diagnosis (negative (N) n = 925, lesion not associated to risk (LNAR) n = 90, low risk lesion (LRL) n = 681, intermediate risk lesion (IRL) n = 638, high risk lesion (HRL) n = 397, carcinoma in situ (CIS) n = 24, and colorectal cancer (CRC) n = 134) considering the top 50 taxa. The green connections are for positively correlated and the red connections are for negatively correlated taxa. The thickness of the arrows represents the strength of the correlations.

S1: *Bacteroides vulgatus*, S2: *Akkermansia muciniphila*, S3: *Akkermansia* spp., S4: *Collinsella aerofaciens*, S5: *Bacteroides* spp., S6: *Agathobacter* spp., S7: *Bacteroides uniformis*, S8: *Faecalibacterium prausnitzii*, S9: *Holdemanella* spp., S10: *Collinsella* spp., S11: *Faecalibacterium_CM04-06* spp., S12: *Ruminococcus bromii*, S13: *Erysipelotrichaceae_UCG-003* spp., S14: *Escherichia* spp., S15: *Faecalibacterium* spp., S16: *Dorea longicatena*, S17: *Alistipes putredinis*, S18: *Phascolarctobacterium* spp., S19: *Ruminococcus* spp., S20: *Blautia* spp., S21: *Subdoligranulum* spp., S22: *Alistipes* spp., S23: *Dorea* spp., S24: *Bifidobacterium* spp., S25: *Bacteroides massiliensis*,

S26: *Streptococcus* spp., S27: *Ruminococcaceae_UCG-002* spp., S28: *F.Lachnospiraceae.UCG*, S29: *Prevotella* spp., S30: *Parabacteroides* spp., S31: *Ruminococcaceae_UCG-014* spp., S32: *Prevotellaceae_NK3B31_group* spp., S33: *F.Ruminococcaceae.UCG*, S34: *Coprococcus* spp., S35: *Anaerostipes* spp., S36: *Dialister* spp., S37: *Roseburia* spp., S38: *Lachnospira* spp., S39: *Barnesiella* spp., S40: *Bacteroides coprocola*, S41: *F.Muribaculaceae.UCG*, S42: *Paraprevotella* spp., S43: *Catenibacterium* spp., S44: *O.Rhodospirillales.UCF*, S45: *Erysipelatoclostridium* spp., S46: *Lachnospiraceae_NK4A136_group* spp., S47: *Christensenellaceae_R-7_group* spp., S48: *Lachnoclostridium* spp., S49: *Ruminiclostridium* spp. and S50: *Alloprevotella* spp.

Of note, some of the specific differences that we detected were that *Akkermansia muciniphila* and *Akkermansia* spp. were found as positively correlated in all the diagnoses, but only in CRC we observed a negative correlation of the *Akkermansia* spp. and *Dorea longicatena* species. In contrast, in LNAR and LRL we found a negative correlation of these species with *Agathobacter* spp. and *Alloprevotella* spp., respectively. Also, we observed a positive correlation between *Collinsella aerofaciens* and *Collinsella* spp. in all the diagnoses except in the CIS group, and only in CRC we observed a negative correlation with another taxon, *Lachnospira* spp.

Co-occurrence networks may reflect underlying microbial communities that may interact metabolically. To obtain functional insights we inferred the functional potential of the microbiota in each sample by exploring metabolic pathways and processes associated with 2927 orthologous groups (OG, i.e., functionally-annotated gene families) in 376 taxa present in our samples (see Materials and Methods, Section 2.6). By studying the variation of abundance of OGs across samples, we identified 184 that were significantly differentially abundant according to the diagnosis (Data S7). The differentially abundant OGs were linked to 23 enriched pathways (containing more than 10 predicted OGs and 10% or more differentially abundant OGs involved), many of which have been linked to CRC in the literature, according to a text-mining approach (Figure 4a).

When performing pairwise comparisons between diagnoses along the path from healthy colon to CRC, we only observed significant differences of OGs in the transition from IRL to HRL (Figure 4b and Data S8). For instance, some of the OGs that we found as significantly differentially abundant between these two diagnoses were: K00850, K00963, K02231, which are involved, respectively, in galactose metabolism, RNA degradation, pentose and glucuronate interconversions, porphyrin and chlorophyll metabolism, peptidoglycan biosynthesis and cell cycle—Caulobacter.

3.4. Development of a Two-Phase Machine Learning Classifier

The observed differences in bacterial composition across samples with varying diagnoses suggest a diagnostic potential for the microbial compositions of FIT-positive samples that could be harnessed to improve the efficiency of current screening programs. With the aim of reducing unnecessary colonoscopies while maintaining a high sensitivity, we explored machine learning approaches to develop a sample classifier able to discriminate samples with clinically-relevant diagnoses (CR, CRC samples and lesions of higher risk). Contrary to most automated classifiers that aim at maximizing accuracy, we intentionally put our focus on achieving high sensitivity at the cost of reduced accuracy. This is justified because, in a clinical context, false negatives (i.e., persons with clinically relevant lesions that do not proceed to colonoscopy) are of higher medical concern as compared to false positives (persons with no lesions that undergo colonoscopy), and because the main aim was to reduce the already high level of false positives in current FIT-based screenings without increasing the amount of false negatives. To derive this predictor, we explored the effect of using different machine learning algorithms, and the use of feature selection to restrict the parameter set to all bacterial taxa showing significant differences, or to a subset of them (see Materials and Methods, Section 2.7). When including more taxa, we observed a better area under the curve (AUC) and specificity (Table S4) This fact can be translated to better reduction of false-positive rates. On the other hand, when restricting to only a panel of taxa, we obtained better recall and sensitivity for CRC and CR samples but poor AUC and specificity (Table 1). However, in the context of the current screening, there is still a satisfactory reduction of the false-positive rate with a good prioritization of relevant cases. We achieved optimal results, in terms of inclusion of clinically relevant samples, with a two-phase classifier trained to classify CRC samples in a first phase and CR samples in a second phase. This final classifier considered information on sex, age and fecal hemoglobin concentration, and abundances from two different subsets of four taxa (first phase: *Akkermansia* spp., *Akkermansia muciniphila, Bacteroides fragilis* and *Bacteroides plebeius* and second phase: *Negativibacillus* spp., *Bacteroides coprocola, Bacteroides caccae* and *Dorea formicigenerans*) (Figure 5). This classifier obtained an average 98.98% sensitivity for CRC samples and 97.98% for clinically relevant samples (Table 1B).

We validated our strategy on two independent datasets. We first constructed a model with all the samples (without including *Bacteroides fragilis*, see Materials and Methods, Section 2.7) and tested it on an independent cohort of 135 FIT-positive samples from the USA [37]. The results of this adjusted model in the USA cohort yielded 100% sensitivity for CRC and 98.46% for CR lesions, reducing 20% of the unnecessary colonoscopies (Table S5A). We also performed an additional validation, in this case including both 4-4 taxa panels, with an independent dataset composed of 100 additional samples from the same Catalan screening detecting all CRC samples, 96% of the CR samples and having a reduction of 12% of the false positives (Table S5B). This last test set was balanced, and it was used for further optimization of the classifier. The corresponding ROC curves are represented at (Figure S7).

We explored how changing some parameters of the classifier affected sensitivity and the number of saved colonoscopies. For instance, by penalizing less the minority class (CR) at the second phase, we obtained better reduction of unnecessary colonoscopies (26%) but at the cost of including less CR samples (90%). Similarly, the number of samples to be tested for the microbial signature can be reduced by applying a FIT-value threshold above which a benefit of colonoscopy is assumed. For instance, applying a value of 954 µg hemoglobin/g feces (3rd quartile in our CR samples) for such a threshold, which is passed by 18% of our samples, would save 14% of unnecessary colonoscopies at the end of the process and reduce the need for microbiome testing. When we combined both approaches, we could reach 30% of saved colonoscopies, at the cost of a reduction of CR detection (87%). However, in all the mentioned cases we detected 100% of the CRC samples. This shows that our algorithm can be fine-tuned to optimize cost-effectiveness (Figure S8). A comparison of our algorithm with the current FIT strategy and other available solutions (GoodGut [47] and ColoGuard [48]) revealed higher sensitivity for both CRC and CR while maintaining a significant reduction of the current false positive rate and, importantly, without the need of collecting a separate sample from the screening (Table S6).

We next assessed possible alternative subsets of species included in the lists of differentially abundant taxa according to the diagnosis (Data S4 and S5) as potential features for the classification (See Materials and Methods, Section 2.7). We tested a total of 948 models and selected 13.5% of them (128/948). The strategy that led to more selected models was the one including subsets of 4 taxa with highest effect size, selecting half of the trained models (Figure S9A). The two *Akkermansia* species were the taxa that were most often included in selected models (Figure S9B) and 96.88% of the selected models included at least one of the 8 taxa used as features in the 4-4 taxa panel classifier (*Akkermansia muciniphila, Akkermansia* spp., *Bacteroides fragilis, Bacteroides plebeius, Bacteroides coprocola, Negativibacillus* spp., *Dorea formicigenerans* or *Bacteroides caccae*). These results suggest that different combinations of biomarkers drawn from the identified differentially abundant taxa can effectively be used to classify samples according to their clinical relevance.

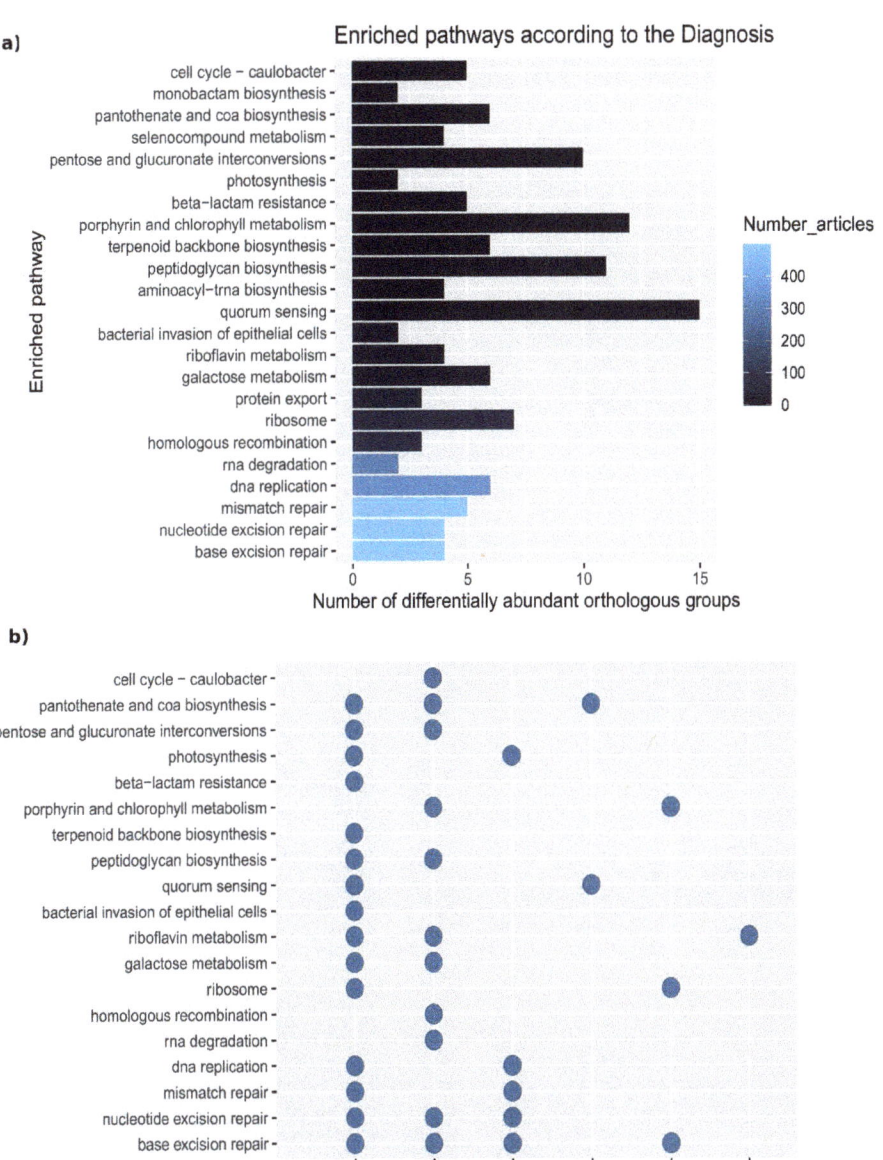

Figure 4. Enriched pathways according to the diagnosis. (**a**) The length of the bar indicates the number of differentially abundant OGs involved. The bars are sorted and colored according to the number of articles for which a given pathway has been linked to CRC. (**b**) Dotplot representing the pairs of diagnoses in which we found differentially abundant OGs involved in the enriched pathways. Of note, monobactam biosynthesis, protein export, selenocompound metabolism and aminoacyl-trna biosynthesis are not represented because multiple comparison tests did not detect involved OG as differentially abundant in any pairwise comparison.

Table 1. Performance of the two-phase machine learning predictor. The reported values are mean values obtained from the 100 random splits and include a panel of four taxa for each of the phases plus sex, age and FIT-value. Samples with missing metadata were discarded from this analysis (n = 2817). (A) Average of area under the curve (AUC), recall and specificity for each of the phases. (B) Average sensitivity for clinically relevant samples and for each of the diagnoses included in this group.

(A)			
	AUC	Recall	Specificity
FIRST PHASE	0.565368	0.8709974	0.2597385
SECOND PHASE	0.5358411	0.8052662	0.2664159
(B)			
			Average sensitivity (%)
CR *			97.98
IRL			97.71
HRL			98.06
CIS			98.54
CRC			98.98

* The average CR sensitivity re-proportionated according to the population (data from the Barcelona colorectal cancer screening, presented at Data S9) is 98.05%.

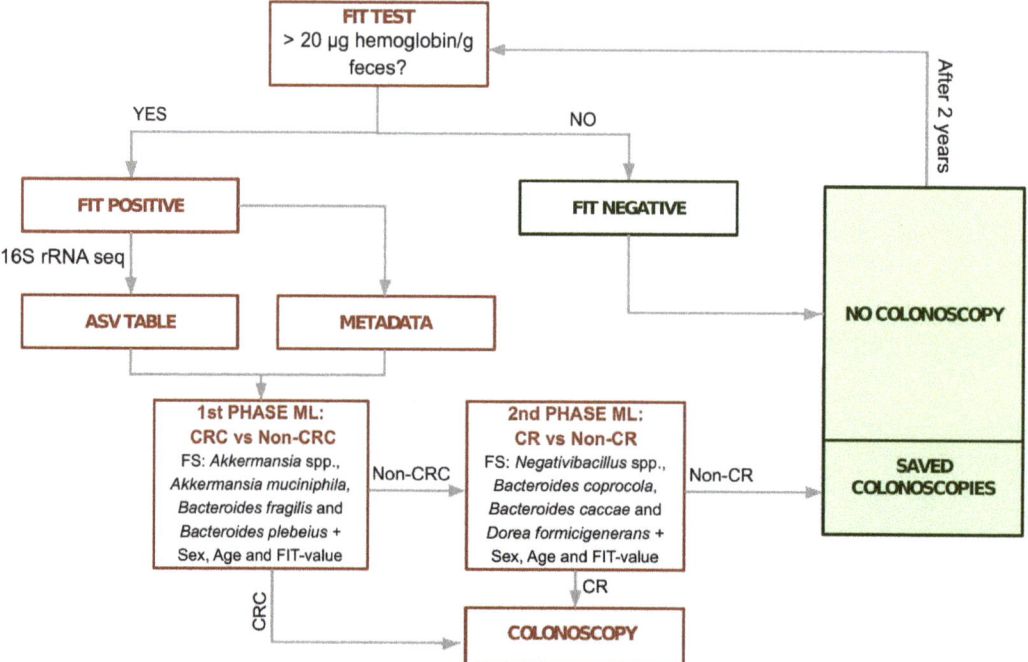

Figure 5. Flow chart of the proposed methodology (4-4 taxa classifier). FIT positive samples are subjected to microbiome profiling by 16S rRNA gene sequencing. Then a two phase classifier is applied. First the algorithm classifies CRC vs. non-CRC samples. Samples that are classified as non-CRC in the first phase are subjected to a second model that classifies CR vs. non-CR samples. FIT: fecal immunochemical test; CRC: colorectal cancer, CR: clinically relevant.

4. Discussion

CRC is a healthcare challenge and one of the leading causes of cancer-related deaths worldwide [49]. Early diagnosis of CRC is key for efficient treatment and for the survival of the patients and, hence, there is a strong interest in implementing diagnostic screenings for populations at risk. Colonoscopy, which is the gold standard for CRC diagnosis, is an expensive, time-consuming, invasive technique with potential complications. To minimize the use of colonoscopy only to cases that are more likely to benefit, population screening programs use less specific, non-invasive tests to pre-screen for risk of CRC. Immunochemical methods, such as FIT, have commonly been used as pre-colonoscopy tests in a two-step approach [50], but they have high false-positive rates, which results in unnecessary colonoscopies. This, in turn, increases healthcare costs and saturates endoscopy units, limiting the efficiency of population screenings. Considering this, there is a need to reduce the false-positive rate of the initial screening step by identifying new biomarkers and developing new risk scores. In this context, the gut microbiome has been suggested as a promising source for biomarkers with diagnostic potential in CRC [51]. In this project, we set out to investigate the potential of FIT samples to identify diagnostic markers and changes in the microbiota along the path from healthy colonic tissue to CRC.

Recent studies have shown the potential of the gut microbiome for CRC screening but these are mainly based on other types of samples [8,41,52,53] (e.g.,: gFOBT or stool samples) and are often focused on the comparison of CRC and healthy controls. In contrast, the focus of this project was on improving current screening programs based on FIT testing, using material from the same samples, and focusing on distinguishing clinically relevant cases (not only CRC) from FIT-positive samples (not the usual healthy baseline but the baseline of the population currently sent for colonoscopy).

Our results support the use of sampled material directly from FIT containers for microbiome analysis, avoiding the complex and costly collection and processing of separate stool samples that are widely and traditionally used to represent the gut microbiome [36]. More importantly, we show that the collected fecal material was enough to perform both the hemoglobin analysis and DNA extraction, and that the DNA was of sufficient quantity and quality to efficiently perform 16S metabarcoding. Earlier studies have also shown good conservation of DNA from frozen samples and close correspondence between microbiome profiles obtained from FIT samples and matching fecal material [54,55]. This is consistent with our results, which showed that the identified taxa and abundances are typically found in studies that use stool samples although observing differences that can be attributed to cohort or methodological particularities. Hence, our study shows that we can use the same fecal sample for both FIT and microbiome analyses, facilitating the implementation of microbiome-based biomarkers in currently ongoing population screening programs.

It is well known that a high percentage of CRCs emerge from premalignant polypoid lesions (i.e., adenomas and serrated lesions), which progress to CRC following a multi-stage development driven by both genetic and environmental risk factors [56]. Diet and lifestyle are key environmental factors associated with the presence of adenomas and their progression to CRC, likely through alterations of the gut microbiome. In our study, we captured differences between the fecal microbiome profiles along the various stages in the path from normal colonic epithelium to CRC. To the best of our knowledge, this is the first large microbiome study considering such a detailed and rigorous diagnostic classification associated with the included samples, which comprises different lesions in addition to healthy and CRC samples (Table S1). We did not observe disparate overall microbiome compositions between different clinical diagnoses but did find significant changes in particular taxa. Thus, different combinations of small but relevant changes may drive microbiome influence on CRC progression. In addition, it must be considered that microbiota alterations might more profoundly affect lesions and surrounding tissues, which may result in only subtle differences in the overall composition of the fecal material contained within FIT tubes.

Expectedly, we observed that CRC was the diagnostic group that had the most distinct microbiome profile. Taxa with the highest deviations in CRC-associated samples were *Akkermansia muciniphila* and an unclassified species from the same genus (*Akkermansia* spp.), which were overrepresented in CRC compared to the other samples, and *Bacteroides fragilis* and *Bacteroides plebeius*, which were underrepresented. Of note, *A. muciniphila* is a mucin-degrading bacterium and mucins such as MUC1 and MUC5AC are known to be overexpressed in CRC patients [57]. Hence, an increase of substrate availability could influence the observed higher abundance of this species. Interestingly, it is known that if microorganisms or their products cross the host epithelial barrier, both the immune and mesenchymal defenses respond with a signaling cascade (e.g., activation of NF-kB and STAT3) in order to maintain epithelial integrity. This fact has a selective impact on the gut microbiome and triggers mucin and antimicrobial peptide secretion [58]. *A. muciniphila* was found as overrepresented in other populations, and it was recently claimed as a potential biomarker for CRC in tissue [59].

Contrary to other studies with fecal and tissue samples that reported an enrichment of *Bacteroides fragilis* in CRC [58], we found this species to be underrepresented in these samples. Previous studies suggested that *B. fragilis* plays a key role in the development of CRC through the action of its toxin (BFT), which can influence colorectal tumorigenesis by disturbance or activation of signaling pathways that produce chronic intestinal inflammation and tissue injury [60]. However, we found this underrepresentation comparing CRC vs. non-CRC (including all the adenomas), as opposed to these other studies which compared CRC vs. healthy samples. Previous studies have shown that there are different strains of *B. fragilis* along the gastrointestinal tract apart from the mentioned BFT-producing strains, such as a non-toxigenic *B. fragilis* which has an immunogenic capsular component, and the Polysaccharide A that promotes mucosal immune development and whose increase has not been associated to CRC [61,62].

We also observed an influence on the differences of the microbiome driven by variables like sex and age and, interestingly, by the number of polyps. As mentioned above, the presence of polyps can be a sign of risk to development or progression of CRC, so the study of the microbiome associated with polyps can serve as a source of predictive biomarkers for CRC. Some of the genera whose abundance correlated with the number of polyps were also reported in previous studies in relation to risk for CRC polyps (e.g., *Bacteroides*, *Blautia* and *Bifidobacterium*). However, the presence of polyps does not necessarily lead to the development of CRC and some patients with particular genetic profiles may present numerous polyps [63].

It is known that the presence of certain metabolites, DNA damage, and inflammation are all factors driving CRC progression [64]. Changes in the microbial composition or functionalities can promote a more optimal microenvironment for the development of CRC. Conversely, CRC progression can alter the surrounding environment and therefore affect microbial communities. In our study, we inferred the potential functionalities of the microbiome profiles associated with each colonoscopy outcome and observed OGs that were significantly differentially abundant across diagnoses. Interestingly, we observed that the transition from intermediate risk lesion to high risk lesion was the stage with the greatest alteration of functional and metabolic capacities. Some examples of enriched pathways were galactose metabolism, RNA degradation, pentose and glucuronate interconversions and quorum sensing. In this regard, it has been reported that microbes can interact with cancer cells through their quorum sensing peptides and influence metastasis [65]. Also of note, many of the pathways found are related to DNA repair. This may reflect a toxic environment for the microbial DNA, perhaps caused by the bacterial metabolism. This same environment could be damaging to the host DNA, supporting a genotoxic pathway connecting the microbiome and CRC development [66]. Our results are based on 16S rRNA sequencing, which is a cost-effective approach that can be applied to many samples. In particular, the presented results related to functional inference should be confirmed using shotgun metagenomics or meta-transcriptomics approaches, which will provide better resolution. However, previous studies demonstrated high correlation of functional profiles predicted from 16S rRNA sequencing data and from metagenomes [67], and we believe the data presented here are a good proxy for generating testable hypotheses.

Metabolic capacities of some microorganisms, such as the mentioned mucin utilization of *A.muciniphila*, can result in sources of nutrients or energy for other microbes in the gut. The study of correlated abundances between different microbes is interesting in this context. We detected distinct taxon co-occurrence patterns in the studied diagnoses that likely reflect changes in microbial ecosystems and their metabolic interactions that accompany the transitions towards CRC development. It is interesting to account for these patterns because of the dominant functional redundancy of the gut microbiome: some bacteria can share functions and exert similar influences on the development and progression of CRC. In addition, it is still unclear how microbes modulate each other, or how they shape the immune environment of the tumor, and these co-occurrence patterns can shed light in this direction [58]. For instance, we observed an exclusive negative association between *Dorea longicatena* and *Akkermansia* spp. only in the CRC group.

The presented machine learning prediction results show a potential role of the microbial composition of FIT samples in CRC screening. We derived a two-phase classifier with high sensitivity for CRC and other CR samples with a small but significant reduction of the false positive rate. In the context of the Barcelona screening program [13], in which there is an average participation of 50%, approximately 5% of participants have a positive FIT result. Of them, around 3–5% have CRC detected during colonoscopy and an additional 30% have a CR lesion associated with CRC risk requiring a more intensive surveillance, whereas around 65% have a normal colonoscopy or only non-CR lesions are detected. Therefore, translating our results to this clinical context and considering the mean participation and diagnosis obtained during the last four available rounds, we would save a range between 423 (12%) to 1057 (30%) unnecessary colonoscopies each year, while maximizing the inclusion of CR individuals (Data S9).

By reducing the number of unnecessary colonoscopies and increasing cost-effectiveness of current population screenings, microbiome-based tests such as the one explored here, could not only save money and time but also increase participation and adherence rates. The present study has some limitations, such as the imbalance in some of the diagnoses, and the lack of more detailed information on polyps or lesion characteristics (e.g., localization, size, histology), genetic profiles, or past treatments, which can be factors influencing the microbiome. However, this lack of information, which is difficult to access beforehand, is also a strength of our study, showing that with just the FIT sample and information on the sex and age of individuals we can draw some conclusions and obtain a classification of the samples with high sensitivity for CRC and CR samples. Further studies are necessary to validate these findings in different cohorts and to properly assess cost-effectiveness in the framework of a health economics analysis that considers direct and indirect costs of colonoscopy and microbiome analysis from FIT samples. Finally, further developments such as a targeted quantification of a species panel by multiplex PCR, or implementations in the FIT tube to accommodate this additional test, will likely further reduce costs and facilitate the adoption of microbiome-based tests.

5. Conclusions

Colorectal cancer (CRC) is a leading cause of cancer deaths worldwide with a substantial challenge in its diagnosis, which if done early could improve overall survival. Our study suggests a potential role of the microbiome in the path from normal epithelia to CRC, revealing taxa, metabolic features and co-occurrence changes along this progression. The proposed classifier and its possible cost-effectivity optimization as well as the addition of other layers of information or current in-use clinical biomarkers such as microRNAs, gene mutations and DNA methylation, that are already stated as potential biomarkers, can be a potential tool for clinical proposes and improvement of current CRC screening.

Patents

A patent covering the use of microbial biomarkers for CRC and CR detection published in this manuscript has been filed.

Supplementary Materials: The following supporting information can be downloaded at: https://www.mdpi.com/article/10.3390/cancers15010120/s1, Supplementary Data (large tables): Data S1. Strengthening The Organization and Reporting of Microbiome Studies (STORMS) checklist; Data S2. Metadata will be available prior to publication; Data S3. Table of the taxa at the species level that we found as differentially abundant according to each of the fixed effects included in the linear model. Only significant p-values are reported. Samples with missing metadata were not considered in this analysis, (n = 2565); Data S4. Table of the taxa at the species level that we found as differentially abundant according to each of the fixed effects included in the linear model when comparing CRC vs. non-CRC. Only significant p-values are reported. Samples with missing metadata were not considered in this analysis, (n = 2565); Data S5. Table of the taxa at the species level that we found as differentially abundant according to each of the fixed effects included in the linear model when comparing clinically relevant (CR) vs. non-Clinically relevant (non-CR) samples. Only significant p-values are reported. Samples with missing metadata were not considered in this analysis, (n = 2565); Data S6. Table of species found as differentially abundant according to the number of polyps, and the significance values (p-value < 0.05). Samples with missing metadata were not considered in this analysis; (n = 2565); Data S7. List of differentially abundant OG according to the diagnosis and the significance values (p-value < 0.05); Data S8. Summary of the significant results obtained when applying multiple comparisons between diagnoses. Significant p values are reported (Tukey test, p.adjusted < 0.05). The p-value has the sign of the corresponding effect size, indicating the direction of the difference; Data S9. Statistics of the last four available rounds of results from the Catalan CRC screening in Barcelona; Supplementary Material (Figures and small tables): Figure S1. Pie chart representing the 10 most abundant genera of studied CRIPREV samples. The other genera were grouped and named as "others"; Figure S2. Comparison of FIT positive 16S samples from the present study and stool 16S samples from an independent study. (A) Multidimensional scaling plot (MDS) representing the Aitchison distance and Shannon index according to the source project. (B) Barplot representing the present phyla. Each column represents a sample; Figure S3. Alpha diversity characterization, (n = 2889). The lines inside the boxplots represent the medians for each of the groups. Statistical test: Kruskall-Wallis or Wilcoxon test, with a significant result when p < 0.05. (A) Observed index according to the diagnosis (carcinoma in situ (CIS), colorectal cancer (CRC), lesion that is not associated to risk (LNAR), high risk lesion (HRL), low risk lesion (LRL), intermediate risk lesion (IRL) or negative (N) samples) and risk (clinically relevant (CR) vs. non-clinically relevant (non-CR) samples) variables. (B) Shannon and Simpson indices according to the diagnosis; Figure S4. MDS plots using Aitchison distance, (n = 2889). The samples are colored according to the diagnosis. 95% confidence ellipses are represented for each of the diagnosed groups; Figure S5. Box plot of the Akkermansia clr according to the different explored diagnosis, (n = 2889). Negative (N), lesion not associated to risk (LNAR), low risk lesion (LRL), intermediate risk lesion (IRL), high risk lesion (HRL), carcinoma in situ (CIS) and colorectal cancer (CRC); Figure S6. Summary of the results of the adonis test, evaluating the effect of lifestyle variables on the overall composition. Only significant (p-value < 0.05) results are colored, including the p-value in each of the cells. The assessment of the individual effect of each variable is in the orange column, while is the impact using as covariate the diagnosis is in the pink column. The explained variability (R2) was used for the color intensity of the cells; Figure S7. ROC curves for each of the phases in the different validations performed. First phase: CRC vs. others, Second phase: clinically relevant vs. non-clinically relevant (a) USA cohort, (b) 100 extra samples from the CRC screening; Figure S8. Percentage of saved colonoscopies and clinically relevant sensitivity according to the different specifications of the proposed classifier; All_taxa: All the intersecting taxa between the CRIPREV and the validation datasets were used as features. DA_taxa: All the intersecting differentially abundant taxa between the CRIPREV and the validation datasets were used as features. 4-4 taxa panel: 4 taxa panel for each of the phases. 4-4 taxa panel, adjW: 4 taxa panel for each of the phases, with less penalization of the CR samples in the second phase. FIT_filter_4-4 taxa panel: samples above 954 of the FIT value (µg hemoglobin/g feces) were directed to colonoscopy and the remaining samples were subjected to the classifier. FIT_filter_4-4 taxa panel_adjW: samples above 954 of the FIT value (µg hemoglobin/g feces) were directed to colonoscopy and the remaining samples were subjected to the classifier. Less penalization of the CR samples in the second phase. Figure S9. (A) Potential selection (number of models selected/number of evaluated models, in %) of the different feature selection methods. (B) Average potential selection of each of the 27 studied taxa (number of selected models in which the taxa were included/number of models in which the taxa were included as a feature); Table S1. Criteria and distribution of the colonoscopy-based diagnosis types considered in this project. Columns indicate, in this order: the diagnosis group, the criteria for classification in the group, the number of samples of this study in the given group, and the clinical relevance; Table S2. Characteristics of the included individuals: sex, median and range age and samples deemed of clinical relevance after colonoscopy. * Samples with 'NA' value for this parameter are excluded from the calculation; Table S3. Table summarizing differential abundance analysis results considering all the diagnoses following the path from healthy colon to colorectal cancer. We used the linear model: tax_element~diagnosis + hospital + sex + age + n_polyps + FIT_value + (1 | run). Samples with missing metadata were not considered in this analysis, (n = 2565); Table S4. Performance of the two-phase machine learning predictor. The reported values are mean values obtained from the 100 random splits. Including 41 and 34 taxa for both phase 1 and phase 2, respectively, plus sex, age and fecal hemoglobin concentration. Samples with missing metadata were discarded from this analysis, (n = 2817). (A) Average of area under the curve (AUC), recall and specificity for each of the phases (B) Average of sensitivity for clinically relevant samples and for each of the diagnosis included in this particular group; Table S5. Performance of the two-phase machine learning predictor on independent datasets. The reported values are obtained by training on all the CriPrev samples (samples with missing metadata were discarded for training the model, n = 2817) and testing on the independent sets. Area under the curve (AUC), recall and specificity for each of the phases and sensitivity for CRC and CR lesions at the end of the two-phase classification were reported. (A) USA cohort. Including a panel of 3 and 4 taxa for phase 1 and 2, respectively, plus sex, age and fecal hemoglobin concentration. (B) 100 extra samples from the Catalan screening; Table S6. Comparison of our algorithm (considering different optimizations, and shadowed cells) with two alternative solutions and the current FIT strategy.

Author Contributions: T.G. designed the study, supervised the work and contributed to the conception, interpretation of the data and drafted the manuscript. E.S. performed the data collection and DNA extraction. S.C.-B. and V.M. collected samples and contributed to data interpretation. O.K.-L. performed the data analysis, interpretation of the data and drafted the manuscript. J.R.W. contributed to the data analysis, interpretation of the data and drafted the manuscript. All authors approved the final manuscript. All authors have read and agreed to the published version of the manuscript.

Funding: This work was supported by the Catalan Government through the Strategic Plan for Research and Innovation in Health (PERIS) (Project CrivPrev SLT002/16/00398). This study was funded by grants from Fondo de Investigación Sanitaria/FEDER (17/00878, 20/00113), CERCA Program (Generalitat de Catalunya) and Agència de Gestió d'Ajuts Universitaris i de Recerca (Generalitat de Catalunya, GRPRE 2017SGR21, GRC 2017SGR653). CIBEREHD, CIBERESP and CIBERINFEC are funded by the Instituto de Salud Carlos III. OKL is supported by the Formación de profesorado universitario (FPU) program from the Spanish Ministerio de Universidades (FPU2020-02907). CAC and JM are supported by a contract from CIBEREHD. LB was supported by a Juan de la Cierva postdoctoral contract (FJCI-2017-32593).

Institutional Review Board Statement: The study was approved by the institutional ethical committees of the involved institutions (Hospital Clínic of Barcelona, Barcelona, Spain; HCB/2017/0193) and informed consent was obtained from the participants.

Informed Consent Statement: Informed consent was obtained from all subjects involved in the study.

Data Availability Statement: The dataset supporting the conclusions of this article is available in the NCBI Sequence Read Archive (SRA) under the BioProject ID PRJNA792716. The study relies on open source software listed in the methodology.

Acknowledgments: We are thankful to all CRC-screening participants that provided consent for the use of their samples in this study.

Conflicts of Interest: A patent has been filed covering the presented results.

Appendix A. Authorship Appendix—CRIPREV Consortium

Fundació Institut d'Investigació Biomèdica de Bellvitge (IDIBELL)—ICO

- Josep M Borràs
- Elisabet Guinó, Gemma Ibañez-Sanz, Mireia Obon-Santacana, Ferran Moratalla-Navarro, Ana Diez-Villanueva, Rebeca Sanz-Pamplona, Victor Moreno

Fundació Clínic per a la Recerca Biomèdica (IRS-IDIBAPS)

- Coral Arnau-Collell, Jenifer Muñoz, Josep M Augé, Laia Bonjoch, Anna Serradesanferm, Àngels Pozo, Leticia Moreira, Marcos Díaz-Gay, Sebastià Franch-Expósito, Cristina Herrera-Pariente, Yasmin Soares de Lima, Lorena Moreno, Teresa Ocaña, Sabela Carballal, Ariadna Sánchez, Francesc Balaguer, Jaume Grau, Antoni Castells, Sergi Castellví-Bel
- Elena Asensio, Sara Lahoz, Carolina Parra, Clàudia Galofré, Iván Archilla, Miriam Cuatrecasas, Jordi Camps

Institut Hospital del Mar d'Investigacions Mèdiques (IMIM)

- Joan Gibert, Raquel Longaron, Clara Montagut
- Xavier Bessa, Beatriz Bellosillo, Carme Márquez Márquez, Rebeca Rueda Miret, Rocio Pérez Berbegal, Gabriel Piquer Velaso, Joan Carles Balboa, Ana Cristina Alvarez Urturi, Ines Ana Ibañez Zafon, Sandra Cordero Cerrudo, Miriam Parrilla Carrasco, Bouchra Alouali Moussakhkhar

Institut de Recerca Biomèdica de Barcelona (IRB)

- Toni Gabaldón, Ester Saus, Olfat Khannous-Lleiffe

Fundació Institut d'Investigació en Ciències de la Salut Germans Trias i Pujol

- Sergio Alonso, Beatriz González, Maria Navarro-Jiménez, Andreu Alibés
- Mar Muñoz, Berta Martin, Miguel A. Peinado

References

1. Bray, F.; Ferlay, J.; Soerjomataram, I.; Siegel, R.L.; Torre, L.A.; Jemal, A. Global cancer statistics 2018: GLOBOCAN estimates of incidence and mortality worldwide for 36 cancers in 185 countries. *CA Cancer J. Clin.* **2018**, *68*, 394–424. [CrossRef] [PubMed]
2. Cancer Genome Atlas Network. Comprehensive molecular characterization of human colon and rectal cancer. *Nature* **2012**, *487*, 330–337. [CrossRef] [PubMed]
3. Murphy, N.; Moreno, V.; Hughes, D.J.; Vodicka, L.; Vodicka, P.; Aglago, E.K.; Gunter, M.J.; Jenab, M. Lifestyle and dietary environmental factors in colorectal cancer susceptibility. *Mol. Aspects Med.* **2019**, *69*, 2–9. [CrossRef] [PubMed]
4. Saus, E.; Iraola-Guzmán, S.; Willis, J.R.; Brunet-Vega, A.; Gabaldón, T. Microbiome and colorectal cancer: Roles in carcinogenesis and clinical potential. *Mol. Aspects Med.* **2019**, *69*, 93–106. [CrossRef] [PubMed]
5. Zackular, J.P.; Baxter, N.T.; Iverson, K.D.; Sadler, W.D.; Petrosino, J.F.; Chen, G.Y.; Schloss, P.D. The gut microbiome modulates colon tumorigenesis. *MBio* **2013**, *4*, e00692-13. [CrossRef] [PubMed]
6. Zackular, J.P.; Rogers, M.A.M.; Ruffin, M.T., 4th; Schloss, P.D. The human gut microbiome as a screening tool for colorectal cancer. *Cancer Prev. Res.* **2014**, *7*, 1112–1121. [CrossRef]
7. Sheng, Q.S.; He, K.X.; Li, J.J.; Zhong, Z.F.; Wang, F.X.; Pan, L.L.; Lin, J.J. Comparison of Gut Microbiome in Human Colorectal Cancer in Paired Tumor and Adjacent Normal Tissues. *Onco Targets Ther.* **2020**, *13*, 635–646. [CrossRef]
8. Yu, J.; Feng, Q.; Wong, S.H.; Zhang, D.; Yi Liang, Q.; Qin, Y.; Tang, L.; Zhao, H.; Stenvang, J.; Li, Y.; et al. Metagenomic analysis of faecal microbiome as a tool towards targeted non-invasive biomarkers for colorectal cancer. *Gut* **2017**, *66*, 70–78. [CrossRef]
9. Winawer, S.J. The history of colorectal cancer screening: A personal perspective. *Dig. Dis. Sci.* **2015**, *60*, 596–608. [CrossRef]
10. Young, G.P.; Rabeneck, L.; Winawer, S.J. The Global Paradigm Shift in Screening for Colorectal Cancer. *Gastroenterology* **2019**, *156*, 843–851.e2. [CrossRef]
11. Zou, S.; Fang, L.; Lee, M.-H. Dysbiosis of gut microbiota in promoting the development of colorectal cancer. *Gastroenterol. Rep.* **2018**, *6*, 1–12. [CrossRef] [PubMed]
12. Vega, P.; Valentín, F.; Cubiella, J. Colorectal cancer diagnosis: Pitfalls and opportunities. *World J. Gastrointest. Oncol.* **2015**, *7*, 422–433. [CrossRef] [PubMed]
13. Inici. [cited 18 May 2021]. Available online: http://www.prevenciocolonbcn.org/ca/ (accessed on 18 May 2021).
14. Quintero, E.; Castells, A.; Bujanda, L.; Cubiella, J.; Salas, D.; Lanas, Á.; Andreu, M.; Carballo, F.; Morillas, J.D.; Hernández, C.; et al. Colonoscopy versus fecal immunochemical testing in colorectal-cancer screening. *N. Engl. J. Med.* **2012**, *366*, 697–706. [CrossRef] [PubMed]

15. Atkin, W.S.; Valori, R.; Kuipers, E.J.; Hoff, G.; Senore, C.; Segnan, N.; Jover, R.; Schmiegel, W.; Lambert, R.; Pox, C. European guidelines for quality assurance in colorectal cancer screening and diagnosis. First Edition—Colonoscopic surveillance following adenoma removal. *Endoscopy* **2012**, *44* (Suppl. 3), SE151–SE163. [CrossRef] [PubMed]
16. Click, B.; Pinsky, P.F.; Hickey, T.; Doroudi, M.; Schoen, R.E. Association of Colonoscopy Adenoma Findings With Long-term Colorectal Cancer Incidence. *JAMA* **2018**, *319*, 2021–2031. [CrossRef] [PubMed]
17. Willis, J.R.; González-Torres, P.; Pittis, A.A.; Bejarano, L.A.; Cozzuto, L.; Andreu-Somavilla, N.; Alloza-Trabado, M.; Valentín, A.; Ksiezopolska, E.; Onywera, H.; et al. Citizen science charts two major "stomatotypes" in the oral microbiome of adolescents and reveals links with habits and drinking water composition. *Microbiome* **2018**, *6*, 218. [CrossRef]
18. Callahan, B.J.; McMurdie, P.J.; Rosen, M.J.; Han, A.W.; Johnson, A.J.; Holmes, S.P. DADA2: High Resolution Sample Inference from Amplicon Data. *Nat Methods* **2016**, *13*, 581–583. [CrossRef]
19. Quast, C.; Pruesse, E.; Yilmaz, P.; Gerken, J.; Schweer, T.; Yarza, P.; Peplies, J.; Glöckner, F.O. The SILVA ribosomal RNA gene database project: Improved data processing and web-based tools. *Nucleic Acids Res.* **2013**, *41*, D590–D596. [CrossRef]
20. Schliep, K.P. phangorn: Phylogenetic analysis in R. *Bioinformatics* **2011**, *27*, 592–593. [CrossRef]
21. Wright, E.; Erik Wright, S. Using DECIPHER v2.0 to Analyze Big Biological Sequence Data in R. *R J.* **2016**, *8*, 352. [CrossRef]
22. McMurdie, P.J.; Holmes, S. phyloseq: An R package for reproducible interactive analysis and graphics of microbiome census data. *PLoS ONE* **2013**, *8*, e61217. [CrossRef] [PubMed]
23. vegan: Community Ecology Package. [cited 20 December 2021]. Available online: https://CRAN.R-project.org/package=vegan (accessed on 20 December 2021).
24. Gloor, G.B.; Reid, G. Compositional analysis: A valid approach to analyze microbiome high-throughput sequencing data. *Can J. Microbiol.* **2016**, *62*, 692–703. [CrossRef] [PubMed]
25. Palarea-Albaladejo, J.; Martín-Fernández, J.A. zCompositions—R package for multivariate imputation of left-censored data under a compositional approach. *Chem. Intell. Lab. Syst.* **2015**, *143*, 85–96. [CrossRef]
26. Gloor, G.B.; Macklaim, J.M.; Pawlowsky-Glahn, V.; Egozcue, J.J. Microbiome Datasets Are Compositional: And This Is Not Optional. *Front. Microbiol.* **2017**, *8*, 2224. [CrossRef] [PubMed]
27. Latorre-Pérez, A.; Hernández, M.; Iglesias, J.R.; Morán, J.; Pascual, J.; Porcar, M.; Vilanova, C.; Collado, L. The Spanish gut microbiome reveals links between microorganisms and Mediterranean diet. *Sci. Rep.* **2021**, *11*, 21602. [CrossRef]
28. Bates, D.; Mächler, M.; Bolker, B.; Walker, S. Fitting Linear Mixed-Effects Models Using lme4. *J. Stat. Softw.* **2015**, *67*, 1–48. Available online: http://www.jstatsoft.org/v67/i01/ (accessed on 20 December 2021). [CrossRef]
29. Fox, J.; Friendly, M.; Weisberg, S. Hypothesis Tests for Multivariate Linear Models Using the car Package. *R J.* **2013**, *5*, 39. [CrossRef]
30. Hothorn, T.; Bretz, F.; Westfall, P. Simultaneous inference in general parametric models. *Biom J.* **2008**, *50*, 346–363. [CrossRef]
31. Rivera-Pinto, J.; Egozcue, J.J.; Pawlowsky-Glahn, V.; Paredes, R.; Noguera-Julian, M.; Calle, M.L. Balances: A New Perspective for Microbiome Analysis. *mSystems* **2018**, *3*, e00053-18. [CrossRef]
32. Kurtz, Z.D.; Müller, C.L.; Miraldi, E.R.; Littman, D.R.; Blaser, M.J.; Bonneau, R.A. Sparse and Compositionally Robust Inference of Microbial Ecological Networks. *PLOS Comput. Biol.* **2015**, *11*, e1004226. [CrossRef]
33. Woloszynek, S.; Mell, J.C.; Zhao, Z.; Simpson, G.; O'Connor, M.P.; Rosen, G.L. Exploring thematic structure and predicted functionality of 16S rRNA amplicon data. *PLoS ONE* **2019**, *14*, e0219235. [CrossRef] [PubMed]
34. easyPubMed: Search and Retrieve Scientific Publication Records from PubMed. [cited 21 December 2021]. Available online: https://CRAN.R-project.org/package=easyPubMed (accessed on 20 December 2021).
35. Kuhn, M. Building Predictive Models in R Using the caret Package. *J. Stat. Softw.* **2008**, *28*, 1–26. Available online: http://www.jstatsoft.org/v28/i05/ (accessed on 20 December 2021). [CrossRef]
36. Krigul, K.L.; Aasmets, O.; Lüll, K.; Org, T.; Org, E. Using fecal immunochemical tubes for the analysis of the gut microbiome has the potential to improve colorectal cancer screening. *Sci. Rep.* **2021**, *11*, 19603. [CrossRef] [PubMed]
37. Baxter, N.T.; Koumpouras, C.C.; Rogers, M.A.M.; Ruffin, M.T., 4th; Schloss, P.D. DNA from fecal immunochemical test can replace stool for detection of colonic lesions using a microbiota-based model. *Microbiome* **2016**, *4*, 59. [CrossRef] [PubMed]
38. Robin, X.; Turck, N.; Hainard, A.; Tiberti, N.; Lisacek, F.; Sanchez, J.C.; Müller, M. pROC: An open-source package for R and S+ to analyze and compare ROC curves. *BMC Bioinform.* **2011**, *12*, 77. [CrossRef] [PubMed]
39. Abrahamson, M.; Hooker, E.; Ajami, N.J.; Petrosino, J.F.; Orwoll, E.S. Successful collection of stool samples for microbiome analyses from a large community-based population of elderly men. *Contemp. Clin. Trials Commun.* **2017**, *7*, 158–162. [CrossRef]
40. Feng, Y.; Duan, Y.; Xu, Z.; Lyu, N.; Liu, F.; Liang, S.; Zhu, B. An examination of data from the American Gut Project reveals that the dominance of the genus Bifidobacterium is associated with the diversity and robustness of the gut microbiota. *Microbiologyopen* **2019**, *8*, e939. [CrossRef] [PubMed]
41. Yang, T.W.; Lee, W.H.; Tu, S.J.; Huang, W.C.; Chen, H.M.; Sun, T.H.; Tsai, M.C.; Wang, C.C.; Chen, H.Y.; Huang, C.C.; et al. Enterotype-based Analysis of Gut Microbiota along the Conventional Adenoma-Carcinoma Colorectal Cancer Pathway. *Sci Rep.* **2019**, *9*, 10923. [CrossRef]
42. Sweeney, T.E.; Morton, J.M. The human gut microbiome: A review of the effect of obesity and surgically induced weight loss. *JAMA Surg.* **2013**, *148*, 563–569. [CrossRef]
43. Rinninella, E.; Raoul, P.; Cintoni, M.; Franceschi, F.; Miggiano, G.A.; Gasbarrini, A.; Mele, M.C. What is the Healthy Gut Microbiota Composition? A Changing Ecosystem across Age, Environment, Diet, and Diseases. *Microorganisms* **2019**, *7*, 14. [CrossRef]

44. Chénard, T.; Malick, M.; Dubé, J.; Massé, E. The influence of blood on the human gut microbiome. *BMC Microbiol.* **2020**, *20*, 1–10. [CrossRef] [PubMed]
45. Shussman, N.; Wexner, S.D. Colorectal polyps and polyposis syndromes. *Gastroenterol. Rep.* **2014**, *2*, 1–15. [CrossRef] [PubMed]
46. Tilg, H.; Adolph, T.E.; Gerner, R.R.; Moschen, A.R. The Intestinal Microbiota in Colorectal Cancer. *Cancer Cell.* **2018**, *33*, 954–964. [CrossRef] [PubMed]
47. Malagón, M.; Ramió-Pujol, S.; Serrano, M.; Amoedo, J.; Oliver, L.; Bahí, A.; Miquel-Cusachs, J.O.; Ramirez, M.; Queralt-Moles, X.; Gilabert, P.; et al. New Fecal Bacterial Signature for Colorectal Cancer Screening Reduces the Fecal Immunochemical Test False-Positive Rate in a Screening Population. *SSRN Electron. J.* **2020**. [CrossRef]
48. Imperiale, T.F.; Ransohoff, D.F.; Itzkowitz, S.H.; Levin, T.R.; Lavin, P.; Lidgard, G.P.; Ahlquist, D.A.; Berger, B.M. Multitarget stool DNA testing for colorectal-cancer screening. *N. Engl. J. Med.* **2014**, *370*, 1287–1297. [CrossRef] [PubMed]
49. Guren, M.G. The global challenge of colorectal cancer. *Lancet Gastroenterol. Hepatol.* **2019**, *4*, 894–895. [CrossRef]
50. Hasegawa, R.; Yashima, K.; Ikebuchi, Y.; Sasaki, S.; Yoshida, A.; Kawaguchi, K.; Isomoto, H. Characteristics of Advanced Colorectal Cancer Detected by Fecal Immunochemical Test Screening in Participants with a Negative Result the Previous Year. *Yonago Acta Med.* **2020**, *63*, 63–69. [CrossRef]
51. Shang, F.-M.; Liu, H.-L. and colorectal cancer: A review. *World J. Gastrointest Oncol.* **2018**, *10*, 71–81. [CrossRef]
52. Young, C.; Wood, H.M.; Fuentes Balaguer, A.; Bottomley, D.; Gallop, N.; Wilkinson, L.; Benton, S.C.; Brealey, M.; John, C.; Burtonwood, C.; et al. Microbiome Analysis of More Than 2,000 NHS Bowel Cancer Screening Programme Samples Shows the Potential to Improve Screening Accuracy. *Clin. Cancer Res.* **2021**, *27*, 2246–2254. [CrossRef]
53. Zeller, G.; Tap, J.; Voigt, A.Y.; Sunagawa, S.; Kultima, J.R.; Costea, P.I.; Amiot, A.; Böhm, J.; Brunetti, F.; Habermann, N.; et al. Potential of fecal microbiota for early-stage detection of colorectal cancer. *Mol. Syst. Biol.* **2014**, *10*, 766. [CrossRef]
54. Nel Van Zyl, K.; Whitelaw, A.C.; Newton-Foot, M. The effect of storage conditions on microbial communities in stool. *PLoS ONE* **2020**, *15*, e0227486. [CrossRef]
55. Zouiouich, S.; Mariadassou, M.; Rué, O.; Vogtmann, E.; Huybrechts, I.; Severi, G.; Boutron-Ruault, M.C.; Senore, C.; Naccarati, A.; Mengozzi, G.; et al. Comparison of Fecal Sample Collection Methods for Microbial Analysis Embedded within Colorectal Cancer Screening Programs. *Cancer Epidemiol. Biomark. Prev.* **2022**, *31*, 305–314. [CrossRef] [PubMed]
56. Vacante, M.; Ciuni, R.; Basile, F.; Biondi, A. Gut Microbiota and Colorectal Cancer Development: A Closer Look to the Adenoma-Carcinoma Sequence. *Biomedicines* **2020**, *8*, 489. [CrossRef] [PubMed]
57. Byrd, J.C.; Bresalier, R.S. Mucins and mucin binding proteins in colorectal cancer. *Cancer Metastasis Rev.* **2004**, *23*, 77–99. [CrossRef] [PubMed]
58. Janney, A.; Powrie, F.; Mann, E.H. Host-microbiota maladaptation in colorectal cancer. *Nature* **2020**, *585*, 509–517. [CrossRef] [PubMed]
59. Osman, M.A.; Neoh, H.M.; Ab Mutalib, N.S.; Chin, S.F.; Mazlan, L.; Raja Ali, R.A.; Zakaria, A.D.; Ngiu, C.S.; Ang, M.Y.; Jamal, R. Parvimonas micra, Peptostreptococcus stomatis, Fusobacterium nucleatum and Akkermansia muciniphila as a four-bacteria biomarker panel of colorectal cancer. *Sci. Rep.* **2021**, *11*, 2925. [CrossRef] [PubMed]
60. Cheng, W.T.; Kantilal, H.K.; Davamani, F. The Mechanism of Toxin Contributes to Colon Cancer Formation. *Malays J. Med. Sci.* **2020**, *27*, 9–21.
61. Zhao, Y.; Wang, C.; Goel, A. Role of gut microbiota in epigenetic regulation of colorectal Cancer. *Biochim. Biophys. Acta (BBA)—Rev. Cancer* **2021**, *1875*, 188490. [CrossRef]
62. Chan, J.L.; Wu, S.; Geis, A.L.; Chan, G.V.; Gomes, T.A.; Beck, S.E.; Wu, X.; Fan, H.; Tam, A.J.; Chung, L.; et al. Non-toxigenic Bacteroides fragilis (NTBF) administration reduces bacteria-driven chronic colitis and tumor development independent of polysaccharide A. *Mucosal Immunol.* **2019**, *12*, 164–177. [CrossRef]
63. Dadkhah, E.; Sikaroodi, M.; Korman, L.; Hardi, R.; Baybick, J.; Hanzel, D.; Kuehn, G.; Kuehn, T.; Gillevet, P.M. Gut microbiome identifies risk for colorectal polyps. *BMJ Open Gastroenterol.* **2019**, *6*, e000297. [CrossRef]
64. Han, S.; Zhuang, J.; Wu, Y.; Wu, W.; Yang, X. Progress in Research on Colorectal Cancer-Related Microorganisms and Metabolites. *Cancer Manag. Res.* **2020**, *12*, 8703–8720. [CrossRef]
65. Wynendaele, E.; Verbeke, F.; D'Hondt, M.; Hendrix, A.; Van De Wiele, C.; Burvenich, C.; Peremans, K.; De Wever, O.; Bracke, M.; De Spiegeleer, B. Crosstalk between the microbiome and cancer cells by quorum sensing peptides. *Peptides* **2015**, *64*, 40–48. [CrossRef] [PubMed]
66. Sepich-Poore, G.D.; Zitvogel, L.; Straussman, R.; Hasty, J.; Wargo, J.A.; Knight, R. The microbiome and human cancer. *Science* **2021**, *371*, eabc4552. [CrossRef] [PubMed]
67. Wemheuer, F.; Taylor, J.A.; Daniel, R.; Johnston, E.; Meinicke, P.; Thomas, T.; Wemheuer, B. Tax4Fun2: Prediction of habitat-specific functional profiles and functional redundancy based on 16S rRNA gene sequences. *Environ. Microbiome* **2020**, *15*, 11. [CrossRef] [PubMed]

Disclaimer/Publisher's Note: The statements, opinions and data contained in all publications are solely those of the individual author(s) and contributor(s) and not of MDPI and/or the editor(s). MDPI and/or the editor(s) disclaim responsibility for any injury to people or property resulting from any ideas, methods, instructions or products referred to in the content.

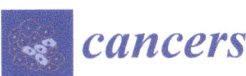

Article

Analysis of Circulating Immune Subsets in Primary Colorectal Cancer

Can Lu [1], Josefine Schardey [1], Ulrich Wirth [1], Viktor von Ehrlich-Treuenstätt [1], Jens Neumann [2], Clemens Gießen-Jung [3], Jens Werner [1,4,5], Alexandr V. Bazhin [1,4,5,†] and Florian Kühn [1,4,5,*,†]

1. Department of General, Visceral, and Transplant Surgery, Ludwig-Maximilians-University Munich, 81377 Munich, Germany
2. Institute of Pathology, Medical Faculty, Ludwig-Maximilians-University Munich, 81377 Munich, Germany
3. Department of Medicine III, University Hospital, Ludwig-Maximilians-University Munich, 81377 Munich, Germany
4. German Cancer Consortium (DKTK), Partner Site Munich, 81377 Munich, Germany
5. Bavarian Cancer Research Center (BZKF), 91054 Erlangen, Germany
* Correspondence: florian.kuehn@med.uni-muenchen.de; Tel.: +49-(0)89-4400-1683535
† These authors contributed equally to this work.

Citation: Lu, C.; Schardey, J.; Wirth, U.; von Ehrlich-Treuenstätt, V.; Neumann, J.; Gießen-Jung, C.; Werner, J.; Bazhin, A.V.; Kühn, F. Analysis of Circulating Immune Subsets in Primary Colorectal Cancer. *Cancers* **2022**, *14*, 6105. https://doi.org/10.3390/cancers14246105

Academic Editors: Rodrigo Barderas-Manchado, Cristina Díaz del Arco, María Jesús Fernández-Aceñero and Javier Martinez Useros

Received: 2 November 2022
Accepted: 10 December 2022
Published: 12 December 2022

Publisher's Note: MDPI stays neutral with regard to jurisdictional claims in published maps and institutional affiliations.

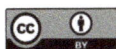

Copyright: © 2022 by the authors. Licensee MDPI, Basel, Switzerland. This article is an open access article distributed under the terms and conditions of the Creative Commons Attribution (CC BY) license (https://creativecommons.org/licenses/by/4.0/).

Simple Summary: The immune system has a vital role in shaping the development and progression of CRC. Circulating immune subsets are the primary resources of tumor-infiltrating immune cells that could directly count against the tumor. The status of the systemic immunity in CRC patients is still unclear. Our study aims to comprehensively evaluate the circulating immune subsets and gene expression profiles of CRC patients. Here, we show that CRC patients have a more prominent systemic immune suppression than healthy controls, as well as NR3C2, CAMK4, and TRAT1, that might involve regulating the number of circulating T helper cells in CRC patients. The distribution of circulating immune subsets in CRC could complement the regional immune status of the tumor microenvironment and contribute to the discovery of immune-related biomarkers, for the diagnosis of CRC.

Abstract: The development and progression of colorectal cancer (CRC) are known to be affected by the interplay between tumor and immune cells. However, the impact of CRC cells on the systemic immunity has yet to be elucidated. We aimed to comprehensively evaluate the circulating immune subsets and transcriptional profiles of CRC patients. In contrast to healthy controls (HCs), CRC patients had a lower percentage of B and T lymphocytes, T helper (Th) cells, non-classical monocytes, dendritic cells, and a higher proportion of polymorphonuclear myeloid-derived suppressor cells, as well as a reduced expression of CD69 on NK cells. Therefore, CRC patients exhibit a more evident systemic immune suppression than HCs. A diagnostic model integrating seven immune subsets was constructed to distinguish CRC patients from HCs with an AUC of 1.000. Moreover, NR3C2, CAMK4, and TRAT1 were identified as candidate genes regulating the number of Th cells in CRC patients. The altered composition of circulating immune cells in CRC could complement the regional immune status of the tumor microenvironment and contribute to the discovery of immune-related biomarkers for the diagnosis of CRC.

Keywords: colorectal cancer; flow cytometry; immunophenotype; diagnostic model; differentially expressed genes

1. Introduction

Colorectal cancer (CRC) is the third most frequent carcinoma and the second leading cause of cancer-associated death globally, accounting for 1.8 million new cases and 900,000 deaths annually [1]. Despite significant advances in diagnostic and therapeutic options in the past decades, nearly 25% of the patients have synchronous metastases at the initial diagnosis, and virtually 50% of primary CRC patients could develop distant metastases during this disease [2]. Furthermore, after receiving a completed resection of CRC, the 5-year survival rate is approximately 60%, while the rate drops to 12% in the metastatic disease [3]. The therapeutic strategies ought to be improved, in terms of the high rate of metastasis and corresponding worse prognosis in patients with primary CRC. Currently, many biomarkers have been proposed to predict the responses to clinical treatment and to stratify CRC patients according to the risk classification, including miRNAs, circulating tumor cells, circulating tumor DNA, and genetic mutations [4]. However, these approaches are virtually characterized by a tumor-cell-centric nature, overlooking the intrinsic heterogeneity of the tumor microenvironment (TME) and immune elements. The accumulating studies indicated that the immune system has a fundamental role in shaping the development and progression of CRC [5–7]. Although most studies focus on tumor-infiltrating lymphocytes (TILs), immune subsets in the peripheral blood are the primary resources for intratumoral immune events. Therefore, the composition and phenotype of circulating immune cell subsets may be linked to the immune response inside the tumor, potentially playing a significant role in predicting the tumor progression and drug responses in CRC. In addition, the impact of CRC on the systemic immunity remains to be elucidated.

Even though acting as the primary effector cell of humoral immunity, B lymphocytes are poorly investigated in the TME because of their controversial role in regulating tumor progression [8]. Conversely, T-cell infiltration of TME has been widely researched in CRC patients [9–13]. Innate immune cells that principally comprise neutrophils, monocytes, dendritic cells (DCs), myeloid-derived suppressor cells (MDSCs), NK, and NKT cells, are also involved in the interplay with tumor cells. Neutrophils are indispensable immune cells to defend against invading microorganisms and facilitate wound healing [14]. Moreover, monocytes are considered critical regulators of cancer development and metastasis, with different subsets performing opposing roles in enabling the tumor growth and preventing the metastatic spread of tumor cells [15]. DCs, one of the essential antigen-presenting cells, could initiate adaptive immune responses and secret the costimulatory molecules to drive the cytotoxic T cells' clonal expansion [16]. Moreover, MDSCs consist of a heterogeneous population of an early-stage (E-MDSC), monocytic (M-MDSC), and polymorphonuclear origin (PMN-MDSCs) that typically arise in chronic inflammatory sites, including cancer [17]. NK and NKT cells are innate-like lymphocyte populations with cytotoxic functions, independent of the MHC molecules on pathogenic cells and tumor cells in the innate immunity. It is worth noting that the composition of the above immune subsets is seldom reported in the peripheral blood of CRC patients.

This study aimed to comprehensively evaluate the circulating immune subsets and gene expression profiles of CRC patients. Furthermore, peripheral blood immune cell profiles were subsequently used to construct a diagnostic model and correlate with the clinical test data. Our study revealed that CRC patients have a significantly suppressed systemic immunity, compared to healthy controls.

2. Materials and Methods

2.1. Study Population

This study included 12 patients with CRC who were diagnosed, according to the 2019 World Health Organization classification, and underwent a curative surgical resection at the Ludwig-Maximilians-University Munich (LMU) hospital (Munich, Germany) between September 2020 and September 2021. Blood samples from these patients were collected within 4 h prior to surgery. The inclusion criteria were a surgical R0 resection, a tumor node metastasis (TNM) stage 0-III, a histologically confirmed colorectal carcinoma, and the provision of written informed consent. The exclusion criteria were a history of chemoradiotherapy treatment, concomitant immune-associated disorders and other carcinomas, and the use of immunomodulating drugs or oral steroids within the past three years. In addition, the pre-operative clinical data of CRC patients were also collected. Peripheral blood samples from 11 healthy donors were obtained from LMU hospital after obtaining written consent, and these samples were considered healthy controls. This study was approved by the local review board.

2.2. Flow Cytometry Data Analysis

The procedure of the flow cytometry antibody staining is depicted in the Supplementary Materials. Circulating B lymphocytes, T lymphocytes, and innate immune subsets from whole blood samples were detected using three multicolor flow cytometry panels, respectively (Table S1). At least 1×10^5 events per sample were acquired promptly after staining by 18-color flow cytometry, using the LSR Fortessa (BD Biosciences) with BD FACSDiva^{TM} software version 8.0.1 (BD Biosciences). For each experiment, the optimal cytometer values were maintained by this software. The flow cytometer setup and performance tracking were conducted using the cytometer setup and tracking beads (BD Biosciences). According to the manufacturer's protocol, the compensation control was carried out with the CompBeads set (BD Biosciences). The positive staining cells were identified using fluorescence minus one (FMO) control, when necessary [18]. The FMO controls were used for IgM, CD38, CD27, CD10, CD24, IgD, and CD20 in flow panel 1. Eight FMO controls were set for flow panel 2, including CD197, CD194, CD38, CD25, CD196, CD127, CD45RO, and HLA-DR. Furthermore, the FMO controls were separately prepared for CD69, HLA-DR, CD14, CD33, CD16, CD11c, CD15, CD11b, CD66b, and CD56 in flow panel 3. The immunophenotyping of the circulating B lymphocytes, T lymphocytes, and innate immune subsets is shown in Table S2. In addition, the sequential gating strategy for each panel was depicted in Figures S1–S3, respectively. The expression levels of the immune markers on the circulating B cells, T cells, and innate immune subsets were evaluated by the percentage of the targeted cells or the median fluorescence intensity (MFI) or the absolute number of immune cells. FlowJo software version 10.4 (Tree Star) was applied to analyze the datasets, and the data were displayed in dot plots.

2.3. Construction of a Diagnostic Model

The univariable logistic regression was conducted to evaluate the predictive ability of each immune subset, in two cohorts. In order to obtain the immune subsets that displayed a relatively higher accuracy with the prediction, we kept those immune subsets with *p*-values less than 0.05. The support vector machine (SVM) learning model was performed to identify the optimal parameters from the above immune subsets to discriminate CRC from the healthy controls. To ensure the stability and reliability of our prediction method, a tenfold cross-validation was applied by the SVM model. The best parameters were identified from the maximum cross-validation results. The selected parameters were fitted into a multivariable logistic regression analysis to construct the diagnostic model. Each parameter would be assigned a logistic regression coefficient, and an immune score was generated using the following formula:

$$Immune\ Score = \sum_{n=1}^{Num} (Composition_n \times LC_n),$$

where Num refers to the number of immune subsets, $Composition_n$ represents the percentage of the immune subset$_n$, and LC_n is the logistic coefficient of the immune subset$_n$.

Furthermore, a nomogram was constructed to visualize this diagnostic model in our cohort. The calibration curve and the Hosmer–Lemeshow test were performed to evaluate the goodness-of-fit of the nomogram model. A decision curve analysis (DCA) was used to assess the model's reliability by calculating the clinical net benefit for patients at each threshold probability. The receiver operating characteristic (ROC) curve was applied to evaluate the discrimination performance of the nomogram.

A logistic regression analysis was performed using the *stats* R package [19]. A SVM model analysis was conducted using the *e1071* R package [20]. The *pROC* and *ggplot2* R packages were used to draw the diagnostic ROC curves [21,22].

2.4. Gene Expression Profile Collection and Processing

The Gene Expression Omnibus (GEO) database was thoroughly searched to find the eligible GEO datasets, based on blood samples with the following searching strategy ("colon" or "colorectal" or "rectal") and ("cancer*" or "neoplas*" or "dysplasia") and ("homo sapiens") and ("gse"). The inclusion criteria of the datasets are listed in Figure S4. A total of two datasets (GSE164191 and GSE46703) representing different independent studies of CRC were enrolled, of which GSE164191 contained 59 CRC and 62 normal samples, and GSE46703 included 14 CRC samples without prior treatment. Moreover, GSE164191 and GSE46703 were derived from GPL570 and GPL6884, respectively. The *GEOquery* R package was used to download the expression matrices of the above datasets [23]. The probes were annotated into gene symbols, based on the corresponding annotation files. When multiple probes matched one gene, the median was calculated as its expression value. Moreover, since GSE164191 and GSE46703 were hybridized into two distinct platforms, the combat function of the *sva* R package was applied to integrate two normalized datasets into a meta-cohort, to remove the batch effects (Figure S5A,B) [24]. Next, the merging datasets were quantile normalized with the normalizeBetweenArrays function of the *limma* R package (Figure S5C,D) [25]. Therefore, the merged GEO datasets were considered the normalized expression profiles of the blood samples for the CRC and healthy controls.

Due to the potential interaction between the colorectal tumors and peripheral blood, the sequencing data of the CRC tissue samples were also obtained from the public repository. The Cancer Genome Atlas (TCGA) projects deposited the largest tissue expression matrices of CRC on the single dataset level. Then the gene expression profiles of 568 CRC patients and 51 non-cancerous samples were downloaded from TCGA through the GDC data portal.

2.5. xCell Algorithm

The *xCell* R package was used to deconvolute the peripheral blood mononuclear cell types, based on the merged GEO datasets. By applying a novel gene signature-based method, the xCell algorithm could reliably estimate the enrichment of 64 stromal and immune cell types from the gene expression data derived from tissue or blood samples, among which 34 cell types are immune subsets [26]. According to the validation results of the extensive in-silico simulations and the cytometry immune profiling, xCell outperformed other digital dissection methodologies, including CIBERSORT [26].

2.6. Differential Expression Analysis

To identify the differentially expressed genes (DEGs) in the blood and tissue samples between the CRC and normal subjects, we performed the differential expression analysis on the merged GEO and TCGA datasets using the *limma* and *DESeq2* R packages, respectively [25,27]. In the GEO dataset, the DEGs were regarded as any gene with adjusted p values of <0.05 and $|\log_2 (\text{Fold change})| > 0.25$. Owing to the entity of colorectal carcinoma, the DEGs of the TCGA dataset were defined as genes with adjusted p values of <0.05 and $|\log_2 (\text{Fold change})| > 1$. Furthermore, DEGs that consistently changed in the above two datasets were identified as the common DEGs.

2.7. Gene Ontology Enrichment Analysis

A gene ontology (GO) enrichment analysis was performed to determine the potential biological function of the identified common DEGs, using the *ClusterProfiler* R package [28]. The GO analysis contained three categories: biological process, molecular function, and cellular components. The cutoff criteria of the p values of <0.05 and the false discovery rate (FDR) < 0.1 were regarded as statistically significant differences for all analyses.

2.8. Correlation Analysis

A correlation analysis was performed to explore the association between the immune cell compositions and genetic expression and to investigate the underlying relationship between the immune cell subsets and clinical test parameters, using the *hmisc* and *corrplot*

R packages. The correlation coefficients and corresponding p values were used to select the significantly correlated pairs.

2.9. Statistical Analysis

The correlation analysis was performed using the Pearson method. The statistical difference between the continuous variables was calculated using the two-sample t-test or the Wilcoxon rank-sum test, depending on the normal distribution. The p-values of the multiple testing were corrected using the Benjamini–Hochberg method. The comparisons between the categorical variables were conducted by applying Fisher's exact test. All statistical analyses were completed using the R software (version 4.1.0). The p-value < 0.05 was regarded as statistically significant.

3. Results

3.1. Patients with CRC Exhibiting a Systemic Immune Suppression

The study was conducted, as depicted in Figure 1. Since chemoradiotherapy could affect the systemic immune system, the blood samples were collected only from patients without neoadjuvant therapy. Table 1 summarizes the clinicopathological characteristics of 12 CRC patients and 11 healthy controls included in the analyses. There was no significant difference in gender between the CRC patients and healthy controls, whereas the CRC patients have a trend towards advanced age, compared to the healthy controls ($p > 0.05$). The detailed data of the immune distributional comparison between these two groups are shown in Table S3.

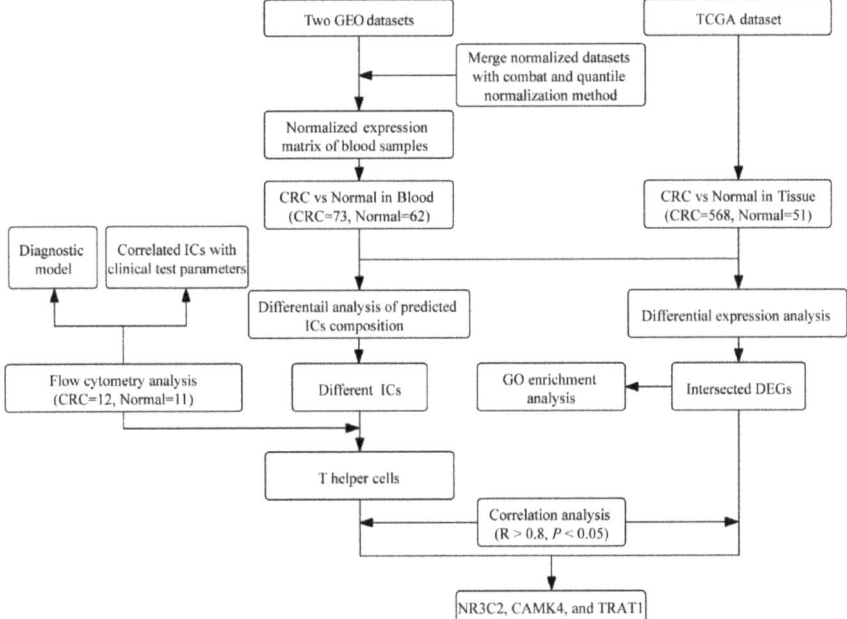

Figure 1. Analysis flow diagram of the study. Abbreviation: GEO, Gene Expression Omnibus; TCGA, The Cancer Genome Atlas; CRC, colorectal cancer; ICs, immune cells; GO, gene ontology; DEGs, differentially expressed genes.

Table 1. Clinical characteristics of healthy controls and CRC patients.

Variables	CRC (*n* = 12)	Healthy Control (*n* = 11)	*p*-Value
Age, year *	75.0 (69.0, 78.0)	58.0 (53.5, 68.0)	0.0600 [a]
Gender			0.6800 [b]
Female	6 (50.0%)	4 (36.4%)	
Male	6 (50.0%)	7 (63.6%)	
Sidedness			
Left side	6 (50.0%)		
Right side	6 (50.0%)		
Elective surgery			
Yes	12 (100.0%)		
Surgery Type			
Open surgery	9 (75.0%)		
Laparoscopic surgery	2 (16.7%)		
Robot-assisted surgery	1 (8.3%)		
T (AJCC 7th)			
T1	1 (8.3%)		
T2	6 (50.0%)		
T3	3 (25.0%)		
T4a	2 (16.7%)		
N (AJCC 7th)			
N0	11 (91.7%)		
N1b	1 (8.3%)		
M (AJCC 7th)			
M0	12 (100.0%)		
Tumor stage (AJCC 7th)			
I	7 (58.4%)		
II	4 (33.3%)		
III	1 (8.3%)		
Residual tumor classification			
R0	12 (100.0%)		
MSI			
No [c]	8 (66.7%)		
Yes [d]	4 (33.3%)		
Bethesda			
No	12 (100.0%)		

Abbreviations: CRC, colorectal cancer; AJCC, American Joint Committee on Cancer; T, tumor; N, lymph node; M, metastasis; MSI, microsatellite instability. Data were represented as n (%) unless otherwise annotated. * Age was presented as the median and confidence interval. [a] represented the Wilcoxon rank-sum test. [b] denoted Fisher's exact test. [c] indicated no protein loss, and [d] suggested the loss of expression of MLH1 and PMS2 in the immunohistochemistry.

At first, compared to the healthy controls, the proportion of B lymphocytes was significantly ($p = 0.0421$) lower in the CRC patients (Figure 2A,C). There was no distributional difference in the two Breg subsets between the CRC patients and the healthy controls (Figure 2A). No differences in other B lymphocyte subsets were detected between the CRC patients and the healthy controls (Figure 2A).

Secondly, the distribution of seven subsets belonging to the T lymphocyte population was statistically different in the two cohorts (Figure 2A,C): remarkably lower proportions of circulating T lymphocytes ($p = 0.0184$), and Th cells ($p = 0.0243$), were observed in the CRC patients. In contrast, the percentage of activated CD8T ($p = 0.0107$) and activated Th ($p = 0.0107$) cells was significantly higher in CRC patients compared to healthy controls. Furthermore, CRC patients presented with an increased percentage of the naïve ($p = 0.0088$) and central memory Th ($p = 0.0088$) cells, but with a decreased proportion of the effector Th ($p = 0.0088$) cells, compared to the healthy controls. In addition, the percentage of Tregs and its subsets was comparable between the CRC patients and healthy controls (Figure 2A).

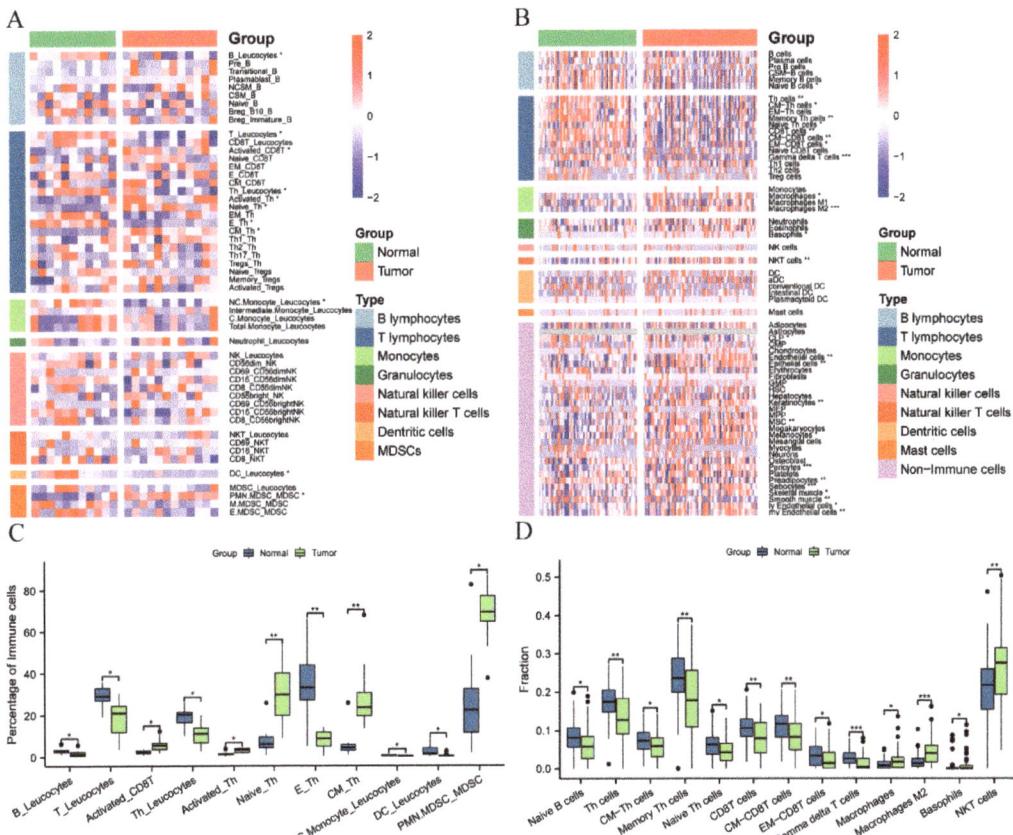

Figure 2. The circulating immune subsets distribution in CRC patients, compared to the healthy controls. (**A**) The heatmap of the immune subsets from a flow cytometry analysis. Each immune subset was expressed as the percentage of the source cells annotated following the underscore; (**B**) The heatmap of the immune and stromal cells computed from the merged GEO datasets using the xCell algorithm; (**C,D**) The boxplot of the significantly different immune subsets from the flow cytometry analysis and xCell algorithm, respectively. The bars show the median values of each immune cell subset and the corresponding 95% confidence interval. Corrected p-values were calculated for each comparison using the Benjamini–Hochberg method. *, $p < 0.05$; **, $p < 0.01$; ***, $p < 0.001$. Abbreviation: NCSM: non-class switched memory; CSM: class switched memory; Breg, regulatory B cells; EM, effector memory; E, effector; CM, central memory; Tregs, regulatory T cells; NC.Monocyte, non-classical monocytes; C. Monocytes, classical monocytes; NK, natural killer; NKT, natural killer T; DC, dendritic cell; PMN.MDSC, polymorphonuclear MDSC; M.MDSC, mononuclear MDSC; E.MDSC, early-stage MDSC; CLP, common lymphoid progenitors; CMP, common myeloid progenitors; GMP, granulocyte-monocyte progenitor; HSC, hematopoietic stem cell; MEP, megakaryocyte-erythroid progenitor cell; MPP, multipotent progenitor; MSC, mesenchymal stem cell; ly, lymphatic; mv, microvascular.

Thirdly, among the four monocyte subsets, only non-classical monocytes were significantly ($p = 0.0125$) lower in CRC patients, compared to the healthy controls. Meanwhile, there was no difference in the percentage of neutrophils between these two groups (Figure 2A).

Fourthly, similar circulating NK and NKT cell percentages were observed in the CRC patients and healthy controls (Figure 2A). No differences were detected in the CD56^{bright}

and $CD56^{dim}$ NK cells (% of NK). Although the CRC patients have a similar distribution of $CD69^+CD56^{dim}$ and $CD69^+CD56^{bright}$ NK cells, to the healthy controls, the expression level (MFI) of CD69 on these two NK subsets was significantly ($p = 0.0277$) lower in the CRC patients than in the healthy controls (Figure S6). No differences in other phenotypic markers on the NK and NKT cells were observed between the CRC patients and healthy controls (Figure S6).

Lastly, in contrast to the healthy controls, the CRC patients also have an increased percentage of the PMN-MDSC ($p = 0.0107$) population (Figure 2C). Moreover, a lower percentage of DCs was detected in the CRC patients than in the healthy controls (Figure 2C).

Furthermore, we applied the digital dissection method of the xCell algorithm to the merged GEO dataset consisting of 73 CRC patients and 62 healthy controls, to estimate the distribution of the circulating immune cells. In total, sixty-four subsets, including thirty-four immune subsets, were calculated for the CRC patients and healthy controls (Figure 2B). Although thirteen immune cell subsets showed a significant difference between the CRC patients and healthy controls (Figure 2D), only the Th cells were consistently changed in the flow cytometry analysis and bioinformatics analysis (Figure 2C,D).

To further characterize the systemic immune status in the different MSI statuses of CRC, we compared the distribution of the circulating fifty-two immune subsets between MSS- and MSI-CRC patients (Figure S7A). No differences were detected in the composition of the peripheral immune cells and phenotypic markers expression on the NK and NKT cells between these two cohorts (Figure S7A,B). Therefore, the MSI status did not influence the systemic immunity of the CRC patients.

3.2. Diagnostic Model Allowed for the Differentiation of the CRC Patients from the Healthy Controls

Eleven immune subsets were identified from the univariable logistic regression on fifty-two immune subsets (Table S4). When the SVM was applied to evaluate the accuracy of the different combinations of the above immune subsets, in discriminating between the CRC individuals and healthy controls, the combination of seven immune subsets was optimal, with an accuracy of 0.936 (Figure 3A), including NC.Monocyte_Leukocytes, E_Th, T_Leukocytes, Activated_Th, Activated_CD8T, Th_Leukocytes, and Naïve_Th (Table S5). Therefore, these seven immune subsets were chosen to construct a diagnostic model using a logistic regression algorithm. The diagnostic formula was determined as follows:

$112.9468 - 44.5381 \times$ Non-Classical Monocyte (% of Leukocytes) $- 3.1629 \times$ Effector Th (% of Th cells) $- 5.8056 \times$ T (% of Leukocytes) $- 6.0697 \times$ Activated Th (% of Th cells) $+ 8.9753 \times$ Activated CD8T (% of CD8T cells) $+ 5.7387 \times$ Th (% of Leukocytes) $+ 0.0072 \times$ Naïve Th (% of Th cells),

Moreover, a nomogram incorporating the above immune subsets was constructed to visualize this diagnostic model and efficiently predict the risk of malignancy (Figure 3B). This study used 12 CRCs and 11 normal samples as the training set. The calibration curve of the nomogram confirmed that the predictive probability of CRC nearly matched the actual probability, which was also supported by the Hosmer–Lemeshow test result ($p = 1.0000$) (Figure 3C). According to the DCA curve, we observed that the diagnostic model acquired the most clinical benefit with the entire range of the threshold probabilities, compared to the individual immune subset (Figure 3D). Furthermore, the ROC analysis in our training cohort suggested that the nomogram model accurately distinguished the CRC and normal subjects with an AUC of 1.000 (95% CI 1.000–1.000), the sensitivity of 1.000, a specificity of 1.000, the positive predictive value of 1.000, and the negative predictive value of 1.000, at the cutoff point of -0.038 (Figure 3E). In addition, each immune cell subset of the model has a good diagnostic performance in distinguishing these two groups with an AUC greater than 0.850 (Figure 3F–H).

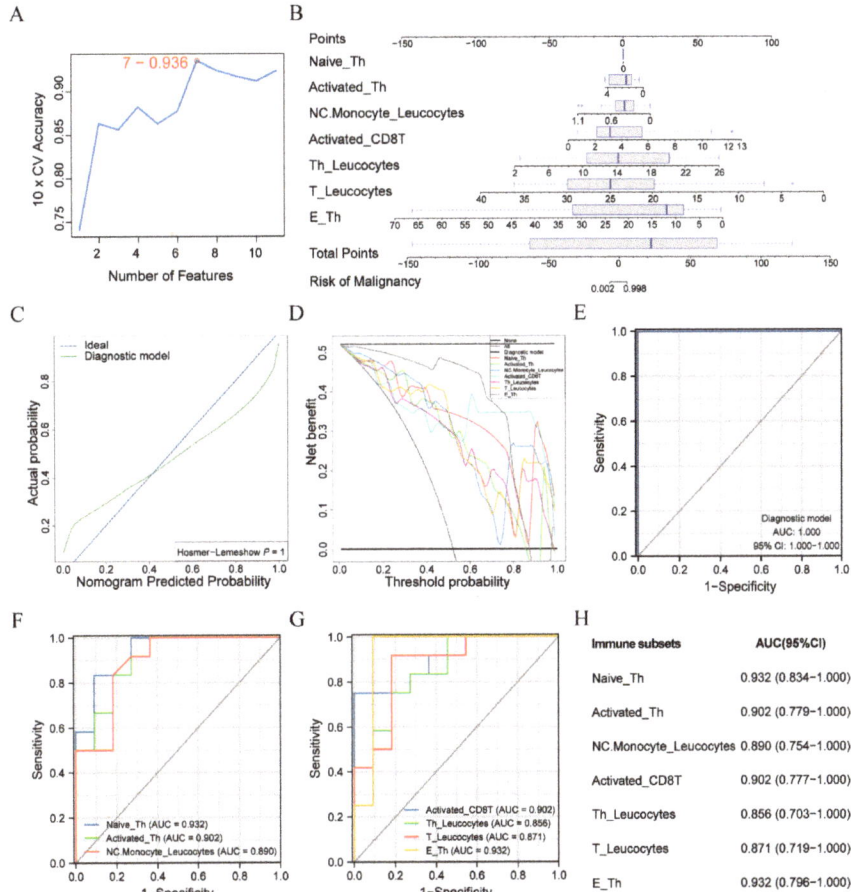

Figure 3. Diagnostic model for differentiating the CRC patients from the healthy controls. (**A**) Tenfold cross-validation accuracy plot of the SVM algorithm; (**B**) Diagnostic nomogram model to predict the risk probability of CRC; (**C**) Calibration curve of the nomogram model; (**D**) DCA curve of the nomogram model and corresponding seven predictive risk factors; (**E**) ROC analysis of the nomogram model; (**F**,**G**) ROC analysis of the seven predictive immune subsets in the model; (**H**) The forest plot of the AUC value and 95% CI for each immune subset. Each immune subset was expressed as the percentage of source cells annotated following the underscore. Abbreviation: Naïve_Th, naïve Th (% of Th); Activated_Th, activated Th (% of Th); NC.Monocyte_Leukocytes, non-classical monocyte (% of Leukocytes); Activated_CD8T, activated CD8T (% of CD8T); Th_Leukocytes, Th (% of Leukocytes); T_Leukocytes, T (% of Leukocytes); E_Th, effector Th (% of Th); Th, T helper, CD8T, CD8+ T; ROC, receiver operating curve; AUC, area under the curve; 95% CI, 95% confidence interval.

3.3. NR3C2, CAMK4, and TRAT1 Associated with the Composition of the Th Cells

To further elucidate the underlying molecular mechanism associated with the distinct circulating immune subsets between the CRC cases and healthy controls, we performed the differential expression analysis on the GEO and TCGA datasets. In the GEO dataset, we identified 398 DEGs in the blood samples of CRC patients, compared to the healthy controls, of which 38 genes and 360 genes were up-regulated and down-regulated, respectively (Figure 4A). Meanwhile, 5245 DEGs were obtained from the gene expression analysis on the CRC and non-cancerous tissue samples in the TCGA dataset, including 2594 upregulated genes and 2651 down-regulated genes (Figure 4B). We performed theintersection of the DEGs between the GEO and TCGA datasets to identify the consistently changed genes in both the blood and tissue samples, regarding the potential interaction between colorectal carcinoma and the systemic immune system. In total, 39 DEGs, consisting of one up-regulated gene and 38 down-regulated genes were identified as the common DEGs (Figure 4C,D). Next, the GO enrichment analysis indicated that these genes were mainly involved in lymphocyte differentiation and purinergic receptor signaling pathway (Figure 4E).

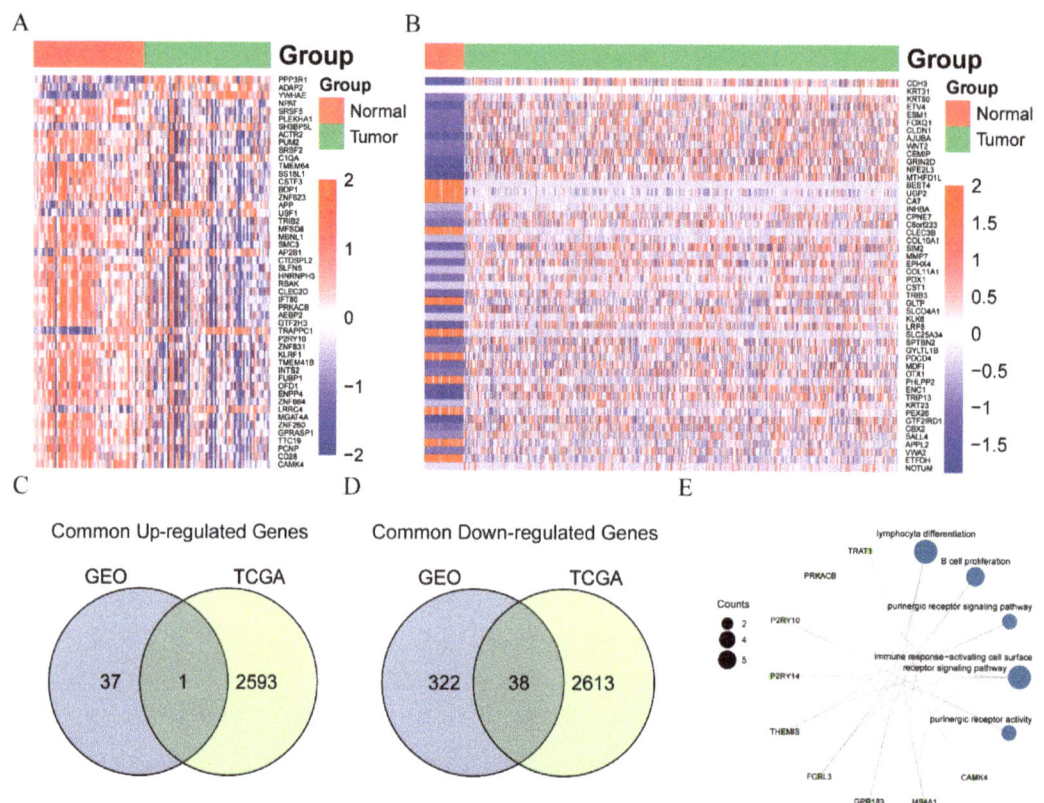

Figure 4. Differentially expressed genes between the normal and CRC in the blood and tissue samples. (**A**) The heatmap of the top 50 DEGs in the GEO dataset; (**B**) The heatmap of the top 50 DEGs in the TCGA dataset; (**C,D**) Common up-regulated and down-regulated DEGs between the GEO and TCGA datasets, respectively; (**E**) GO enrichment analysis of the common DEGs. Abbreviation: GEO, Gene Expression Omnibus; TCGA, The Cancer Genome Atlas. DEG, differentially expressed genes.

In order to study the relationship between the different distributional immune subsets and the regulated genes, the correlation analysis between the immune cell subsets and common DEGs was conducted in the healthy controls and CRC patients, respectively (Figure 5A,B). Furthermore, the details of the correlation results are depicted in Tables S6 and S7. To ensure the robustness of the selection on the potential genes associated with the composition of the Th cells, the correlation pairs between the immune cell subsets and DEGs were used to filter the genes with a coefficient greater than 0.8 and a p-value less than 0.05 in both the healthy controls and the CRC patients. Three genes: NR3C2, CAMK4, and TRAT1, were identified as the candidate genes that may involve the regulation of the composition of circulating Th cells in patients with CRC (Figure 5C–H).

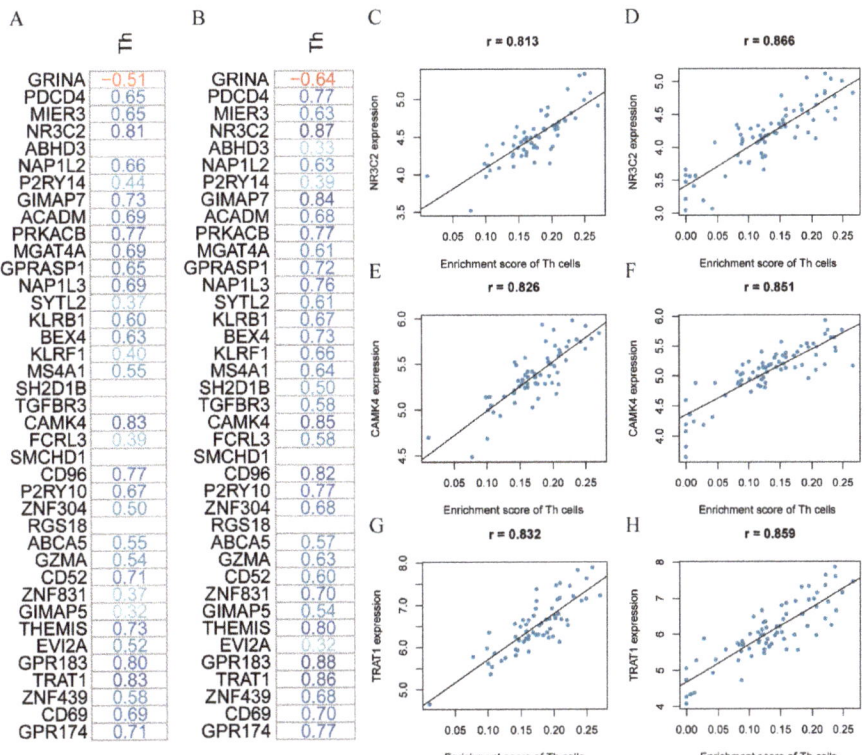

Figure 5. Identification of the candidate genes associated with the composition of the circulating Th cells. (**A,B**) The heatmap of the correlation coefficient between the common DEGs and the Th cells in the healthy controls and CRC patients, respectively. Blank cells represented the *p*-value of the correlation greater than 0.05. Blue color and red color referred to the positive and negative correlations, respectively; (**C,D**) Correlation plot of NR3C2 with the Th cells in the healthy controls and CRC patients, respectively; (**E,F**) Correlation plot of CAMK4 with the Th cells in the healthy controls and CRC patients, respectively; (**G,H**) Correlation plot of TRAT1 with the Th cells in the healthy controls and CRC patients, respectively. Abbreviation: Th, T helper.

3.4. Correlation of the Clinical Test Parameters with the Immune Subsets in the CRC Patients

To further study the relationship between the fifty-two immune cell subsets and the twelve clinical test parameters, the correlation analysis was performed for the CRC patients using the absolute number of the respective immune subsets from a flow cytometry detection (Figure 6). In order to find the reliable biomarkers associated with the immune cell composition in the peripheral blood, the correlated pairs with the coefficient greater than 0.8 and a *p*-value less than 0.05 were selected from the above analysis. Three parameters were strongly associated with the distribution of the immune subsets in the CRC patients (Table 2). Firstly, the gamma-glutamyltransferase was positively correlated with the level of circulating DCs. Five positively correlated pairs involving the aspartate aminotransferase (AST) were identified, including plasmablasts, activated CD8T cells, effector CD8T cells, class-switched memory B cells, and CD8T cells. In contrast to AST, only two immune subsets, T lymphocytes, and memory Treg cells, were positively associated with the alanine aminotransferase (ALT).

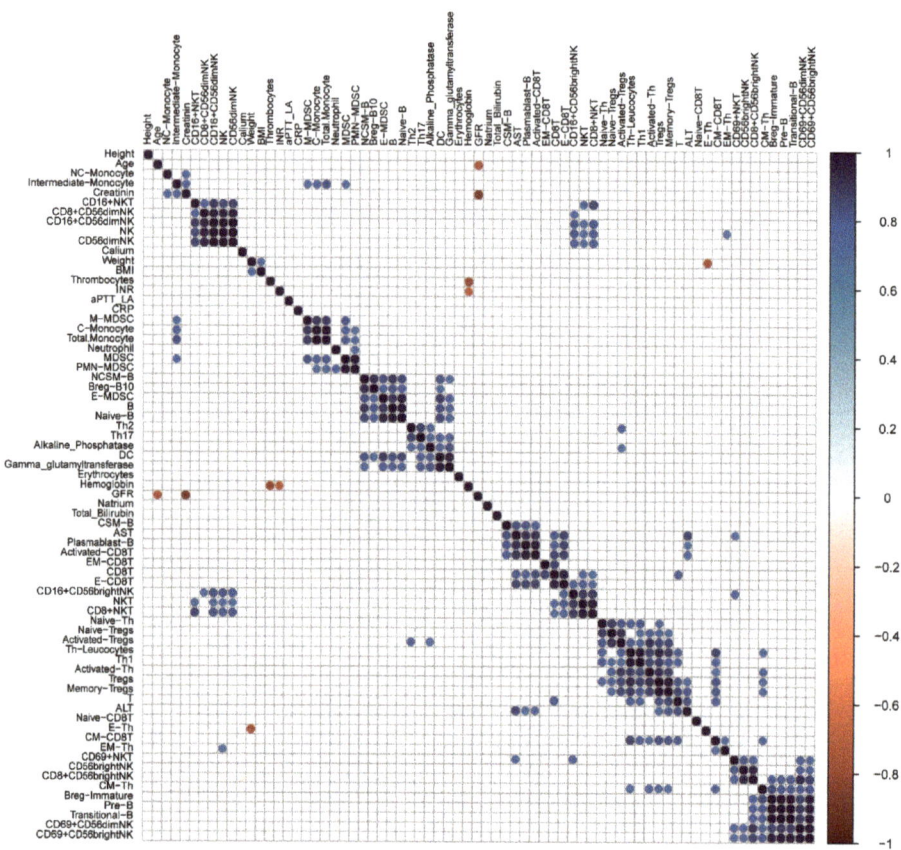

Figure 6. Correlation analysis between the circulating immune subsets and the clinical test parameters. Each immune subset was expressed as the absolute cell number in 200 uL of peripheral blood. Blank cells represented the *p*-value of the correlation greater than 0.05. Blue circles and red circles referred to positive and negative correlations, respectively. Abbreviation: NCSM: non-class switched memory; CSM: class switched memory; Breg, regulatory B cells; EM, effector memory; E, effector; CM, central memory; Tregs, regulatory T cells; NC.Monocyte, non-classical monocytes; C.Monocytes, classical monocytes; NK, natural killer; NKT, natural killer T; DC, dendritic cell; PMN.MDSC, polymorphonuclear MDSC; M.MDSC, mononuclear MDSC; E-MDSC, early-stage MDSC.

Table 2. Clinical test parameters correlated with the immune subsets.

Clinical Parameters	Immune Cells	Coefficient	*p*-Value
Gamma-glutamyltransferase	Dendritic cells	0.96	1.31×10^{-6}
AST	Plasmablasts	0.95	1.55×10^{-6}
AST	Activated CD8T cells	0.91	4.91×10^{-5}
AST	Effector CD8T cells	0.87	2.60×10^{-4}
ALT	T lymphocytes	0.84	6.60×10^{-4}
AST	CSM-B cells	0.83	7.29×10^{-4}
ALT	Memory Treg cells	0.82	1.19×10^{-3}
AST	CD8T cells	0.81	1.34×10^{-3}

Abbreviation: AST, aspartate aminotransferase; ALT, alanine aminotransferase; CSM, class-switched memory; Treg, regulatory T; CD8T, CD8$^+$ T.

4. Discussion

The immunoscore, based on the quantification of the CD3+ and CD8+ tumor-infiltrating lymphocytes at the invasive margin and at the core of the carcinoma, has been proven to be more reliable than tumor-node-metastasis (TNM) staging, as a prognostic marker in patients with CRC [29,30]. Meanwhile, cancer immunity is considered a combination of the intratumoral immune system and the systemic immune response [31]. Until now, most publications regarding the systemic immune status of patients with CRC focused on specific cell subtypes and did not consider investigating the majority of the immune cell subsets, simultaneously. To characterize the peripheral blood immune features of the CRC patients, we analyzed fifty-two subsets of circulating immune cells, including B and T lymphocytes, monocytes, neutrophils, NK cells, NKT cells, DCs, and MDSCs. Furthermore, these immune subsets were used to construct the diagnostic model to differentiate the CRC patients from the healthy controls and were further correlated with the clinical test data.

We first demonstrated that the CRC patients have a lower percentage of B lymphocytes than the healthy controls, which is in line with a recent study [32]. However, this finding contradicted Shimabukuro-Vornhagen et al., which showed a comparable proportion of B lymphocytes in the peripheral blood of CRC patients, compared to healthy controls [33]. Since chemoradiotherapy before surgery can potentially change the circulating immune landscape by stimulating the systemic immune response, this discrepancy may be attributed to the different inclusion criteria of patients with CRC. Meanwhile, we observed that multiple subsets of T lymphocytes have different compositional features in CRC patients, than in the healthy controls. T lymphocytes, Th cells, and effector Th cells have a decreased proportion in CRC patients, whereas activated CD8T cells, activated Th cells, naïve Th cells, and central memory Th cells, were significantly increased in those patients. Although evidence reported that the CRC patients have a similar distribution of naïve T cells, central memory T cells, and effector memory T cells with healthy controls [34], they failed to discriminate between the two major subpopulations of T cells, namely CD8T and Th cells. Conflicting results have been reported on circulating Treg cell levels in CRC patients. Dylag-Trojanowska et al. indicated that Treg cells were significantly decreased in CRC patients [35], whereas the opposite trend of Treg cells was reported in another study [34]. Interestingly, our results showed that Treg cells have similar distributional characteristics in CRC patients and healthy controls. In addition, Krijgsman et al. reported no statistical difference in the distribution of T lymphocytes and Th cells, between CRC patients and healthy controls, which is not in line with our study [14]. Due to the critical role of T lymphocytes in the systemic immune reaction, it is fundamental to focus on the dynamic distributional changes of circulating T cells, in the context of leukocytes. Compared to leukocytes as the denominator for T lymphocytes and Th cells in our study, Krijgsman et al. [14] used the lymphocytes or T lymphocytes as the denominator of the above immune cell subsets, partially explaining the discrepant results between the two studies. Due to the low percentage of B and T lymphocytes, and Th cells in the leukocyte population of the peripheral blood, CRC patients have an immune suppression in the adaptive immune response.

To our knowledge, this is the first study comparing circulating DCs of CRC patients and healthy controls. We found that those were significantly less frequent than healthy controls. Furthermore, we demonstrated that CRC patients presented an altered distribution of monocytes, compared to healthy controls, characterized by the reduced proportions of circulating non-classical monocytes. These findings are partially consistent with one clinical study that showed no significant compositional differences in the total monocytes, classical monocytes, intermediate monocytes, and non-classical monocytes, between CRC patients and healthy controls [36]. The explanation for the difference was that in their study $CD14^+CD16^{++}$ was used to identify non-classical monocytes, whereas we regarded $CD14^{low/+}CD16^+$ as the immunophenotype of these cells. Regarding DCs and non-classical monocytes belonging to antigen-presenting cells, CRC patients may have an impaired immune activation on the adaptive immune response, due to the low number of these two immune cell subsets in the peripheral blood.

Neutrophils are regarded as critical effector cells in the innate arm of the immune system by counting against the invading microorganisms [37]. Nevertheless, studies on circulating neutrophils are virtually scarce. Our study showed that CRC patients have a similar proportion of circulating neutrophils to healthy controls. Furthermore, it is widely accepted that MDSCs exert immune suppressive effects mostly via inhibiting the T-cell proliferation and stimulating the Treg development [38]. In contrast to several studies that reported that circulating MDSCs were significantly increased in CRC patients [39,40], we found no difference in the distribution of MDSCs between CRC patients and healthy controls. Moreover, our study explicitly indicated that CRC patients had an increased percentage of PMN-MDSCs, compared to healthy controls. Accumulating studies have reported that PMN-MDSCs are the main components of circulating MDSCs and have a more prominent immune suppressive function than M-MDSC [38]. Hence, the high proportions of PMN-MDSCs within the MDSCs population could present a stronger immune suppression on the systemic immune response of CRC patients, than healthy controls.

Additionally, compared to the healthy controls, we demonstrated that CRC patients have an altered phenotype of circulating $CD56^{dim}$ and $CD56^{bright}$ NK cells, characterized by the reduced expression of CD69. Due to CD69 being regarded as the stimulatory membrane receptor of the NK cells [41], both $CD56^{dim}$ and $CD56^{bright}$ NK cells may have a compromised cytotoxic activity in patients with CRC. These findings align with a recent study that showed a reduced expression of activating receptors on the NK cells in CRC patients [34]. Furthermore, Krijgsman et al. proved that the immune suppression of the circulating NK cells could be removed by tumor resection in patients with colon carcinoma [42]. Therefore, CRC could inhibit the immune function of the circulating NK cells via downregulating the expression of the cytotoxic activation receptors.

Furthermore, through bioinformatics analyses on the gene expression profiles of the peripheral blood samples, only the Th cells were consistently identified as the differential immune cells in CRC patients between the flow cytometry detection and xCell algorithm analysis. To explore the underlying molecular mechanism involving the regulation of the Th cells in the peripheral blood, we identified genes differentially expressed, not only in the blood samples, but also in tissue samples of CRC patients, compared to the normal controls, with the consideration of the potential effects of the colorectal tumor on the systemic immune system. Next, we pinpointed three genes that have a strong positive correlation with the level of Th cells in the peripheral blood of both the healthy controls and CRC patients, namely NR3C2, CAMK4, and TRAT1. NR3C2, known as a mineralocorticoid receptor (MR), it has a critical role in mediating a cardiovascular injury induced by the activation of MR. Recent studies revealed that the MR activation could facilitate inflammation by inducing the T lymphocyte differentiation into the pro-inflammatory Th1 and Th17 subsets, while inhibiting the formation of the anti-inflammatory Tregs [43]. CAMK4, a serine/threonine kinase family member, could regulate the gene expression via activating the transcription factors in the cells of immune systems [44]. Previous studies reported that CAMK4, highly expressed in the T cells, was an essential molecule mediating the differentiation of the Th17 cells from the T lymphocytes [45,46]. TRAT1, also referred to as TRIM, can stabilize the T cell receptor (TCR) levels by working as the integral component of TCR [47]. Although lacking studies reported the influence of TRAT1 on the proliferation of T cells, TRAT1 could elevate the expression level of surface CTLA-4 via accelerating its transport from the cytoplasm [48], which may result in the inhibition of the Th cell proliferation. Therefore, NR3C2, CAMK4, and TRAT1, have the potential to be candidate genes involving regulating the number of Th cells in the peripheral blood.

Meanwhile, we established a 7-immune subsets classifier to differentiate the CRC patients from the healthy controls in our cohort. This 7-immune subsets classifier has an excellent performance in diagnosing patients with CRC, according to the corresponding

AUC value and the Hosmer–Lemeshow test result. Due to the limited number of CRC patients in our study, we could not conduct the internal validation of our diagnostic model. However, to maximally increase the stability and reliability of this model, we applied the tenfold cross-validation method of the SVM model, to select the best combination of parameters, to build the final diagnostic model. Nevertheless, a large cohort study is needed to validate the diagnostic accuracy of this classifier in the early diagnosis of CRC.

When investigating the associations between the circulating immune cell subsets and the clinical test parameters, eight positively correlated pairs involving three parameters were identified in CRC patients: AST, ALT, and gamma-glutamyltransferase. Although there were scarcely reports about these relationships in CRC, the above clinical parameters could indirectly reflect the status of the systemic immune profiles, which may contribute to predicting surgery-related complications.

The primary limitation of this study is that the number of patients is low, which could compromise the validity of our diagnostic model. However, recently, several robust studies constructed the diagnostic model, based on a comparable size of subjects [49–51]. In terms of the advanced age in CRC patients, compared to healthy controls, it is difficult to completely eradicate the potential age-related bias in immune cells. Although we failed to validate the expression of NR3C2, CAMK4, and TRAT1 in the Th cells between CRC patients and healthy controls, our study hinted that colorectal carcinoma might affect the expression of these genes, to mediate further the regulation of the circulating Th cells via a direct or indirect interaction. The tumor cell shedding from CRC could directly contact the hematopoietic stem cells, progenitor cells, and circulating lymphocytes, to cause a systemic immunosuppression for the development and progression of the regional CRC, even for metastasis. Moreover, CRC could regulate the systemic immunity via the secretion of soluble biological molecules and extracellular particles. Furthermore, our study characterized the distribution of a broad spectrum of circulating immune subsets and opened new avenues to underlie the molecular mechanisms regulating the composition of the Th cells in the peripheral blood of CRC patients.

5. Conclusions

CRC patients displayed profound distinctions in the immune cell subsets' distribution and their phenotype, compared to the healthy controls, showing that CRC patients have an evident immune suppression in the systemic immune response. Moreover, NR3C2, CAMK4, and TRAT1 were identified as the candidate genes regulating the level of the circulating Th cells in CRC patients, which will be the focus of future studies in our laboratory. These findings are of importance for deciphering the unique features of the circulating immune cell subsets in CRC, which could complement the regional immune status of the TME and contribute to the discovery of immune-related biomarkers for the diagnosis of CRC.

Supplementary Materials: The following supporting information can be downloaded at: https://www.mdpi.com/article/10.3390/cancers14246105/s1, Figure S1: Flow cytometry gating strategy applied for the identification of circulating 891 B lymphocyte subsets; Figure S2: Flow cytometry gating strategy applied for the identification of circulating 902 T lymphocytes subsets; Figure S3: Flow cytometry gating strategy applied for the identification of circulating 914 innate immune cell subsets; Figure S4: Flow diagram of identifying and selecting eligible GEO datasets; Figure S5: The pre-processing of merged GEO datasets; Figure S6: The peripheral blood immunophenotype of NK and NKT cells in CRC 935 patients compared to healthy controls; Table S1: Flow cytometry panels applied to identify peripheral blood B-, T-, and Innate immune subsets; Table S2: Immunophenotyping of B lymphocytes, T lymphocytes, and Innate immune subsets; Table S3: Comparison of circulating immune subsets between CRC patients and healthy controls; Table S4: Identification of circulating immune subsets to differentiate CRC patients from healthy controls through univariable logistic regression; Table S5: The accuracy of individual immune subset or the combination of different immune subsets as the classifier to distinguish CRC patients from healthy controls by Support Vector Machine learning algorithm; Table S6: Correlation analysis between circulating Th cells and common

DEGs in healthy controls; Table S7: Correlation analysis between circulating Th cells and common DEGs in CRC patients.

Author Contributions: Conceptualization, C.L., A.V.B. and F.K.; data curation, C.L., J.S., U.W. and V.v.E.-T.; formal analysis, A.V.B.; investigation, C.L., V.v.E.-T. and F.K.; methodology, A.V.B.; supervision, C.L., J.S., U.W., J.N., C.G.-J., J.W., A.V.B. and F.K.; validation, A.V.B.; visualization, C.L.; writing—original draft, C.L.; writing—review & editing, J.S., U.W., V.v.E.-T., J.N., C.G.-J., J.W., A.V.B. and F.K. All authors have read and agreed to the published version of the manuscript.

Funding: Can Lu was financially supported by the China Scholarship Council (201906230312) for his doctoral study.

Institutional Review Board Statement: This study was conducted according to the guidelines of the Declaration of Helsinki and approved by the Institutional Review Board of the Ludwig-Maximilians-University Munich, Germany (approval number: 0476, 2020).

Informed Consent Statement: Consent to participate and consent for publication were obtained from all of the patients included in the study.

Data Availability Statement: The original flow cytometry data can be provided by the corresponding author. The public datasets presented in this study are openly available in the GEO (https://www.ncbi.nlm.nih.gov/geo/, accessed on 15 January 2022) and TCGA (https://portal.gdc.cancer.gov/, accessed on 25 January 2022) databases.

Acknowledgments: The authors want to thank Nadine Gesse for her excellent technical support. The administrative assistance of Elvira Krause is highly appreciated.

Conflicts of Interest: The authors declare no conflict of interest.

References

1. Keum, N.; Giovannucci, E. Global burden of colorectal cancer: Emerging trends, risk factors and prevention strategies. *Nat. Rev. Gastroenterol. Hepatol.* **2019**, *16*, 713–732. [CrossRef] [PubMed]
2. Van Cutsem, E.; Cervantes, A.; Nordlinger, B.; Arnold, D. Metastatic colorectal cancer: ESMO Clinical Practice Guidelines for diagnosis, treatment and follow-up. *Ann. Oncol.* **2014**, *25*, iii1–iii9. [CrossRef] [PubMed]
3. Siegel, R.L.; Miller, K.D.; Jemal, A. Cancer statistics, 2019. *CA Cancer J. Clin.* **2019**, *69*, 7–34. [CrossRef] [PubMed]
4. Van Cutsem, E.; Cervantes, A.; Adam, R.; Sobrero, A.; Van Krieken, J.H.; Aderka, D.; Aranda Aguilar, E.; Bardelli, A.; Benson, A.; Bodoky, G.; et al. ESMO consensus guidelines for the management of patients with metastatic colorectal cancer. *Ann. Oncol.* **2016**, *27*, 1386–1422. [CrossRef] [PubMed]
5. Markman, J.L.; Shiao, S.L. Impact of the immune system and immunotherapy in colorectal cancer. *J. Gastrointest. Oncol.* **2015**, *6*, 208–223. [CrossRef]
6. Ferrone, C.; Dranoff, G. Dual roles for immunity in gastrointestinal cancers. *J. Clin. Oncol.* **2010**, *28*, 4045–4051. [CrossRef]
7. Fletcher, R.; Wang, Y.-J.; Schoen, R.E.; Finn, O.J.; Yu, J.; Zhang, L. Colorectal cancer prevention: Immune modulation taking the stage. *Biochim. Biophys. Acta Rev. Cancer* **2018**, *1869*, 138–148. [CrossRef]
8. Xie, Y.; Xie, F.; Zhang, L.; Zhou, X.; Huang, J.; Wang, F.; Jin, J.; Zhang, L.; Zeng, L.; Zhou, F. Targeted Anti-Tumor Immunotherapy Using Tumor Infiltrating Cells. *Adv. Sci.* **2021**, *8*, e2101672. [CrossRef]
9. Fridman, W.H.; Pagès, F.; Sautès-Fridman, C.; Galon, J. The immune contexture in human tumours: Impact on clinical outcome. *Nat. Rev. Cancer* **2012**, *12*, 298–306. [CrossRef]
10. Tosolini, M.; Kirilovsky, A.; Mlecnik, B.; Fredriksen, T.; Mauger, S.; Bindea, G.; Berger, A.; Bruneval, P.; Fridman, W.-H.; Pagès, F.; et al. Clinical Impact of Different Classes of Infiltrating T Cytotoxic and Helper Cells (Th1, Th2, Treg, Th17) in Patients with Colorectal Cancer. *Cancer Res.* **2011**, *71*, 1263–1271. [CrossRef]
11. Galon, J.; Costes, A.; Sanchez-Cabo, F.; Kirilovsky, A.; Mlecnik, B.; Lagorce-Pagès, C.; Tosolini, M.; Camus, M.; Berger, A.; Wind, P.; et al. Type, density, and location of immune cells within human colorectal tumors predict clinical outcome. *Science* **2006**, *313*, 1960–1964. [CrossRef] [PubMed]
12. Liu, J.; Duan, Y.; Cheng, X.; Chen, X.; Xie, W.; Long, H.; Lin, Z.; Zhu, B. IL-17 is associated with poor prognosis and promotes angiogenesis via stimulating VEGF production of cancer cells in colorectal carcinoma. *Biochem. Biophys. Res. Commun.* **2011**, *407*, 348–354. [CrossRef] [PubMed]
13. Yoshida, N.; Kinugasa, T.; Miyoshi, H.; Sato, K.; Yuge, K.; Ohchi, T.; Fujino, S.; Shiraiwa, S.; Katagiri, M.; Akagi, Y.; et al. A High RORγT/CD3 Ratio is a Strong Prognostic Factor for Postoperative Survival in Advanced Colorectal Cancer: Analysis of Helper T Cell Lymphocytes (Th1, Th2, Th17 and Regulatory T Cells). *Ann. Surg. Oncol.* **2016**, *23*, 919–927. [CrossRef] [PubMed]
14. Coffelt, S.B.; Wellenstein, M.D.; de Visser, K.E. Neutrophils in cancer: Neutral no more. *Nat. Rev. Cancer* **2016**, *16*, 431–446. [CrossRef] [PubMed]

15. Olingy, C.E.; Dinh, H.Q.; Hedrick, C.C. Monocyte heterogeneity and functions in cancer. *J. Leukoc. Biol.* **2019**, *106*, 309–322. [CrossRef] [PubMed]
16. Banchereau, J.; Steinman, R.M. Dendritic cells and the control of immunity. *Nature* **1998**, *392*, 245–252. [CrossRef]
17. Ma, T.; Renz, B.W.; Ilmer, M.; Koch, D.; Yang, Y.; Werner, J.; Bazhin, A.V. Myeloid-Derived Suppressor Cells in Solid Tumors. *Cells* **2022**, *11*, 310. [CrossRef]
18. Maecker, H.T.; Trotter, J. Flow cytometry controls, instrument setup, and the determination of positivity. *Cytom. Part A* **2006**, *69A*, 1037–1042. [CrossRef]
19. R Core Team. *R: A Language and Environment for Statistical Computing*; R Foundation for Statistical Computing: Vienna, Austria, 2021. Available online: https://www.R-project.org/ (accessed on 3 January 2022).
20. Meyer, D.; Dimitriadou, E.; Hornik, K.; Weingessel, A.; Leisch, F. e1071: Misc Functions of the Department of Statistics, Probability Theory Group (Formerly: E1071), TU Wien. R Package Version 1.7-9. 2021. Available online: https://CRAN.R-project.org/package=e1071 (accessed on 3 January 2022).
21. Robin, X.; Turck, N.; Hainard, A.; Tiberti, N.; Lisacek, F.; Sanchez, J.-C.; Müller, M. pROC: An open-source package for R and S+ to analyze and compare ROC curves. *BMC Bioinform.* **2011**, *12*, 77. [CrossRef]
22. Wickham, H. *ggplot2: Elegant Graphics for Data Analysis*; Springer: New York, NY, USA, 2016. Available online: https://ggplot2.tidyverse.org (accessed on 3 January 2022).
23. Davis, S.; Meltzer, P.S. GEOquery: A bridge between the Gene Expression Omnibus (GEO) and BioConductor. *Bioinformatics* **2007**, *23*, 1846–1847. [CrossRef]
24. Leek, J.T.; Johnson, W.E.; Parker, H.S.; Jaffe, A.E.; Storey, J.D. The sva package for removing batch effects and other unwanted variation in high-throughput experiments. *Bioinformatics* **2012**, *28*, 882–883. [CrossRef] [PubMed]
25. Ritchie, M.E.; Phipson, B.; Wu, D.; Hu, Y.; Law, C.W.; Shi, W.; Smyth, G.K. limma powers differential expression analyses for RNA-sequencing and microarray studies. *Nucleic Acids Res.* **2015**, *43*, e47. [CrossRef] [PubMed]
26. Aran, D.; Hu, Z.; Butte, A.J. xCell: Digitally portraying the tissue cellular heterogeneity landscape. *Genome Biol.* **2017**, *18*, 220. [CrossRef] [PubMed]
27. Love, M.I.; Huber, W.; Anders, S. Moderated estimation of fold change and dispersion for RNA-seq data with DESeq2. *Genome Biol.* **2014**, *15*, 550. [CrossRef]
28. Yu, G.; Wang, L.G.; Han, Y.; He, Q.Y. clusterProfiler: An R package for comparing biological themes among gene clusters. *Omics A J. Integr. Biol.* **2012**, *16*, 284–287. [CrossRef]
29. Pages, F.; Mlecnik, B.; Marliot, F.; Bindea, G.; Ou, F.S.; Bifulco, C.; Lugli, A.; Zlobec, I.; Rau, T.T.; Berger, M.D.; et al. International validation of the consensus Immunoscore for the classification of colon cancer: A prognostic and accuracy study. *Lancet* **2018**, *391*, 2128–2139. [CrossRef]
30. Anitei, M.G.; Zeitoun, G.; Mlecnik, B.; Marliot, F.; Haicheur, N.; Todosi, A.M.; Kirilovsky, A.; Lagorce, C.; Bindea, G.; Ferariu, D.; et al. Prognostic and predictive values of the immunoscore in patients with rectal cancer. *Clin. Cancer Res. Off. J. Am. Assoc. Cancer Res.* **2014**, *20*, 1891–1899. [CrossRef]
31. Choi, J.; Maeng, H.G.; Lee, S.J.; Kim, Y.J.; Kim, D.W.; Lee, H.N.; Namgung, J.H.; Oh, H.M.; Kim, T.J.; Jeong, J.E.; et al. Diagnostic value of peripheral blood immune profiling in colorectal cancer. *Ann. Surg. Treat. Res.* **2018**, *94*, 312–321. [CrossRef]
32. Waidhauser, J.; Nerlinger, P.; Arndt, T.T.; Schiele, S.; Sommer, F.; Wolf, S.; Löhr, P.; Eser, S.; Müller, G.; Claus, R.; et al. Alterations of circulating lymphocyte subsets in patients with colorectal carcinoma. *Cancer Immunol. Immunother. CII* **2021**, *71*, 1937–1947. [CrossRef]
33. Shimabukuro-Vornhagen, A.; Schlosser, H.A.; Gryschok, L.; Malcher, J.; Wennhold, K.; Garcia-Marquez, M.; Herbold, T.; Neuhaus, L.S.; Becker, H.J.; Fiedler, A.; et al. Characterization of tumor-associated B-cell subsets in patients with colorectal cancer. *Oncotarget* **2014**, *5*, 4651–4664. [CrossRef]
34. Krijgsman, D.; de Vries, N.L.; Skovbo, A.; Andersen, M.N.; Swets, M.; Bastiaannet, E.; Vahrmeijer, A.L.; van de Velde, C.J.H.; Heemskerk, M.H.M.; Hokland, M.; et al. Characterization of circulating T-, NK-, and NKT cell subsets in patients with colorectal cancer: The peripheral blood immune cell profile. *Cancer Immunol. Immunother. CII* **2019**, *68*, 1011–1024. [CrossRef] [PubMed]
35. Dylag-Trojanowska, K.; Rogala, J.; Pach, R.; Siedlar, M.; Baran, J.; Sierzega, M.; Zybaczynska, J.; Lenart, M.; Rutkowska-Zapala, M.; Szczepanik, A.M. T Regulatory CD4(+)CD25(+)FoxP3(+) Lymphocytes in the Peripheral Blood of Left-Sided Colorectal Cancer Patients. *Medicina* **2019**, *55*, 307. [CrossRef]
36. Krijgsman, D.; De Vries, N.L.; Andersen, M.N.; Skovbo, A.; Tollenaar, R.A.E.M.; Møller, H.J.; Hokland, M.; Kuppen, P.J.K. CD163 as a Biomarker in Colorectal Cancer: The Expression on Circulating Monocytes and Tumor-Associated Macrophages, and the Soluble Form in the Blood. *Int. J. Mol. Sci.* **2020**, *21*, 5925. [CrossRef] [PubMed]
37. Rosales, C. Neutrophil: A Cell with Many Roles in Inflammation or Several Cell Types? *Front. Physiol.* **2018**, *9*, 113. [CrossRef] [PubMed]
38. Gabrilovich, D.I.; Nagaraj, S. Myeloid-derived suppressor cells as regulators of the immune system. *Nat. Rev. Immunol.* **2009**, *9*, 162–174. [CrossRef]
39. Zhang, B.; Wang, Z.; Wu, L.; Zhang, M.; Li, W.; Ding, J.; Zhu, J.; Wei, H.; Zhao, K. Circulating and tumor-infiltrating myeloid-derived suppressor cells in patients with colorectal carcinoma. *PLoS ONE* **2013**, *8*, e57114. [CrossRef]

40. Solito, S.; Falisi, E.; Diaz-Montero, C.M.; Doni, A.; Pinton, L.; Rosato, A.; Francescato, S.; Basso, G.; Zanovello, P.; Onicescu, G.; et al. A human promyelocytic-like population is responsible for the immune suppression mediated by myeloid-derived suppressor cells. *Blood* **2011**, *118*, 2254–2265. [CrossRef]
41. Borrego, F.; Robertson, M.J.; Ritz, J.; Peña, J.; Solana, R. CD69 is a stimulatory receptor for natural killer cell and its cytotoxic effect is blocked by CD94 inhibitory receptor. *Immunology* **1999**, *97*, 159–165. [CrossRef]
42. Krijgsman, D.; De Vries, N.L.; Andersen, M.N.; Skovbo, A.; Tollenaar, R.A.E.M.; Bastiaannet, E.; Kuppen, P.J.K.; Hokland, M. The effects of tumor resection and adjuvant therapy on the peripheral blood immune cell profile in patients with colon carcinoma. *Cancer Immunol. Immunother.* **2020**, *69*, 2009–2020. [CrossRef]
43. Bene, N.C.; Alcaide, P.; Wortis, H.H.; Jaffe, I.Z. Mineralocorticoid receptors in immune cells: Emerging role in cardiovascular disease. *Steroids* **2014**, *91*, 38–45. [CrossRef]
44. Racioppi, L.; Means, A.R. Calcium/calmodulin-dependent kinase IV in immune and inflammatory responses: Novel routes for an ancient traveller. *Trends Immunol.* **2008**, *29*, 600–607. [CrossRef] [PubMed]
45. Koga, T.; Hedrich, C.M.; Mizui, M.; Yoshida, N.; Otomo, K.; Lieberman, L.A.; Rauen, T.; Crispín, J.C.; Tsokos, G.C. CaMK4-dependent activation of AKT/mTOR and CREM-α underlies autoimmunity-associated Th17 imbalance. *J. Clin. Investig.* **2014**, *124*, 2234–2245. [CrossRef] [PubMed]
46. Koga, T.; Kawakami, A. The role of CaMK4 in immune responses. *Mod. Rheumatol.* **2018**, *28*, 211–214. [CrossRef]
47. Kirchgessner, H.; Dietrich, J.; Scherer, J.; Isomäki, P.; Korinek, V.; Hilgert, I.; Bruyns, E.; Leo, A.; Cope, A.P.; Schraven, B. The transmembrane adaptor protein TRIM regulates T cell receptor (TCR) expression and TCR-mediated signaling via an association with the TCR zeta chain. *J. Exp. Med.* **2001**, *193*, 1269–1284. [CrossRef]
48. Valk, E.; Leung, R.; Kang, H.; Kaneko, K.; Rudd, C.E.; Schneider, H. T cell receptor-interacting molecule acts as a chaperone to modulate surface expression of the CTLA-4 coreceptor. *Immunity* **2006**, *25*, 807–821. [CrossRef] [PubMed]
49. Vacchi, E.; Burrello, J.; Burrello, A.; Bolis, S.; Monticone, S.; Barile, L.; Kaelin-Lang, A.; Melli, G. Profiling Inflammatory Extracellular Vesicles in Plasma and Cerebrospinal Fluid: An Optimized Diagnostic Model for Parkinson's Disease. *Biomedicines* **2021**, *9*, 230. [CrossRef]
50. Vacchi, E.; Burrello, J.; Di Silvestre, D.; Burrello, A.; Bolis, S.; Mauri, P.; Vassalli, G.; Cereda, C.W.; Farina, C.; Barile, L.; et al. Immune profiling of plasma-derived extracellular vesicles identifies Parkinson disease. *Neurol Neuroimmunol. Neuroinflamm.* **2020**, *7*. [CrossRef] [PubMed]
51. Yang, X.; Song, X.; Zhang, X.; Shankar, V.; Wang, S.; Yang, Y.; Chen, S.; Zhang, L.; Ni, Y.; Zare, R.N.; et al. In situ DESI-MSI lipidomic profiles of mucosal margin of oral squamous cell carcinoma. *EBioMedicine* **2021**, *70*, 103529. [CrossRef]

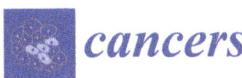

Article

Identification of a Twelve-microRNA Signature with Prognostic Value in Stage II Microsatellite Stable Colon Cancer

Ferran Moratalla-Navarro [1,2,3,4], Anna Díez-Villanueva [1,2], Ainhoa Garcia-Serrano [5], Adrià Closa [6], David Cordero [1,2], Xavier Solé [7,8], Elisabet Guinó [1,2], Rebeca Sanz-Pamplona [1,2,3,9], Xavier Sanjuan [2,10], Cristina Santos [2,11,12], Sebastiano Biondo [2,4,13], Ramón Salazar [2,4,11,12] and Victor Moreno [1,2,3,4,*]

[1] Oncology Data Analytics Program, Catalan Institute of Oncology (ICO), 08908 Barcelona, Spain
[2] Colorectal Cancer Group, Bellvitge Biomedical Research Institute (IDIBELL), 08908 Barcelona, Spain
[3] Consortium for Biomedical Research in Epidemiology and Public Health (CIBERESP), 28029 Madrid, Spain
[4] Department of Clinical Sciences, Faculty of Medicine, University of Barcelona (UB), 08907 Barcelona, Spain
[5] Department of Clinical Science, Intervention and Technology (CLINTEC), Karolinska Institutet, 14186 Stockholm, Sweden
[6] Department of Pathology, Netherlands Cancer Institute, 1066 CX Amsterdam, The Netherlands
[7] Molecular Biology CORE, Center for Biomedical Diagnostics, Hospital Clinic de Barcelona, 08036 Barcelona, Spain
[8] Translational Genomic and Targeted Therapeutics in Solid Tumors, August Pi i Sunyer Biomedical Research Institute (IDIBAPS), 08036 Barcelona, Spain
[9] Lozano Blesa University Hospital, Aragon Health Research Institute (IISA), Aragon I+D Foundation (ARAID), Government of Aragon, 50009 Zaragoza, Spain
[10] Department of Pathology, Bellvitge University Hospital, 08907 Barcelona, Spain
[11] Oncology Service, Catalan Institute of Oncology (ICO), 08908 Barcelona, Spain
[12] Consortium for Biomedical Research in Oncology (CIBERONC), 28029 Madrid, Spain
[13] Department of General and Digestive Surgery, Bellvitge University Hospital, 08907 Barcelona, Spain
* Correspondence: v.moreno@iconcologia.net

Simple Summary: Colorectal cancer (CRC) is one of the most prevalent cancers, and approximately a quarter of patients diagnosed at stage II exhibit a significant risk of recurrence. In this study, we successfully identified a microRNA (miRNA) signature allowing the recognition of patients at high recurrence risk. The validity of these findings has been confirmed through an entirely separate group of patients diagnosed with stage II microsatellite stability (MSS) colon adenocarcinoma (COAD). Most of the miRNAs present in the signature have demonstrated prognostic relevance in various other cancer types. Upon examining their gene targets, we discovered that some of these miRNAs are intricately involved in pivotal pathways of cancer progression.

Abstract: We aimed to identify and validate a set of miRNAs that could serve as a prognostic signature useful to determine the recurrence risk for patients with COAD. Small RNAs from tumors of 100 stage II, untreated, MSS colon cancer patients were sequenced for the discovery step. For this purpose, we built an miRNA score using an elastic net Cox regression model based on the disease-free survival status. Patients were grouped into high or low recurrence risk categories based on the median value of the score. We then validated these results in an independent sample of stage II microsatellite stable tumor tissues, with a hazard ratio of 3.24, (CI$_{95\%}$ = 1.05–10.0) and a 10-year area under the receiver operating characteristic curve of 0.67. Functional analysis of the miRNAs present in the signature identified key pathways in cancer progression. In conclusion, the proposed signature of 12 miRNAs can contribute to improving the prediction of disease relapse in patients with stage II MSS colorectal cancer, and might be useful in deciding which patients may benefit from adjuvant chemotherapy.

Keywords: colorectal cancer; microRNA; prognosis; biomarker

1. Introduction

CRC is the third most newly diagnosed cancer type worldwide. Although systematic screening programs have reduced the incidence of CRC in Western countries [1], it is still the second leading cause of cancer-related deaths worldwide for both men and women [2], with millions of cases being reported each year. Currently, stage at diagnosis is the most relevant predictor of prognosis. It is known that about a quarter of patients with CRC are diagnosed in stage II, with localized disease and no evidence of regional lymph node invasion [3]. Nevertheless, disease will recur or progress to distant metastasis in about 20–25% of these patients. Clinical and pathological risk factors, such as the size and location of the tumor, are used to identify patients at high risk of recurrence, but they are not always reliable. As a result, there has been growing interest in the use of biomarkers to improve the accuracy of prognostic and predictive testing for CRC patients [4–8]. However, these approaches are limited by small populations or accuracy [9,10]. Molecular biomarkers could be used to identify patients who are at high risk of disease recurrence or improve stratification of patients who could benefit from adjuvant chemotherapy or immunotherapy.

miRNAs are short, double-stranded, non-coding RNA molecules, typically between 19 and 24 nucleotides in length, which play a critical role in the regulation of gene expression. MiRNAs are involved in post-transcriptional regulation of multiple protein coding genes, mainly by binding to the 3' untranslated regions (UTRs) of target genes, leading to inhibition of messenger RNA (mRNA) transcription [11]. Changes in miRNA expression affect target genes regulation, and consequently, their deregulation can lead to irregular cell processes related to tumor development and progression [12]. To date, several miRNAs have been proposed to be either oncogenic or tumor suppressors [13–15], and there have been some miRNA signatures proposed as molecular biomarkers in CRC for both diagnosis and prognosis, as well as treatment decisions [16–19].

In this study, we aimed to identify and validate a signature of miRNAs with prognostic value in stage II COAD patients. We used next-generation sequencing (NGS) techniques to obtain miRNA expression values for a set of tumor samples, and we tried to validate the findings in an independent sample series.

2. Materials and Methods

2.1. Subjects and Samples

In the discovery series, we included Colonomics (CLX): 98 tumor tissue samples, MSS stage II patients with a new diagnosis of COAD at the University Hospital of Bellvitge in Barcelona (Spain) between January 1996 and December 2000. Patients were selected from those that had donated fresh tissue to the biobank and had undergone a complete surgical resection of the tumor, but had not received adjuvant chemotherapy. In addition, a minimum of 3 years of follow-up was required.

The validation series included public independent samples of 130 COAD patients (stage II) from The Cancer Genome Atlas (TCGA) study.

The study was performed in accordance with relevant ethics guidelines and regulations. The Clinical Research Ethics Committee of the Bellvitge Hospital approved the study protocol (PR178/11). Individuals provided written informed consent to participate and for genetic analysis to be carried out on their samples. Additional information about the study can be found at www.colonomics.org (accessed on 15 May 2023). This study carefully follows the recommendations for reporting proposed by the REMARK guidelines [20].

2.2. Sample Processing

Tumor samples were cut by the pathologist from the surgical specimen during the first hour after removal and kept frozen at −80 °C in the hospital's tumor bank. Total RNA was isolated from tissue samples using the miRCURY^{TM} RNA isolation kit (Exiqon, Vedbaek, Denmark) according to the manufacturer's protocol, quantified using a NanoDrop® ND-1000 Spectrophotometer (Nanodrop technologies, Wilmington, DE, USA) and stored at −80 °C. The quality of these RNA samples was assessed with the RNA 6000 Nano Assay

(Agilent Technologies, Santa Clara, CA, USA) following the manufacturer's recommendations. The RNA integrity number (RIN) showed high quality values for all the samples (mean = 7.89, sd = 0.86). The RNA purity was measured with the ratio of absorbance at 260 nm and 280 nm (mean = 1.96, sd = 0.04). The quality control for the small RNA fraction was assessed with the Small RNA Assay in the Agilent 2100 Bioanalyzer (Agilent Technologies, Santa Clara, CA, USA) following the manufacturer's recommendations.

2.3. Small RNA-Seq Analysis of the Discovery Series

The small RNA-seq was performed through the SOLiD platform. The PureLink miRNA isolation kit was used to construct the libraries of compatible fragments with SOLiD from an enriched fraction of small RNA. Sequencing microspheres were obtained by applying an emulsion PCR into an equimolar mixture of 48 libraries followed by an enrichment process before charging in the reaction chamber. Finally, the reaction to obtain the sequences (35 nucleotides + 10 nucleotides barcode) from the small RNA fraction was performed with the Applied Biosystems SOLiD 4 System. Samples were randomly distributed among the different sequencing slides to minimize batch effects. The data quality was estimated using the SOLiD Experimental Tracking System (SETS) software.

2.4. Expression Data of the Discovery Series

CLX is a multiomics experiment design with different high-throughput sequencing data. In addition to small RNA-seq, it has microarray expression data for the same subjects. Sample processing, quality control and normalization are described elsewhere [21].

2.5. Bioinformatics Analysis

Quality control of sequenced reads was ensured using specially designed bioinformatics framework for the SOLiD system [22]. Total number of reads, proportion of miscalled reads and low-average-quality-score proportion reads were evaluated. All samples passed the quality control criteria and were selected for further analysis. Next, quantification of specific miRNAs was performed by mapping reads to the reference of mature miRNA sequences annotated in miRBase release 22 [23], containing 2641 human mature miRNA sequences. The FASTX-toolkit [24] was used to preprocess miRNA data and provide compatible sequences for mapping with Bowtie aligner. Read adapters were trimmed with cutadapt [25], and finally, a table of counts was generated with SAMtools [26]. A principal component analysis (PCA) was computed to detect possible outliers. A filter based on low variability of miRNAs across all samples was performed to remove unwanted noisy data (standard deviation < 0.1). Data normalization was performed using DESeq2 package [27], after which it was transformed with a logarithmic function to reduce positive skewness. MiRNAs with normalized expression values not detected in more than 90% of samples were filtered out due to low expression. This criterion was mandatory for both discovery and validation datasets.

2.6. Statistical Analysis of Prognosis

For this study, disease-free survival (DFS) was assessed, and disease progression, defined as local tumor recurrence, metastasis or cancer-related death, was the event of interest. First, we wanted to inspect miRNA profiles based on possible sources of confounding variables. For this purpose, differential miRNA expression analysis (DEA) was carried out with the DESeq2 package for sex and tumor site. In addition, a proportional hazards assumption test was performed to assess possible sources of analysis bias from common covariates: age, sex and tumor site (left or right colon). Univariate Cox proportional hazard models were computed for each miRNA and adjusted for age, sex, tumor site and sub-stage. Kaplan–Meier survival curves were used to graph the results, which were split by median normalized expression values. Next, in order to identify an miRNA signature that could capture disease progression, a regularized Cox regression model was performed with an alpha parameter ($\alpha = 0.5$) and leave-one-out cross-validation. Adjustment variables were included in all models, and we selected the model that minimized the cross-validation error. The coefficients for the miRNAs that were not shrunk in the optimal model were used to compute an miRNA prognosis risk score (RS) as follows:

$$\sum_{i=1}^{n} = \beta_i * expr_i$$

where n is the total number of active miRNAs in the model, β_i is the coefficient for each active miRNA, and $expr_i$ is the expression value of each active miRNA. The score obtained was ranked and split into two equal groups by the median value. The performance of the model was assessed with Cox proportional hazard models (selecting miRNA (RS) and adjustment variables, as mentioned before) and Kaplan–Meier survival curves. Univariate Cox proportional hazard models and Kaplan–Meier estimates were obtained with the *survival* R package [28]. Regularized Cox regression models were computed with the *glmnet* R package [29]. All statistical analysis was performed in R version 3.5 [30].

2.7. Validation Analysis

For the validation dataset, TCGA COAD samples were filtered in order to obtain similar clinical characteristics and reproducible analysis. Sample exclusion criteria included no clinical information for disease-free survival status or microsatellite instability (MSI) subtype, the latter of which was assessed in cBioPortal [31,32]. Normalization of miRNA expression values and filtering was identical in discovery and validation series. Independent prognosis analysis for stage II was assessed. The same coefficients and cutoffs obtained in the training dataset were used for the validation.

2.8. Functional Characterization

We conducted two separate approaches to characterize the resulting miRNA signature and score. On the one hand, for the signature study, two different miRNA–mRNA interaction resources were interrogated to extract high-confidence gene targets for each miRNA present in our signature. Only common interactions present in mirDB (release 6.0) [33,34] and miRTarBase (release 9.0) [35] were included to define the functional role of miRNAs associated with prognosis. mirDB annotates predicted miRNA–target interactions (MTI) while miRTarBase captures experimentally validated MTIs from research articles. Network analysis was carried out with igraph [36] to identify hub miRNAs; next, we performed an enrichment analysis with the ReactomePA [37] R package based on the REACTOME pathway database, including direct targets for each selected miRNA. On the other hand, we wanted to study the relationship between miRNA prognosis RS and the abundance of tissue-infiltrating immune cell populations that could potentially play different roles in the tumor microenvironment. For this purpose, a deconvolution method [38] was used to estimate cell population proportions (immune and non-immune stromal) from average gene expression signals. Non-parametric Spearman's rank-order correlations were computed to evaluate correlation patterns between each of the ten different cell types and miRNA prognosis RS.

3. Results

3.1. Study Population Characteristics and Quality Control of Samples

The CLX small-RNA sequencing dataset comprised 100 tumor tissues, stage II MSS, and 2641 different miRNAs were initially identified. The first filter removed 153 miRNAs due to low variability. The second filter was applied to remove low-expression features. A total of 928 miRNAs passed the filtering criteria. Two samples were filtered out after PCA analysis (see Supplementary Figure S1). The same procedure was performed for the validation dataset, which lowered the number of different miRNAs from 2117 to 796. Finally, 605 miRNAs were determined to be present in both datasets and were selected for the next analysis. Table 1 summarizes the main characteristics of the patients included in both datasets. DEA comparing tumor location resulted in only 10 significant miRNAs with different profiles between the left and right sides (seven overexpressed on the right side, three overexpressed on the left side). All of them had an absolute log2-fold change greater than 0.5. When comparing expression profiles between sex, only two significant miRNAs were observed (Supplementary Table S1 and Figure S2). None of the inspected covariates violated the proportional hazards assumption of the Cox model (p-values > 0.05, Supplementary Table S2). Univariate Cox proportional hazard models, adjusted by sex, age, site and stage, identified 55 miRNAs associated with disease-free survival (p-value < 0.05). However, none of them passed the false discovery rate (Benjamini–Hochberg-adjusted p-value < 0.05) (Supplementary Table S3).

Table 1. Summary of characteristics of the patients included in the study.

	Colonomics n (%)	TCGA n (%)
Number of Patients	98	130
Gender		
Male	70 (71.43%)	69 (53.08%)
Female	28 (28.57%)	61 (46.92%)
Median Age (Years)	71	69
Tumor Site		
Right	38 (38.78%)	75 (57.69%)
Left	60 (61.22%)	50 (38.46%)
Stage		
II-A	90 (91.84%)	99 (76.15%)
II-B	8 (8.16%)	6 (4.62%)
Disease-Free Survival		
No Event	76 (77.55%)	104 (80.00%)
Event	22 (22.45%)	26 (20.00%)
Microsatellite Instability		
MSS	98 (100%)	101 (77.69%)
MSI	0 (0%)	20 (15.38%)
Median Metastatic Lymph Nodes	0 (100%)	0 (100%)
Median Isolated Lymph Nodes	18.5	20.0
Lymphatic Invasion		
Yes	7 (0.07%)	26 (20.00%)
No	86 (87.76%)	92 (70.77%)
Perineural Invasion		
Yes	2 (2.04%)	13 (10.00%)
No	83 (84.69%)	38 (29.23%)

3.2. miRNA Signature and Score

The regularized Cox regression model resulted in a 12-miRNA signature computed in the discovery dataset (Table 2). Of note, all miRNAs present in the signature were statistically significant according to the univariate models ($p < 0.05$), and all of them showed the same trend at the individual coefficient signs, suggesting low collinearity between all of them (Supplementary Table S4), which was confirmed with a Spearman's correlation matrix (absolute Spearman's $r \leq 0.43$ for all pairwise comparisons (Supplementary Figure S3).

The RS formula obtained was:

miRNA RS = hsa-miR-1185-5p × (−0.185) + hsa-miR-16-5p × (−0.111) + hsa-miR-181a-2-3p × 0.181 + hsa-miR-204-5p × 0.003 + hsa-miR-2355-3p × 0.242 + hsa-miR-29b-2-5p × (−0.306) + hsa-miR-331-3p × 0.153 + hsa-miR-423-3p × (−0.355) + hsa-miR-432-5p × (−0.187) + hsa-miR-497-5p × (−0.183) + hsa-miR-656-3p × (−0.526) + hsa-miR-935 × (−0.136)

Kaplan–Meier curves demonstrated a good performance of the model, clearly differentiating low- and high-risk patient log-rank p-values = 1.62×10^{-6}. Patients in the high-risk group were found to have higher recurrence rates (HR = 33.59, 4.34–244.8, $p < 0.001$) (Figure 1a,c). Three-, five- and ten-year disease-free survival (DFS) were selected to compute the area under the ROC curve (AUC). AUCs of 0.89, 0.92 and 0.94 were obtained for three-, five- and ten-year DFS, respectively (Figure 2a).

Table 2. List of miRNAs present in the signature and the coefficient extracted from the elastic net Cox regression model.

miRNA	Coefficient
hsa-miR-1185-5p	−0.185
hsa-miR-16-5p	−0.111
hsa-miR-181a-2-3p	0.181
hsa-miR-204-5p	0.003
hsa-miR-2355-3p	0.242
hsa-miR-29b-2-5p	−0.306
hsa-miR-331-3p	0.153
hsa-miR-423-3p	−0.355
hsa-miR-432-5p	−0.187
hsa-miR-497-5p	−0.183
hsa-miR-656-3p	−0.526
hsa-miR-935	−0.136

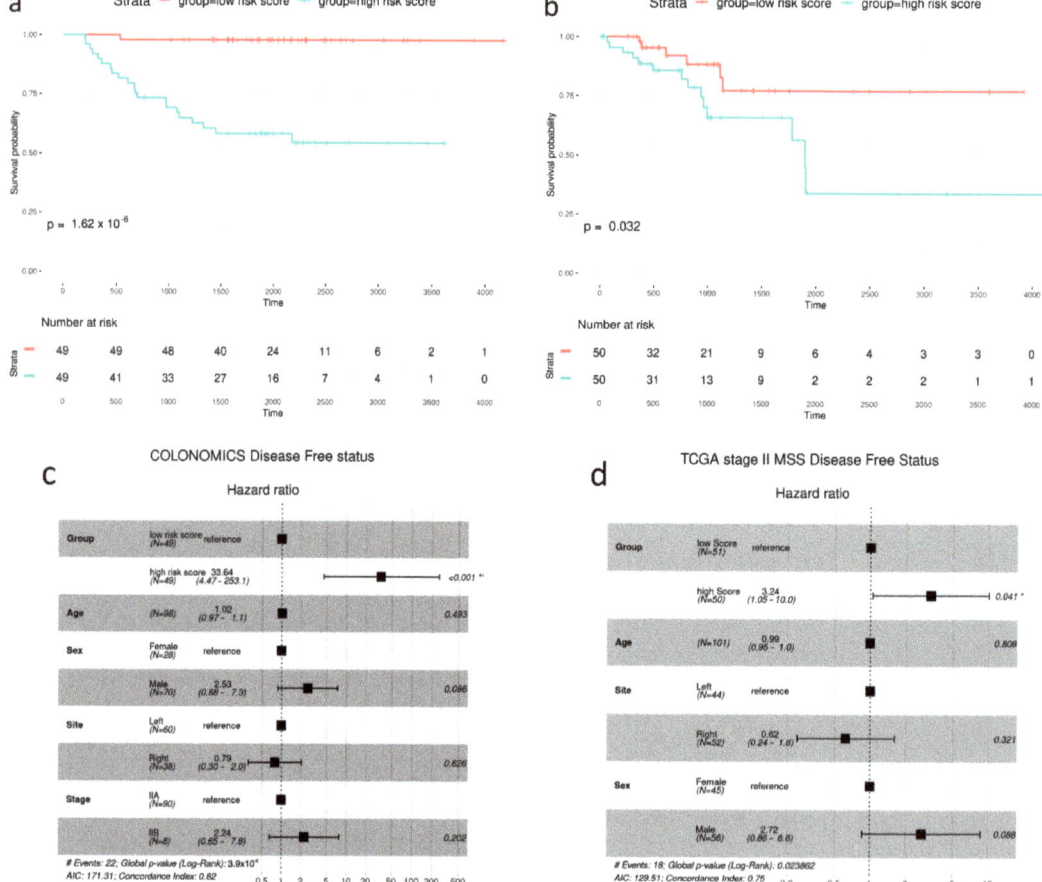

Figure 1. Comparison of the prognostic value with stratification analysis by miRNA risk group using Kaplan–Meier disease-free survival curves. (**a**) Discovery series (Colonomics). (**b**) Validation series (TCGA stage II MSS). Multivariate COX regression hazard models. (**c**) Discovery series (Colonomics). (**d**) Validation series (TCGA stage II MSS). Statistically significant HRs denoted with *.

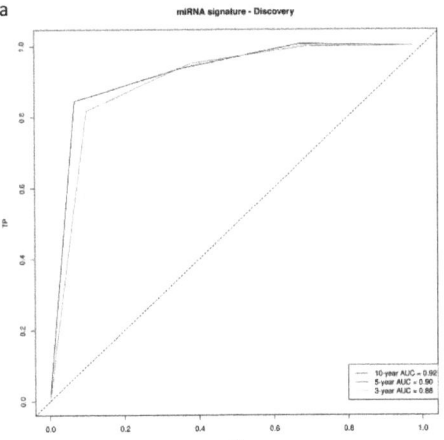 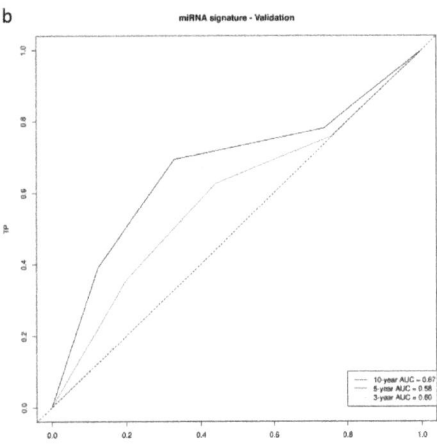

Figure 2. ROC curves at 3-, 5- and 10-year disease-free survival. (**a**) Discovery series (Colonomics). (**b**) Validation series (TCGA stage II MSS).

3.3. Validation

CLX miRNA signatures were tested on an independent COAD dataset from TCGA. Overall, the miRNA predictive capacity was poor, which is mainly explained by the poor performance on stage II MSI tumor samples. However, it improved substantially when only stage II MSS samples were analyzed (n = 100). A similar trend to that in CLX was observed; the miRNA risk group had an HR of 3.24, with a range of 1.05–10.0, and $p = 0.041$ (Figure 1d), and the low- versus high-risk patient log-rank p-value was 0.034, as assessed using KM curves (Figure 1b). The AUCs were 0.60, 0.59 and 0.67 for three-, five- and ten-year DFS, respectively (Figure 2b).

3.4. Functional Characterization

Gene target candidates for each miRNA present in our signature were retrieved from mirDB and mirTarBase (10,352 and 3673, respectively). Overall, common MTIs from both datasets revealed 1015 MTIs. Network analysis showed three hub miRNAs: hsa-miR-16-5p (483 gene interactions), hsa-miR-497-5p (252 gene interactions) and hsa-miR-204-5p (119 gene interactions). Of note, the first two miRNAs shared 242 common gene interactions (Figure 3). Next, Reactome pathway analysis identified relevant cancer pathways associated with both hsa-miR-16-5p and hsa-miR -497-5p, such as signaling by the TGF-beta receptor complex ($p = 1.84 \times 10^{-7}$, $p = 1.76 \times 10^{-5}$, respectively), regulation of RUNX1 expression and activity ($p = 2.82 \times 10^{-7}$, 1.47×10^{-7}, respectively) and aberrant regulation of the mitotic G1/S transition in cancer due to RB1 defects ($p = 2.82 \times 10^{-7}$, 1.46×10^{-7}, respectively). The complete results of the enrichment analysis are available in Supplementary Tables S5–S13.

MCP-counter was applied to gene expression data from the discovery series. Abundances of reported immune-infiltrating cell populations, as well as other non-immune cell types, are summarized in Supplementary Figure S4. B-cell infiltrates (Spearman's r = -0.34, p-value = 6.24×10^{-4}), myeloid dendritic cell infiltrates (Spearman's r = -0.32, p-value = 1.51×10^{-3}) and T-cell infiltrates (Spearman's r = -0.29, p-value = 3.79×10^{-3}) appeared with a moderate inverse association with miRNA RS (Supplementary Figure S5). It is worth mentioning that all tested cell population abundances were inversely correlated with miRNA RS, suggesting an overall increase in immune infiltration in tumors with lower values for the computed RS.

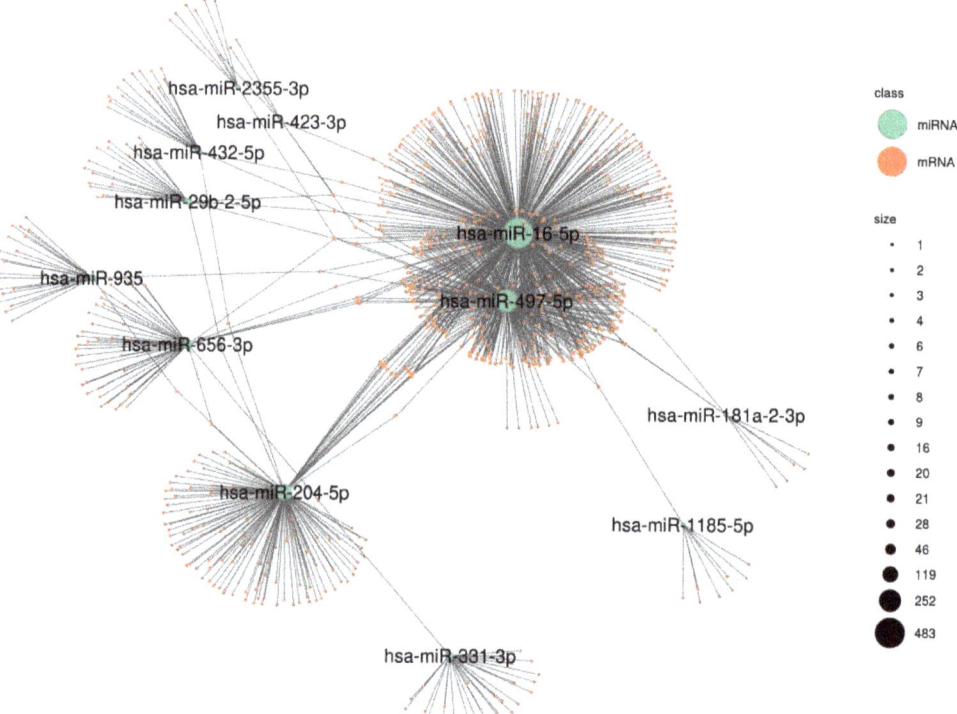

Figure 3. mRNA–miRNA interaction network representation. Light-green nodes represent miRNAs present in the signature, and orange nodes represent their direct target mRNAs. Gray lines represent an interaction present between an miRNA and an mRNA (validated in miRTarBase and also predicted by mirDB). Node size is proportional to its degree centrality measure (number of direct interactors).

4. Discussion

A comprehensive analysis has been conducted in order to identify an miRNA signature with potential value for stratifying patients into different disease progression risk groups in stage II MSS colon cancer.

Similar to other prognostic signatures previously published [16–18,39], our signature demonstrated a significant association. However, its ability to accurately predict which patients will experience recurrence was limited [40]. Nevertheless, this does not imply that the signature is not valuable since it can be used to classify patients into distinct risk groups.

To the best of our knowledge, only 2 of the 12 miRNAs included in the proposed signature have been previously included in other CRC miRNA signatures [41,42]. However, several of them have been associated with CRC development and/or prognosis; some of them have also been associated with tumoral progression in other tissues. Our findings agree with current knowledge concerning the miRNAs present in our signature. Recently, it has been found that overexpression of hsa-miR-16-5p can inhibit CRC cell proliferation, migration, immune modulation and invasion [43,44]. Another recent publication pointed out the relationship between the down-regulation of hsa-miR-16-5p and hsa-miR-497-5p and the progression of endometrial cancer mediated by circular RNA hsa-circ-0011324 [45]. Both miRNAs appeared to have lower expression values in the CLX series high-risk group, as reported in univariate Cox proportional hazard models. hsa-miR-656-3p was also included in one miRNA classifier for tumor recurrence in stage II CRC [42]. Interestingly, it has also been identified as an inhibitor of CRC cell migration in vitro [46]. In contrast, hsa-miR-204-5p has been identified to be negatively associated with CRC progression and chemoresistance [47,48]. This specific miRNA goes in the opposite direction both in the discovery and validation series. Another miRNA present in the signature, hsa-miR-935, has been studied in different cancer types and seems to have different behaviors depending on the targeted tissue, inhibiting or promoting tumor development in glioblastoma, liver and gastric cancer [49–51]. Hsa-miR-423-3p was seen to be down-regulated in hepatocellular carcinoma compared to healthy and liver cirrhosis samples [52]. In a recent study conducted on bladder urothelial carcinoma patients, hsa-miR-432-5p was found to be a good biomarker for diagnosis, being under-expressed in tumoral samples [53]. Regarding the remnant miRNAs, one study suggested opposite effects from what we have reported for hsa-miR-181a-2-3p in glioblastoma [54], and two studies found hsa-miR-331-3p to be under-expressed in prostate cancers [55] and CRC [56] compared to healthy groups. Higher levels of hsa-29b-2-5p expression were associated with the staging of esophageal and gastric cancer [57] in TCGA. However, this association was not observed in TCGA COAD stage II samples. No previous studies were found for hsa-miR-2355-3p and hsa-miR-1185-5p related to cancer.

To assess the complex functional interrelationships between the miRNAs and their putative target mRNAs, we analyzed a network of validated miRNA–target gene associations. Our results show a significant enrichment of genes involved in cellular processes relevant for cancer progression, such as cell cycle regulation, interleukin signaling and cell migration [58,59]. Since the information on validated target genes for miRNA is still incomplete, these results might be biased because more well-known miRNAs share more interactions with important cancer genes. However, this behavior is expected to be minimized with the release of the latest updated versions. In addition, to further evaluate the possible effects of the miRNA signature, the immune profile analysis of the miRNA risk groups revealed an overall increased abundance of all types of immune cell populations as measured through deconvolution analyses, suggesting a protective effect of immune infiltration in tumors [60]. Although the role of immune cell infiltrates in cancer progression is complex and context-dependent [61], it is thought that in early CRC stages, immune cells could help to control the growth and spread of cancer cells. However, as the tumor progresses, these immune cells can adapt a pro-tumorigenic role, promoting tumor growth and metastasis [62,63].

Besides the considerable efforts to generate biomarkers for risk assessment based on miRNA expression levels [16–18,42], other emerging tools are being investigated as potential prognostic factors for stage II CRC. One such approach involves examining molecular characteristics, including mutations or expression profile alterations in BRAF, KRAS or PIK3CA. These molecular features can aid in determining more targeted treatment strategies for patients [64–66]. Another emerging tool, circulating tumor DNA (ctDNA) analysis, has shown promise in identifying minimal residual disease [67], which results in a higher risk of recurrence for patients and may require closer surveillance or additional treatment options. Furthermore, the study of the gut microbiome is also a recent topic of interest for the assessment of both tumor onset and recurrent disease [68,69]. Lastly, exploring the tumor microenvironment [40,70], such as TILs, tumor-associated fribroblasts and stromal characteristics, and understanding the interactions between tumor cells and their microenvironment might provide valuable prognostic information.

This study has several limitations. The most important is the low number of events in both the discovery and the validation series, which is probably related to the good prognosis for early COAD diagnosis. In addition, our results may have been underestimated due to the lack of information regarding the administration of adjuvant chemotherapy or radiation therapy in the validation series. The low number of events together with the limited sample size reduces the statistical power for this kind of analysis; as a result, we saw a trend in the validation cohort with borderline statistical significance. Another limitation of the study is the lack of microsatellite instability (MSI) patients. The proportion of MSI in our hospital was low, around 8%; thus, the CLX series was only composed of MSS patients.

Overall, based on the reported results, this signature could be valuable to stratify MSS stage II COAD patients and identify those that require adjuvant chemotherapy. Additionally, the individual miRNA prognostic data provided in the discovery series contribute to increasing the knowledge on these markers in CRC.

5. Conclusions

In summary, we have identified a panel of 12 miRNAs that can be used to stratify prognosis in MSS stage II COAD. These miRNAs have been described to regulate a large list of genes involved in relevant cancer pathways, which reinforces the validity of the panel. Further studies with larger samples sizes are needed to improve our ability to classify patients with recurrence risk in a more general way.

Supplementary Materials: The following supporting information can be downloaded at: https://www.mdpi.com/article/10.3390/cancers15133301/s1.Supplementary Figure S1: PCA representation for the first two components of CLX normalized miRNA. Supplementary Figure S2: Volcano plots for DEA miRNA for tumor side (a) and sex (b). Supplementary Figure S3: Correlation plot of the 12 miRNA presents in the signature. Supplementary Figure S4: Histogram of ten cell populations abundance detected by MPC counter method. Supplementary Figure S5: Scatter plots for significant correlation between miRNA prognostic RS and B-cells, T-cells and myeloid Dendritic cells detected by MCP-counter. Supplementary Table S1: Differential miRNA expression analysis. Supplementary Table S2: Cox Proportional Hazards assumption test. Supplementary Table S3: Univariate Cox regression models for discovery series, adjusted by age, sex, site and stage. Supplementary Table S4: Univariate Cox regression models for validation series adjusted by age, sex and site. Supplementary Table S5: hsa-miR-16-5p target gene Enrichment. Supplementary Table S6: hsa-miR-432-5p target gene Enrichment. Supplementary Table S7: hsa-miR-497-5p target gene Enrichment. Supplementary Table S8: hsa-miR-432-5p target gene Enrichment. Supplementary Table S9: hsa-miR-181-a-2-3p target gene Enrichment. Supplementary Table S10: hsa-miR-204-5p target gene Enrichment. Supplementary Table S11: hsa-miR-2355-3p target gene Enrichment. Supplementary Table S12: hsa-miR-656-3p target gene Enrichment. Table S13: hsa-miR-935 target gene Enrichment.

Author Contributions: Conceptualization and methodology V.M., F.M.-N. and A.C.; formal analysis, F.M.-N., A.C., A.D.-V., A.S., D.C., X.S. (Xavier Solé) and E.G.; resources C.S., R.S., S.B. and X.S. (Xavier Sanjuan); writing—original draft preparation F.M.-N. and A.C.; writing—review and editing, F.M.-N., A.C., V.M. and R.S.-P. All authors have read and agreed to the published version of the manuscript.

Funding: This study received funding from Instituto de Salud Carlos III and was co-funded by FEDER funds—a way to build Europe—under the grant PI17-00092; the Spanish Association Against Cancer (AECC) Scientific Foundation under the grant GCTRA18022MORE; Consortium for Biomedical Research in Epidemiology and Public Health (CIBERESP), action Genrisk. ADV received funding from the Catalan Government, under fellowship PERIS SLT017/20/00042.

Institutional Review Board Statement: The study was conducted in accordance with the Declaration of Helsinki, and approved by the Clinical Research Ethics Committee of Bellvitge Hospital (PR178/11).

Informed Consent Statement: Informed consent was obtained from all subjects involved in the study.

Data Availability Statement: Full normalized miRNA expression data matrix of the training set and its associated clinical data are available at the project site: https://www.colonomics.org/data (accessed on 15 May 2023). Raw small RNA seq data are available upon request at the European Genome-Phenome Archive under the study ID: EGAS00001002453; dataset ID: EGAD00001004827.

Acknowledgments: The authors would like to thank Isabel Padrol and Carmen Atencia for their technical assistance. The "Xarxa de Bancs de Tumors de Catalunya (XBTX)" sponsored by "Pla Director d'Oncologia de Catalunya" and the ICO Biobank and PLATAFORMA BIOBANCOS PT13/0010/0013 helped with simple collection.

Conflicts of Interest: VM, co-investigator, received grants from Aniling SL.

References

1. Navarro, M.; Nicolas, A.; Ferrandez, A.; Lanas, A. Colorectal Cancer Population Screening Programs Worldwide in 2016: An Update. *World J. Gastroenterol.* **2017**, *23*, 3632. [CrossRef] [PubMed]
2. Sung, H.; Ferlay, J.; Siegel, R.L.; Laversanne, M.; Soerjomataram, I.; Jemal, A.; Bray, F. Global Cancer Statistics 2020: GLOBOCAN Estimates of Incidence and Mortality Worldwide for 36 Cancers in 185 Countries. *CA. Cancer J. Clin.* **2021**, *71*, 209–249. [CrossRef] [PubMed]
3. AJCC Cancer Staging Manual | SpringerLink. Available online: https://link.springer.com/book/9783319406176 (accessed on 4 January 2023).
4. Guo, W.; Cai, Y.; Liu, X.; Ji, Y.; Zhang, C.; Wang, L.; Liao, W.; Liu, Y.; Cui, N.; Xiang, J.; et al. Single-Exosome Profiling Identifies ITGB3+ and ITGAM+ Exosome Subpopulations as Promising Early Diagnostic Biomarkers and Therapeutic Targets for Colorectal Cancer. *Research* **2023**, *6*, 0041. [CrossRef] [PubMed]
5. Levy, J.J.; Zavras, J.P.; Veziroglu, E.M.; Nasir-Moin, M.; Kolling, F.W.; Christensen, B.C.; Salas, L.A.; Barney, R.E.; Palisoul, S.M.; Ren, B.; et al. Identification of Spatial Proteomic Signatures of Colon Tumor Metastasis: A Digital Spatial Profiling Approach. *Am. J. Pathol.* **2023**, *193*, 778–795. [CrossRef]
6. Ciocan, A.; Ciocan, R.A.; Al Hajjar, N.; Benea, A.M.; Pandrea, S.L.; Cătană, C.S.; Drugan, C.; Oprea, V.C.; Dîrzu, D.S.; Bolboacă, S.D. Exploratory Evaluation of Neopterin and Chitotriosidase as Potential Circulating Biomarkers for Colorectal Cancer. *Biomedicines* **2023**, *11*, 894. [CrossRef] [PubMed]
7. Linke, C.; Hunger, R.; Reinwald, M.; Deckert, M.; Mantke, R. Quantification of Mitochondrial CfDNA Reveals New Perspectives for Early Diagnosis of Colorectal Cancer. *BMC Cancer* **2023**, *23*, 291. [CrossRef]
8. Hosseini, F.A.; Rejali, L.; Zabihi, M.R.; Salehi, Z.; Daskar-Abkenar, E.; Taraz, T.; Fatemi, N.; Hashemi, M.; Asadzadeh-Aghdaei, H.; Nazemalhosseini-Mojarad, E. Long Non-coding RNA LINC00460 Contributes as a Potential Prognostic Biomarker through Its Oncogenic Role with ANXA2 in Colorectal Polyps. *Mol. Biol. Rep.* **2023**, *50*, 4505–4515. [CrossRef]
9. Cortes-Ciriano, I.; Lee, S.; Park, W.-Y.; Kim, T.-M.; Park, P.J. A Molecular Portrait of Microsatellite Instability across Multiple Cancers. *Nat. Commun.* **2017**, *8*, 15180. [CrossRef]
10. Gibney, G.T.; Weiner, L.M.; Atkins, M.B. Predictive Biomarkers for Checkpoint Inhibitor-Based Immunotherapy. *Lancet Oncol.* **2016**, *17*, e542–e551. [CrossRef]
11. Bartel, D.P. MicroRNAs: Genomics, Biogenesis, Mechanism, and Function. *Cell* **2004**, *116*, 281–297. [CrossRef]
12. MacFarlane, L.-A.; Murphy, P.R. MicroRNA: Biogenesis, Function and Role in Cancer. *Curr. Genom.* **2010**, *11*, 537–561. [CrossRef]
13. Yu, W.; Liang, X.; Li, X.; Zhang, Y.; Sun, Z.; Liu, Y.; Wang, J. MicroRNA-195: A Review of Its Role in Cancers. *OncoTargets Ther.* **2018**, *11*, 7109–7123. [CrossRef] [PubMed]
14. Chen, D.; Sun, Y.; Yuan, Y.; Han, Z.; Zhang, P.; Zhang, J.; You, M.J.; Teruya-Feldstein, J.; Wang, M.; Gupta, S.; et al. MiR-100 Induces Epithelial-Mesenchymal Transition but Suppresses Tumorigenesis, Migration and Invasion. *PLoS Genet.* **2014**, *10*, e1004177. [CrossRef] [PubMed]
15. Wang, X.; Zhang, H.; Yang, H.; Bai, M.; Ning, T.; Deng, T.; Liu, R.; Fan, Q.; Zhu, K.; Li, J.; et al. Exosome-Delivered CircRNA Promotes Glycolysis to Induce Chemoresistance through the MiR-122-PKM2 Axis in Colorectal Cancer. *Mol. Oncol.* **2020**, *14*, 539–555. [CrossRef]
16. Wang, Y.; Huang, L.; Shan, N.; Ma, H.; Lu, S.; Chen, X.; Long, H. Establishing a Three-MiRNA Signature as a Prognostic Model for Colorectal Cancer through Bioinformatics Analysis. *Aging* **2021**, *13*, 19894–19907. [CrossRef] [PubMed]
17. Ma, R.; Zhao, Y.; He, M.; Zhao, H.; Zhang, Y.; Zhou, S.; Gao, M.; Di, D.; Wang, J.; Ding, J.; et al. Identifying a Ten-MicroRNA Signature as a Superior Prognosis Biomarker in Colon Adenocarcinoma. *Cancer Cell Int.* **2019**, *19*, 360. [CrossRef]
18. Zhang, J.-X.; Song, W.; Chen, Z.-H.; Wei, J.-H.; Liao, Y.-J.; Lei, J.; Hu, M.; Chen, G.-Z.; Liao, B.; Lu, J.; et al. Prognostic and Predictive Value of a MicroRNA Signature in Stage II Colon Cancer: A MicroRNA Expression Analysis. *Lancet Oncol.* **2013**, *14*, 1295–1306. [CrossRef]
19. Slattery, M.L.; Herrick, J.S.; Mullany, L.E.; Valeri, N.; Stevens, J.; Caan, B.J.; Samowitz, W.; Wolff, R.K. An Evaluation and Replication of MiRNAs with Disease Stage and Colorectal Cancer-Specific Mortality. *Int. J. Cancer* **2015**, *137*, 428–438. [CrossRef] [PubMed]
20. McShane, L.M.; Altman, D.G.; Sauerbrei, W.; Taube, S.E.; Gion, M.; Clark, G.M.; Statistics Subcommittee of the NCI-EORTC Working Group on Cancer Diagnostics. REporting Recommendations for Tumour MARKer Prognostic Studies (REMARK). *Br. J. Cancer* **2005**, *93*, 387–391. [CrossRef]
21. Díez-Villanueva, A.; Sanz-Pamplona, R.; Solé, X.; Cordero, D.; Crous-Bou, M.; Guinó, E.; Lopez-Doriga, A.; Berenguer, A.; Aussó, S.; Paré-Brunet, L.; et al. COLONOMICS—Integrative Omics Data of One Hundred Paired Normal-Tumoral Samples from Colon Cancer Patients. *Sci. Data* **2022**, *9*, 595. [CrossRef]
22. Sasson, A.; Michael, T.P. Filtering Error from SOLiD Output. *Bioinformatics* **2010**, *26*, 849–850. [CrossRef] [PubMed]
23. Kozomara, A.; Birgaoanu, M.; Griffiths-Jones, S. MiRBase: From MicroRNA Sequences to Function. *Nucleic Acids Res.* **2019**, *47*, D155–D162. [CrossRef]
24. FASTX-Toolkit. Available online: http://hannonlab.cshl.edu/fastx_toolkit/ (accessed on 11 April 2023).
25. Martin, M. Cutadapt Removes Adapter Sequences from High-Throughput Sequencing Reads. *EMBnet. J.* **2011**, *17*, 10. [CrossRef]
26. Danecek, P.; Bonfield, J.K.; Liddle, J.; Marshall, J.; Ohan, V.; Pollard, M.O.; Whitwham, A.; Keane, T.; McCarthy, S.A.; Davies, R.M.; et al. Twelve Years of SAMtools and BCFtools. *GigaScience* **2021**, *10*, giab008. [CrossRef] [PubMed]

27. Love, M.I.; Huber, W.; Anders, S. Moderated Estimation of Fold Change and Dispersion for RNA-Seq Data with DESeq2. *Genome Biol.* **2014**, *15*, 550. [CrossRef] [PubMed]
28. Therneau, T. A Package for Survival Analysis in R. Available online: https://cran.r-project.org/web/packages/survival/vignettes/survival.pdf (accessed on 20 April 2023).
29. Simon, N.; Friedman, J.H.; Hastie, T.; Tibshirani, R. Regularization Paths for Cox's Proportional Hazards Model via Coordinate Descent. *J. Stat. Softw.* **2011**, *39*, 1–13. [CrossRef] [PubMed]
30. R core team. R: The R Project for Statistical Computing. Available online: https://www.r-project.org/ (accessed on 25 April 2023).
31. Cerami, E.; Gao, J.; Dogrusoz, U.; Gross, B.E.; Sumer, S.O.; Aksoy, B.A.; Jacobsen, A.; Byrne, C.J.; Heuer, M.L.; Larsson, E.; et al. The CBio Cancer Genomics Portal: An Open Platform for Exploring Multidimensional Cancer Genomics Data. *Cancer Discov.* **2012**, *2*, 401–404. [CrossRef]
32. Gao, J.; Aksoy, B.A.; Dogrusoz, U.; Dresdner, G.; Gross, B.; Sumer, S.O.; Sun, Y.; Jacobsen, A.; Sinha, R.; Larsson, E.; et al. Integrative Analysis of Complex Cancer Genomics and Clinical Profiles Using the CBioPortal. *Sci. Signal.* **2013**, *6*, pl1. [CrossRef]
33. Chen, Y.; Wang, X. MiRDB: An Online Database for Prediction of Functional MicroRNA Targets. *Nucleic Acids Res.* **2020**, *48*, D127–D131. [CrossRef] [PubMed]
34. Liu, W.; Wang, X. Prediction of Functional MicroRNA Targets by Integrative Modeling of MicroRNA Binding and Target Expression Data. *Genome Biol.* **2019**, *20*, 18. [CrossRef]
35. Huang, H.-Y.; Lin, Y.-C.-D.; Cui, S.; Huang, Y.; Tang, Y.; Xu, J.; Bao, J.; Li, Y.; Wen, J.; Zuo, H.; et al. MiRTarBase Update 2022: An Informative Resource for Experimentally Validated MiRNA-Target Interactions. *Nucleic Acids Res.* **2022**, *50*, D222–D230. [CrossRef]
36. Csardi, G.; Nepusz, T. The Igraph Software Package for Complex Network Research. *InterJ. Complex Syst.* **2005**, *1695*, 1–9.
37. Yu, G.; He, Q.-Y. ReactomePA: An R/Bioconductor Package for Reactome Pathway Analysis and Visualization. *Mol. Biosyst.* **2016**, *12*, 477–479. [CrossRef]
38. Becht, E.; Giraldo, N.A.; Lacroix, L.; Buttard, B.; Elarouci, N.; Petitprez, F.; Selves, J.; Laurent-Puig, P.; Sautès-Fridman, C.; Fridman, W.H.; et al. Estimating the Population Abundance of Tissue-Infiltrating Immune and Stromal Cell Populations Using Gene Expression. *Genome Biol.* **2016**, *17*, 218. [CrossRef] [PubMed]
39. Jiang, S.; Xie, X.; Jiang, H. Establishment of a 7-MicroRNA Prognostic Signature and Identification of Hub Target Genes in Colorectal Carcinoma. *Transl. Cancer Res.* **2022**, *11*, 367. [CrossRef]
40. Sanz-Pamplona, R.; Berenguer, A.; Cordero, D.; Riccadonna, S.; Solé, X.; Crous-Bou, M.; Guinó, E.; Sanjuan, X.; Biondo, S.; Soriano, A.; et al. Clinical Value of Prognosis Gene Expression Signatures in Colorectal Cancer: A Systematic Review. *PLoS ONE* **2012**, *7*, e48877. [CrossRef]
41. Yang, Z.; Lu, S.; Wang, Y.; Tang, H.; Wang, B.; Sun, X.; Qu, J.; Rao, B. A Novel Defined Necroptosis-Related MiRNAs Signature for Predicting the Prognosis of Colon Cancer. *Int. J. Gen. Med.* **2022**, *15*, 555–565. [CrossRef]
42. Jacob, H.; Stanisavljevic, L.; Storli, K.E.; Hestetun, K.E.; Dahl, O.; Myklebust, M.P. A Four-MicroRNA Classifier as a Novel Prognostic Marker for Tumor Recurrence in Stage II Colon Cancer. *Sci. Rep.* **2018**, *8*, 6157. [CrossRef] [PubMed]
43. Huang, X.; Xu, X.; Ke, H.; Pan, X.; Ai, J.; Xie, R.; Lan, G.; Hu, Y.; Wu, Y. MicroRNA-16-5p Suppresses Cell Proliferation and Angiogenesis in Colorectal Cancer by Negatively Regulating Forkhead Box K1 to Block the PI3K/Akt/MTOR Pathway. *Eur. J. Histochem. EJH* **2022**, *66*, 3333. [CrossRef] [PubMed]
44. Zhu, T.; Lin, Z.; Han, S.; Wei, Y.; Lu, G.; Zhang, Y.; Xiao, W.; Wang, Z.; Jia, X.; Gong, W. Low MiR-16 Expression Induces Regulatory CD4+NKG2D+ T Cells Involved in Colorectal Cancer Progression. *Am. J. Cancer Res.* **2021**, *11*, 1540–1556. [PubMed]
45. Liu, D.; Bi, X.; Yang, Y. Circular RNA Hsa_circ_0011324 Is Involved in Endometrial Cancer Progression and the Evolution of Its Mechanism. *Bioengineered* **2022**, *13*, 7485–7499. [CrossRef] [PubMed]
46. Zhang, B.; Gao, S.; Bao, Z.; Pan, C.; Tian, Q.; Tang, Q. MicroRNA-656-3p Inhibits Colorectal Cancer Cell Migration, Invasion, and Chemo-Resistance by Targeting Sphingosine-1-Phosphate Phosphatase 1. *Bioengineered* **2022**, *13*, 3810–3826. [CrossRef] [PubMed]
47. Yao, S.; Yin, Y.; Jin, G.; Li, D.; Li, M.; Hu, Y.; Feng, Y.; Liu, Y.; Bian, Z.; Wang, X.; et al. Exosome-Mediated Delivery of MiR-204-5p Inhibits Tumor Growth and Chemoresistance. *Cancer Med.* **2020**, *9*, 5989–5998. [CrossRef] [PubMed]
48. Bian, Z.; Jin, L.; Zhang, J.; Yin, Y.; Quan, C.; Hu, Y.; Feng, Y.; Liu, H.; Fei, B.; Mao, Y.; et al. LncRNA—UCA1 Enhances Cell Proliferation and 5-Fluorouracil Resistance in Colorectal Cancer by Inhibiting MiR-204-5p. *Sci. Rep.* **2016**, *6*, 23892. [CrossRef]
49. Huang, Y.; Xiao, W.; Jiang, X.; Li, H. MicroRNA-935 Acts as a Prognostic Marker and Promotes Cell Proliferation, Migration, and Invasion in Colorectal Cancer. *Cancer Biomark.* **2019**, *26*, 229–237. [CrossRef]
50. Zhang, D.; Ma, S.; Zhang, C.; Li, P.; Mao, B.; Guan, X.; Zhou, W.; Peng, J.; Wang, X.; Li, S.; et al. MicroRNA-935 Directly Targets FZD6 to Inhibit the Proliferation of Human Glioblastoma and Correlate to Glioma Malignancy and Prognosis. *Front. Oncol.* **2021**, *11*, 566492. [CrossRef]
51. Yang, M.; Cui, G.; Ding, M.; Yang, W.; Liu, Y.; Dai, D.; Chen, L. MiR-935 Promotes Gastric Cancer Cell Proliferation by Targeting SOX7. *Biomed. Pharmacother. Biomed. Pharmacother.* **2016**, *79*, 153–158. [CrossRef] [PubMed]
52. de Oliveira, A.R.C.P.; Castanhole-Nunes, M.M.U.; Biselli-Chicote, P.M.; Pavarino, É.C.; da Silva, R.C.M.A.; da Silva, R.F.; Goloni-Bertollo, E.M. Differential Expression of Angiogenesis-Related MiRNAs and VEGFA in Cirrhosis and Hepatocellular Carcinoma. *Arch. Med. Sci. AMS* **2020**, *16*, 1150–1157. [CrossRef]
53. Yerukala Sathipati, S.; Tsai, M.-J.; Shukla, S.K.; Ho, S.-Y.; Liu, Y.; Beheshti, A. MicroRNA Signature for Estimating the Survival Time in Patients with Bladder Urothelial Carcinoma. *Sci. Rep.* **2022**, *12*, 4141. [CrossRef] [PubMed]

54. Plata-Bello, J.; Fariña-Jerónimo, H.; Betancor, I.; Salido, E. High Expression of FOXP2 Is Associated with Worse Prognosis in Glioblastoma. *World Neurosurg.* **2021**, *150*, e253–e278. [CrossRef]
55. Luedemann, C.; Reinersmann, J.-L.; Klinger, C.; Degener, S.; Dreger, N.M.; Roth, S.; Kaufmann, M.; Savelsbergh, A. Prostate Cancer-Associated MiRNAs in Saliva: First Steps to an Easily Accessible and Reliable Screening Tool. *Biomolecules* **2022**, *12*, 1366. [CrossRef] [PubMed]
56. Wang, S.; Xiang, J.; Li, Z.; Lu, S.; Hu, J.; Gao, X.; Yu, L.; Wang, L.; Wang, J.; Wu, Y.; et al. A Plasma MicroRNA Panel for Early Detection of Colorectal Cancer. *Int. J. Cancer* **2015**, *136*, 152–161. [CrossRef]
57. Chen, Z.; Shen, Z.; Zhang, Z.; Zhao, D.; Xu, L.; Zhang, L. RNA-Associated Co-Expression Network Identifies Novel Biomarkers for Digestive System Cancer. *Front. Genet.* **2021**, *12*, 659788. [CrossRef] [PubMed]
58. Ruan, X.-J.; Ye, B.-L.; Zheng, Z.-H.; Li, S.-T.; Zheng, X.-F.; Zhang, S.-Z. TGFβ1I1 Suppressed Cell Migration and Invasion in Colorectal Cancer by Inhibiting the TGF-β Pathway and EMT Progress. *Eur. Rev. Med. Pharmacol. Sci.* **2020**, *24*, 7294–7302. [CrossRef]
59. Amirkhah, R.; Schmitz, U.; Linnebacher, M.; Wolkenhauer, O.; Farazmand, A. MicroRNA-MRNA Interactions in Colorectal Cancer and Their Role in Tumor Progression. *Genes Chromosomes Cancer* **2015**, *54*, 129–141. [CrossRef] [PubMed]
60. Wu, X.; Li, J.; Zhang, Y.; Cheng, Y.; Wu, Z.; Zhan, W.; Deng, Y. Identification of Immune Cell Infiltration Landscape for Predicting Prognosis of Colorectal Cancer. *Gastroenterol. Rep.* **2023**, *11*, goad014. [CrossRef] [PubMed]
61. Xiong, Y.; Wang, K.; Zhou, H.; Peng, L.; You, W.; Fu, Z. Profiles of Immune Infiltration in Colorectal Cancer and Their Clinical Significant: A Gene Expression-Based Study. *Cancer Med.* **2018**, *7*, 4496–4508. [CrossRef]
62. Fridman, W.H.; Pagès, F.; Sautès-Fridman, C.; Galon, J. The Immune Contexture in Human Tumours: Impact on Clinical Outcome. *Nat. Rev. Cancer* **2012**, *12*, 298–306. [CrossRef]
63. Teng, M.W.L.; Ngiow, S.F.; Ribas, A.; Smyth, M.J. Classifying Cancers Based on T-Cell Infiltration and PD-L1. *Cancer Res.* **2015**, *75*, 2139–2145. [CrossRef]
64. Potocki, P.M.; Wójcik, P.; Chmura, Ł.; Goc, B.; Fedewicz, M.; Bielańska, Z.; Swadźba, J.; Konopka, K.; Kwinta, Ł.; Wysocki, P.J. Clinical Characterization of Targetable Mutations (BRAF V600E and KRAS G12C) in Advanced Colorectal Cancer-A Nation-Wide Study. *Int. J. Mol. Sci.* **2023**, *24*, 9073. [CrossRef]
65. Ma, Z.; Qi, Z.; Gu, C.; Yang, Z.; Ding, Y.; Zhou, Y.; Wang, W.; Zou, Q. BRAFV600E Mutation Promoted the Growth and Chemoresistance of Colorectal Cancer. *Am. J. Cancer Res.* **2023**, *13*, 1486–1497. [PubMed]
66. Mirzapoor Abbasabadi, Z.; Hamedi Asl, D.; Rahmani, B.; Shahbadori, R.; Karami, S.; Peymani, A.; Taghizadeh, S.; Samiee Rad, F. KRAS, NRAS, BRAF, and PIK3CA Mutation Rates, Clinicopathological Association, and Their Prognostic Value in Iranian Colorectal Cancer Patients. *J. Clin. Lab. Anal.* **2023**, *37*, e24868. [CrossRef] [PubMed]
67. Mo, S.; Ye, L.; Wang, D.; Han, L.; Zhou, S.; Wang, H.; Dai, W.; Wang, Y.; Luo, W.; Wang, R.; et al. Early Detection of Molecular Residual Disease and Risk Stratification for Stage I to III Colorectal Cancer via Circulating Tumor DNA Methylation. *JAMA Oncol.* **2023**, *9*, 770–778. [CrossRef] [PubMed]
68. Debelius, J.W.; Engstrand, L.; Matussek, A.; Brusselaers, N.; Morton, J.T.; Stenmarker, M.; Olsen, R.S. The Local Tumor Microbiome Is Associated with Survival in Late-Stage Colorectal Cancer Patients. *Microbiol. Spectr.* **2023**, *11*, e0506622. [CrossRef] [PubMed]
69. Xu, Y.; Zhao, J.; Ma, Y.; Liu, J.; Cui, Y.; Yuan, Y.; Xiang, C.; Ma, D.; Liu, H. The Microbiome Types of Colorectal Tissue Are Potentially Associated with the Prognosis of Patients with Colorectal Cancer. *Front. Microbiol.* **2023**, *14*, 1100873. [CrossRef]
70. Kamal, Y.; Dwan, D.; Hoehn, H.J.; Sanz-Pamplona, R.; Alonso, M.H.; Moreno, V.; Cheng, C.; Schell, M.J.; Kim, Y.; Felder, S.I.; et al. Tumor Immune Infiltration Estimated from Gene Expression Profiles Predicts Colorectal Cancer Relapse. *Oncoimmunology* **2021**, *10*, 1862529. [CrossRef]

Disclaimer/Publisher's Note: The statements, opinions and data contained in all publications are solely those of the individual author(s) and contributor(s) and not of MDPI and/or the editor(s). MDPI and/or the editor(s) disclaim responsibility for any injury to people or property resulting from any ideas, methods, instructions or products referred to in the content.

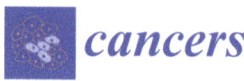

Article

High OCT4 Expression Might Be Associated with an Aggressive Phenotype in Rectal Cancer

Lina Lambis-Anaya [1,†], Mashiel Fernández-Ruiz [1,†], Yamil Liscano [2] and Amileth Suarez-Causado [1,*]

1. Grupo Prometeus & Biomedicina Aplicada a las Ciencias Clínicas, Facultad de Medicina, Universidad de Cartagena, Cartagena 130014, Colombia; llambisa1@unicartagena.edu.co (L.L.-A.); mfernandezr1@unicartagena.edu.co (M.F.-R.)
2. Grupo de Investigación en Salud Integral (GISI), Departamento Facultad de Salud, Universidad Santiago de Cali, Cali 760035, Colombia; yamil.liscano00@usc.edu.co
*   Correspondence: asuarezc1@unicartagena.edu.co; Tel.: +57-301-3240462
†   These authors contributed equally to this work.

Simple Summary: The oncofetal protein OCT4 is a factor that promotes self-renewal and maintenance of pluripotency of embryonic stem cells and induced stem cells, which has been linked to neoplastic processes, but its role and clinical significance in rectal cancer are unknown. Therefore, the aim of this study was to evaluate the expression of the stem cell marker OCT4 related to clinical-pathological characteristics and its clinical significance in rectal cancer patients. Protein expression of the stem cell marker OCT4 was found in rectal tumor tissue but not in adjacent non-tumor tissue, and high expression was significantly associated with phenotypical characteristics of more aggressive rectal cancer.

Abstract: Rectal cancer (RC) is one of the most common malignant neoplasms, and cancer stem cells (CSCs) of the intestinal tract have been implicated in its origin. The oncofetal protein OCT4 has been linked to neoplastic processes, but its role and clinical significance in RC are unknown. This study investigates the expression of the stem cell marker OCT4 related to clinical-pathological characteristics and its clinical significance in RC patients. The expression level of stem cell marker OCT4 was analyzed in 22 primary rectal tumors by western blot. The association between OCT4 protein expression and the clinical-pathological features of tumors was evaluated by χ^2 test and Fisher's exact test. We demonstrated that the expression of the stem cell marker OCT4 was observed in tumor tissue but not adjacent non-tumor tissue. High expression of the stem cell marker OCT4 was significantly associated with histological differentiation grade ($p = 0.039$), tumor invasion level ($p = 0.004$), lymph node involvement ($p = 0.044$), tumor-node-metastasis (TNM) stage ($p = 0.002$), and clinical stage ($p = 0.021$). These findings suggest that high OCT4 expression is associated with a more aggressive RC phenotype, with a greater likelihood of progression and metastasis. These results shed light on the importance of targeting this CSC marker to attenuate RC progression.

Keywords: rectal cancer; colorectal cancer; cancer stem cells; OCT4; oncofetal protein

Citation: Lambis-Anaya, L.;
Fernández-Ruiz, M.; Liscano, Y.;
Suarez-Causado, A. High OCT4
Expression Might Be Associated with
an Aggressive Phenotype in Rectal
Cancer. *Cancers* **2023**, *15*, 3740.
https://doi.org/10.3390/
cancers15143740

Academic Editors: María Jesús
Fernández-Aceñero, Rodrigo
Barderas-Manchado, Javier Martinez
Useros and Cristina Díaz del Arco

Received: 16 June 2023
Revised: 17 July 2023
Accepted: 18 July 2023
Published: 23 July 2023

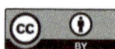

Copyright: © 2023 by the authors.
Licensee MDPI, Basel, Switzerland.
This article is an open access article
distributed under the terms and
conditions of the Creative Commons
Attribution (CC BY) license (https://
creativecommons.org/licenses/by/
4.0/).

1. Introduction

Colorectal cancer (CRC) is the second leading cause of cancer-related deaths and the third most common cancer worldwide. Rectal cancer (RC) represents 63% of all CRC cases and approximately 58% of deaths caused by this disease globally [1]. Although often considered the same pathological entity, colon and rectal cancers have anatomical and biological differences that affect the prognosis [2,3]. Despite advances in surgical treatment, radiation therapy, chemotherapy, and adjuvant therapies, the prognosis for RC patients is unsatisfactory due to the high rate of local recurrence, treatment resistance, and distant metastasis, which are strongly related to mortality [4].

Cancer stem cells (CSCs) represent a subpopulation of tumor cells characterized by their ability to self-renew, heterogeneity, plasticity, and infinite proliferation. These characteristics, together with scientific evidence, have closely linked this cell population to tumor development, therapy resistance, metastasis, and recurrence after primary treatment [5,6].

Among the transcription factors described as regulators of pluripotency and maintenance of CSCs is the octamer-binding protein 4 (OCT4; also known as POU domain, class 5, transcription factor 1 (POU5F1)), an oncofetal protein that promotes self-renewal and maintenance of pluripotency of embryonic stem cells and induced stem cells, and which has been found to be involved in the progression and poor prognosis of various cancers [7], including gastric [8–10], pancreatic [11], breast [12], bladder [13], ovarian [14], prostate [15], and hepatocellular carcinoma [16]. However, few studies have included OCT4 evaluation in RC [17,18], and even fewer have evaluated its clinical significance in these patients [19]. The few existing reports on OCT4 expression have been developed in in vitro models of CRC [20] or in intestinal tumor tissues that have evaluated colon and rectal cancer as the same pathological entity [21,22]. Therefore, the purpose of this study was to investigate the expression of the stem cell marker OCT4 related to clinical-pathological features and its clinical significance in RC patients.

2. Materials and Methods

2.1. Participants and Sample Collection

A cross-sectional study was conducted that included samples of tumor tissue and adjacent non-tumor tissue obtained from 63 patients diagnosed with primary RC who were treated at two tertiary referral centers in the city of Cartagena, Colombia. A total of 22 samples that met the appropriate size criteria were used for molecular analysis. None of the patients had received neoadjuvant therapy or had a history of other tumors or serious infections. The collected fresh tissues were embedded in RNAlater™ and stored at −80 °C for subsequent analysis. This study was approved by the Ethics Committee of the Universidad de Cartagena (Minutes No. 108, 10 May 2018) and was conducted in accordance with the principles of the Helsinki Declaration. Each eligible participant signed an informed consent form.

2.2. Data Collection

Sociodemographic, pathological, and clinical characteristics were collected from medical records and a structured survey. Data such as age, sex, symptoms and clinical history, tumor differentiation grade, lymph node involvement, presence of metastasis, and TNM stage were collected. TNM stage was evaluated according to the seventh edition of the cancer staging manual of the American Joint Committee on Cancer (AJCC) [23].

2.3. Western Blot Analysis

The OCT4 protein was isolated using the western blot technique. The tissues were thawed and resuspended in lysis buffer [20 mM Tris-HCl (pH 7.4), 150 mM NaCl, 10% glycerol, 0.2% Nonidet P-40, 1 mM EDTA, 1 mM EGTA, 1 mM phenylmethylsulfonyl fluoride (Sigma-Aldrich, St. Louis, MO, USA), 10 mM NaF, 5 mg/mL aprotinin (Sigma-Aldrich), 20 mM leupeptin (Sigma-Aldrich, St. Louis, MO, USA), and 1 mM sodium orthovanadate (Sigma-Aldrich, St. Louis, MO, USA)]. The concentration of total protein in the supernatant was quantified using a spectrophotometric method [24]. The absorbance at 595 nm was calculated using a standard curve previously prepared with bovine serum albumin (BSA). The samples were prepared with Laemmli loading buffer and denatured by heating at 95 °C for 5 min. A total of 30 μg of protein was loaded onto a 10% polyacrylamide gel prepared with sodium dodecyl sulfate (SDS-PAGE) and subjected to electrophoresis in the presence of an electrophoresis buffer at a constant voltage [25]. After electrophoresis, the proteins were transferred from the gel to a PVDF membrane (iBlot™ Transfer Stack, PVDF Invitrogen™ Thermo Waltham, MA, USA) using the iBlot™ 2 Gel Transfer Device dry transfer technology (Thermo Scientific™, Waltham, MA, USA). Ponceau staining was performed to confirm that the transfer was successful. Subsequently, the membrane was treated with a blocking solution of 5% skim milk in TTBS 1X [10 mM Tris/HCl, 150 mM NaCl, 0.05% Tween-20 (pH 7.5)] and then incubated overnight with the primary antibody anti-OCT4 diluted 1:2000 (Abcam, Cambridge, UK) [EPR2054] (ab109183). After the incubation period, the membrane was washed with TTBS 1X to remove excess antibody. The membrane was then incubated with a horseradish peroxidase-conjugated secondary antibody for 2 h. Finally, the membrane was washed with TTBS 1X and immunodetection was performed using the SuperSignal™ West Pico chemiluminescent substrate (Thermo Scientific™, Waltham, MA, USA). The results were validated using anti-beta glucuronidase (GUSB) antibody 1:2000 (Abcam Cambridge, UK) [EPR10616] (ab166904) as a housekeeping antibody. The PVDF membranes were analyzed using an imaging documentation system, using the iBright CL1000 equipment (Thermo Scientific™ Waltham, MA, USA). The iBright analysis software desktop version (Thermo Scientific™ Waltham, MA, USA) was used to measure the band densitometry to determine OCT4 expression.

2.4. Statistical Analysis

Statistical data were analyzed using SPSS for Windows, version 21.0 (IBM Corp., Armonk, NY, USA), and GraphPad Prism 8.0.2 (Graphpad Software Inc., San Diego, CA, USA). The normality of the data distribution was evaluated using the Kolmogorov-Smirnov test. Descriptive data are presented as mean ± standard deviation (SD) or frequency and percentage. Student's *t*-test was used to determine statistical significance when comparing two groups. To evaluate the association between OCT4 expression and clinical and pathological characteristics, Pearson's chi-square test or Fisher's exact test was used. A $p < 0.05$ was considered statistically significant.

3. Results

3.1. Characteristics of the Studied Population

The average age of the participants was 61.7 years (range between 22 and 90 years), 60.3% ($n = 38$) were women, and 39.7% ($n = 25$) were men, mainly residing in urban areas (74.6%, $n = 47$). The most frequent clinical characteristics were rectal bleeding (52.4%; $n = 33$) and exophytic lesions detected by colonoscopy (57.1%; $n = 36$). The most frequent histological type, histological grade, clinical stage, and TNM were adenocarcinoma (87.5%; $n = 55$), moderately differentiated grade (44.4%; $n = 28$), advanced/regional stage (65.1%; $n = 41$), and classification IIIB (22.2%; $n = 14$) and IVA (17.5%; $n = 11$), respectively (Table 1).

Table 1. Sociodemographic, clinical, and pathological characteristics of the studied population.

Characteristics	N = 63	
	n	%
Age		
≤50 years	17	27
>50 years	46	73
Sex		
Female	38	60.3
Male	25	39.7
Residential area		
Urban	47	74.6
Rural	16	25.4
Main sign/symptom		
Rectal bleeding	33	52.4
Change in bowel habits	10	15.9
Weight loss	1	1.6
Anemia	2	3.2
Acute abdominal pain	10	15.9
Intestinal obstruction	6	9.5
Other	1	1.6

Table 1. *Cont.*

Characteristics	N = 63	
	n	%
Finding during colonoscopy		
Ulcerative lesion	3	4.8
Multiple polyps	3	4.8
Single polyp	4	6.3
Exophytic lesion	36	57.1
Stenosing lesion	17	27
Histological type		
Adenocarcinoma	55	87.3
Mucinous adenocarcinoma	3	4.8
Neuroendocrine carcinoma	5	7.9
Histological grade		
Well-differentiated	24	38.1
Moderately differentiated	28	44.4
Poorly differentiated	11	17.5
Clinical stage		
Early/local	22	34.9
Advanced/regional	41	65.1
TNM		
0	1	1.6
I	8	12.7
IIA	7	11.1
IIB	3	4.8
IIC	4	6.3
IIIA	7	11.1
IIIB	14	22.2
IIIC	5	7.9
IVA	11	17.5
IVB	3	4.8
Local invasion		
TIs	4	6.3
T1	6	9.5
T2	21	33.3
T3	11	17.5
T4a	20	31.7
T4b	1	1.6
Lymph node involvement		
N1a	30	47.6
N1b	15	23.8
N1c	4	6.3
N2a	11	17.5
N2b	1	1.6
Unknown	2	3.2
Metastasis		
M0	49	77.8
M1a	11	17.5
M1b	3	4.8
Vascular invasion		
Si	15	23.8
No	29	46
Unknown	19	30.2

3.2. Molecular Determination of OCT4 in Tumor Tissue and Adjacent Non-Tumor Tissue

The expression of OCT4 protein was higher in tumors with some degree of undifferentiation (Figure 1a,b) and in advanced clinical stages (Figure 1c,d). No protein expression of OCT4 was observed in adjacent non-tumor tissue.

Bivariate analysis showed higher levels of OCT4 expression in tumors with some degree of undifferentiation (moderately and poorly differentiated) compared to well-differentiated tumors ($p = 0.046$) (Figure 2a). In advanced clinical stages, there was also higher OCT4 expression compared to early stages ($p = 0.0356$) (Figure 2b).

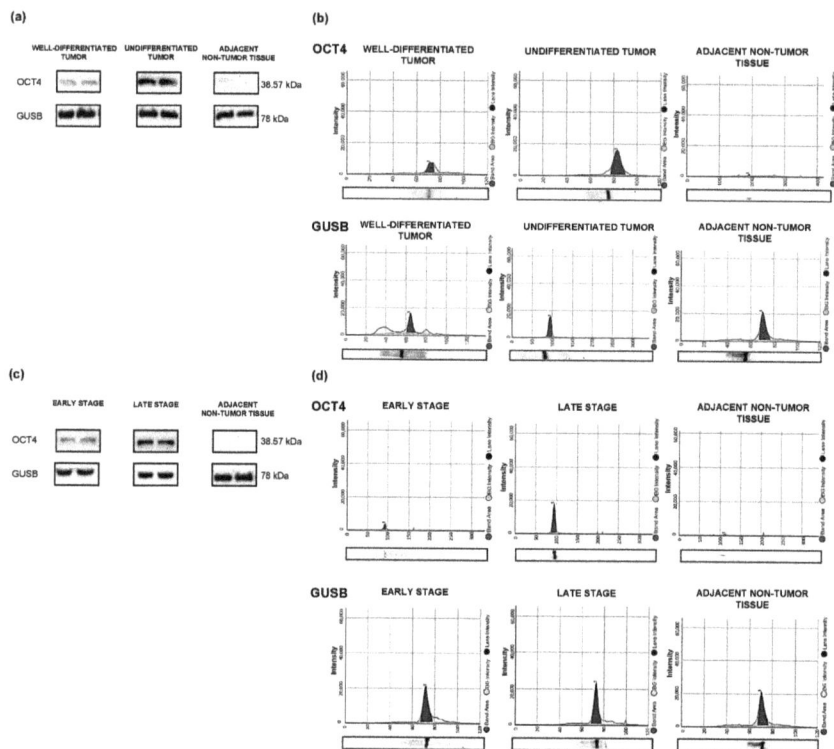

Figure 1. Expression of OCT4 protein in RC tissue and adjacent non-tumor tissue according to the histological differentiation grade and tumor stage. (**a**) Western blot analysis of OCT4 protein expression according to the histological differentiation grade. (**b**) Immunoelectrophoretic analysis of OCT4 protein expression according to the histological differentiation grade. (**c**) Western blot analysis of OCT4 protein expression according to the tumor stage. (**d**) Immunoelectrophoretic analysis of OCT4 protein expression according to the tumor stage. The expression of GUSB was used as a normalizer. See Supplementary Material for the original image of the Western Blots.

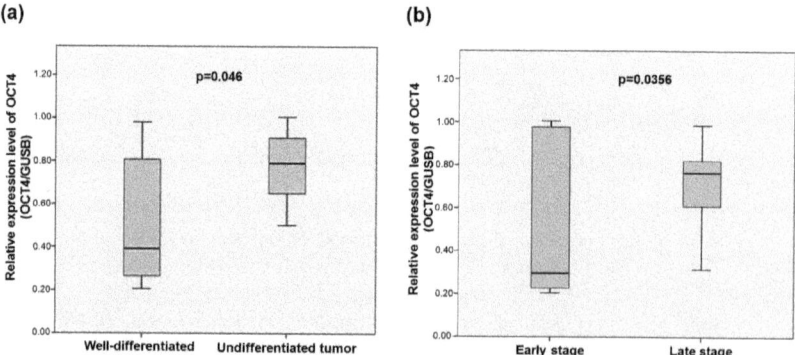

Figure 2. Protein expression levels of OCT4 in rectal tumors. (**a**) OCT4 expression levels in rectal tumors according to histological differentiation grade. (**b**) OCT4 expression levels in rectal tumors according to clinical-pathological stage. Results are the ratio of OCT4 expression normalized to GUSB protein levels. Statistical differences between groups were evaluated by two-tailed Student's t-test.

3.3. Association between OCT4 Expression and Clinical and Pathological Characteristics

The results showed a significant association between the expression (high/low) of OCT4 and the degree of histological differentiation ($p = 0.039$), invasion level ($p = 0.004$), and lymph node involvement ($p = 0.044$). No association was found between OCT4 expression and tumor metastasis. Significant differences were found in relation to TNM stage ($p = 0.002$) and early clinical stage compared to advanced stage ($p = 0.021$) (Table 2).

Table 2. Association between OCT4 expression and clinical and pathological variables of the studied samples ($n = 22$).

	Total Samples	OCT4 Expression		*p*-Value
		High	Low	
		n (%)	n (%)	
Histological grade				
Well-differentiated	8 (36.4)	4 (18.2)	4 (18.2)	0.039 *
Undifferentiated	14 (63.6)	13 (59.1)	1 (4.5)	
Local invasion				
TIs	2 (9.1)	0	2 (9.1)	
T1	3 (13.6)	1 (4.5)	2 (9.1)	
T2	9 (40.9)	9 (40.9)	0	0.004 **
T3	4 (18.2)	3 (13.6)	1 (4.5)	
T4a	3 (13.6)	3 (13.6)	0	
T4b	1 (4.5)	1 (4.5)	0	
Lymph node involvement				
N1a	12 (54.5)	7 (31.8)	5 (22.7)	
N1b	2 (9.1)	2 (9.1)	0	
N1c	3 (13.6)	3 (13.6)	0	0.044 *
N2a	4 (18.2)	4 (18.2)	0	
N2b	1 (4.5)	1 (4.5)	0	
Metastasis				
M0	20 (90.9)	15 (68.2)	5 (22.7)	
M1a	1 (4.5)	1 (4.5)	0	0.458
M1b	1 (4.5)	1 (4.5)	0	
TNM				
I	5 (22.7)	1 (4.5)	4 (18.2)	
II	2 (9.1)	2 (9.1)	0	0.002 **
III	13 (59.1)	12 (54.5)	1 (4.5)	
IVA	2 (9.1)	2 (9.1)	0	
Clinical stage				
Early/local	7 (31.8)	3 (13.6)	4 (18.2)	0.021 *
Late/regional	15 (68.2)	14 (63.6)	1 (4.5)	

* $p < 0.05$; ** $p < 0.01$.

4. Discussion

Association between stem cell molecules and their derived signals with the evolution of the tumorigenic process is widely accepted [26,27]. It has been proposed that intestinal stem cells represent an important part of the origin of CRC [28,29]. Embryonic stem cells express diverse proteins, including the octamer-binding protein 4 (OCT4), an oncofetal protein that plays a significant role in self-renewal and pluripotency [30]. Recent evidence shows increasing numbers of early-onset RC [31], as well as a high frequency of RC among individuals diagnosed with CRC in the Colombian Caribbean region, as we have previously reported [32]. Therefore, it is pertinent to have more knowledge of the development of this disease to provide new therapeutic targets that allow better management of patients. This study is the first in Colombia to evaluate the relationship between OCT4 expression and clinical-pathological characteristics in primary rectal tumors.

The samples collected for this study were from individuals with an average age of 61.75 years, similar to the mean age reported in epidemiological studies that have evaluated colon and rectal cancer together [33]. Recent studies show increasing incidence rates in adults under 50 years old (early-onset tumors) [34], and in RC, the behavior is similar, including the population of Latin America and the Caribbean [31,35,36]. Our study reports 27% of individuals with RC under 50 years old, which could be supported by the adoption of dietary patterns characterized by high consumption of processed and refined foods and a sedentary lifestyle, among other unhealthy habits that are considered risk factors for the appearance of RC. We found that the incidence was higher in females, consistent with the research of Vargas Moranth et al. in a population of the Colombian Caribbean [37]. Similarly, most individuals were of black race, a characteristic that, beyond being related to a genetic component, is likely to be a consequence of the predominance of this race in the region where the study was carried out, where there was historically African settlement during the colonial period. All these conditions associated with lifestyle and environmental or hormonal factors can impact the clinical characteristics of the population and influence the behavior of the disease. However, it must be borne in mind that all these data related to the epidemiological characteristics of the population should be interpreted with caution, considering that the sample size limits the statistical efficiency of the results.

Our results showed an absence of modulation of the expression of the stem cell marker OCT4 in adjacent non-tumor tissue, but did show OCT4 expression in tumor tissue consistent with other authors, who have reported OCT4 protein expression in various human cancer tissues such as stomach [9], pancreas [11], bladder [13], ovary [14], prostate [15], and CRC, but not in normal somatic tissues [38]. It is believed, then, that OCT4 reactivation occurs in cells that have undergone malignancy [30], in which the expression of pluripotency genes by stem cells has been related to tumor proliferation, metastasis, and poor prognosis [10]. In this sense, our findings suggest that the OCT4 protein may have a relevant role in the development and progression of the tumor.

Likewise, our work shows increased expression of the intestinal oncofetal protein OCT4 in tumors with some degree of undifferentiation (moderately and poorly differentiated), which could lead to progression and even metastasis in RC, considering that it has been reported that the level of stem cell protein expression may be related to the content of these cells in the tumor and suggests its aggressiveness according to the degree of histological differentiation [39]. Similar observations to our data have been described in RC [19], in a case report of CRC [40], as well as in cervical tumors [41] and gastric cancer [8], which could indicate the role of this cell subpopulation in the loss of colonic identity and poorer prognosis [42].

For its part, the data from this study revealed a close association between the expression of the oncofetal protein OCT4 and the stage of the tumors. In this regard, Shaheen et al. stated that higher expression of OCT4 is associated with more advanced stages of CRC and distant metastasis [38]. In line with this, Roudi et al. evaluated, through immunohistochemical staining, the expression of CSCs markers OCT4 and NANOG, reporting a trend between low OCT4 expression and absence of metastasis or lymph node involvement, which could indicate that increased OCT4 expression would contribute to the malignant behavior of CRC and be related to advanced disease [21]. Similarly, several studies have confirmed the association between OCT4 and TNM staging in other types of cancer, such as gastric cancer [9] and lung cancer [43]. Likewise, in gastric cancer, high levels of CSC biomarkers have been strongly associated with TNM staging, lymph node metastasis, and poor survival [44]. In contrast, Fujino et al. did not find a significant correlation between OCT4 expression and TNM staging; however, it is important to note that this study evaluated the expression of OCT4 mRNA, which was significantly correlated with poor metastasis-free survival [22].

There is evidence that points to the expression of OCT4 in the regulation of various signaling pathways associated with tumor formation and malignant transformation and increased recurrence, such as p38 mitogen-activated protein kinase (MAPK)/caspase-3, Wnt/β-catenin, AKT, and Janus Kinase (JAK)/signal transducer and activator of transcription (STAT)3 signal pathways [45–47]. Therefore, our results regarding the presence of OCT4 in RC at its various stages increase the possibility that CSCs are involved in resistance to conventional radiotherapy and chemotherapy treatments, increasing recurrences. It has previously been reported in patients with RC who underwent preoperative chemoradiotherapy that the CD133, OCT4, and SOX2 markers could be useful for predicting distant recurrence and poor prognosis, in addition to their possible association with tumor regrowth and metastases after chemoradiotherapy. [48]. Consequently, the data generated by our study could point towards the oncogenic role of OCT4 in RC, supported by the fact that the aberrant expression of this transcription factor and abnormal biological behavior of signaling pathways in stem cells during the development of RC may contribute to the promotion of tumorigenesis, its progression and aggressiveness, and the promotion of recurrences.

The major limitation of this study was the small sample size; however, we consider the obtained results valuable, taking into account the scarcity of recent data referring to clinicopathological and molecular aspects of RC in our population. We believe that a larger study population would allow us to validate our results; furthermore, it would be relevant to verify the data obtained through other molecular techniques, as well as to analyze the behavior of this marker over time, in order to analyze its clinical potential in the diagnosis, prognosis, and treatment follow-up in patients with RC.

5. Conclusions

We demonstrated expression of the stem cell marker OCT4 in tumor tissue of RC and the absence of modulation of this protein in adjacent non-tumor tissue; furthermore, we found that high expression of OCT4 was associated with undifferentiated histological grade, a greater degree of tumor invasion, lymph node involvement, and advanced or regional clinical stage, and higher TNM grades. Therefore, our results suggest that high expression of OCT4 is associated with a more aggressive phenotype of RC, with a greater likelihood of progression and metastasis. These findings shed light on the importance of focusing on this CSC marker and directing further studies aimed at investigating the mechanisms involved in its probable role in the initiation and progression of RC.

Supplementary Materials: The following supporting information can be downloaded at: https://www.mdpi.com/article/10.3390/cancers15143740/s1. File S1: The original image of the Western Blots.

Author Contributions: Conceptualization, A.S.-C.; methodology, A.S.-C.; validation, A.S.-C., L.L.-A., M.F.-R. and Y.L.; formal analysis, A.S.-C., L.L.-A., M.F.-R. and Y.L.; investigation, A.S.-C., L.L.-A., M.F.-R., and Y.L.; resources, A.S.-C. and Y.L.; data curation, A.S.-C., L.L.-A., M.F.-R., and Y.L.; writing—original draft preparation, A.S.-C., L.L.-A., and M.F.-R.; writing—review and editing, A.S.-C., L.L.-A., M.F.-R., and Y.L.; visualization, A.S.-C., L.L.-A., and M.F.-R.; supervision, A.S.-C. and Y.L.; project administration, A.S.-C. and Y.L.; funding acquisition, A.S.-C. and Y.L. All authors have read and agreed to the published version of the manuscript.

Funding: This research was funded by COLCIENCIAS (nowadays MINCIENCIAS—Ministerio de Ciencia, Tecnología e Innovación), Centro De Diagnóstico Citopatológico del Caribe CENDIPAT and Universidad de Cartagena, through the 807 national grant for science, technology and innovation in health projects 2018 (project code 110780763299 contract 804-2018). This publication was funded by MINCIENCIAS and Dirección General de Investigaciones de la Universidad Santiago de Cali (Convocatoria Interna No. 02-2023).

Institutional Review Board Statement: The study was conducted in accordance with the Declaration of Helsinki and approved by the Institutional Ethics Committee of the Universidad de Cartagena (Minutes No. 108, 10 May 2018).

Informed Consent Statement: Informed consent was obtained from all subjects involved in the study.

Data Availability Statement: All data are contained within the manuscript. Raw data are available upon reasonable request from the corresponding author.

Acknowledgments: The authors are grateful to the Universidad de Cartagena and MINCIENCIAS for funding this study through the 807 national grant for science, technology and innovation in health projects and the Young Researchers program, Dirección General de Investigaciones de la Universidad Santiago de Cali for supporting publication of this manuscript, the students of the Prometeus & Biomedicina aplicada a las ciencias clínicas research group, the medical team of the gastroenterology unit of the Hospital Universitario del Caribe de Cartagena, Gastrolap IPS, and Centro de Diagnóstico Citopatológico del Caribe CENDIPAT, for their valuable help during the development of the study.

Conflicts of Interest: The authors declare no conflict of interest. The funders had no role in the design of the study; in the collection, analyses, or interpretation of data; in the writing of the manuscript; or in the decision to publish the results.

References

1. Ferlay, J.; Ervik, M.; Lam, F.; Colombet, M.; Mery, L.; Piñeros, M.; Znaor, A.; Soerjomataram, I.; Bray, F. Global Cancer Observatory (GLOBOCAN): Cancer Today. Available online: https://gco.iarc.fr/today/data/factsheets/populations/900-world-fact-sheets.pdf (accessed on 19 April 2022).
2. Schlechter, B.L. Management of Rectal Cancer. *Hematol Oncol. Clin. N. Am.* **2022**, *36*, 521–537. [CrossRef] [PubMed]
3. Paschke, S.; Jafarov, S.; Staib, L.; Kreuser, E.D.; Maulbecker-Armstrong, C.; Roitman, M.; Holm, T.; Harris, C.C.; Link, K.H.; Kornmann, M. Are Colon and Rectal Cancer Two Different Tumor Entities? A Proposal to Abandon the Term Colorectal Cancer. *Int. J. Mol. Sci.* **2018**, *19*, 2577. [CrossRef] [PubMed]
4. Zhao, X.; Han, P.; Zhang, L.; Ma, J.; Dong, F.; Zang, L.; He, Z.; Zheng, M. Prolonged neoadjuvant chemotherapy without radiation versus total neoadjuvant therapy for locally advanced rectal cancer: A propensity score matched study. *Front. Oncol.* **2022**, *12*, 953790. [CrossRef] [PubMed]
5. Chen, B.; Sun, H.; Xu, S.; Mo, Q. Long Non-coding RNA TPT1-AS1 Suppresses APC Transcription in a STAT1-Dependent Manner to Increase the Stemness of Colorectal Cancer Stem Cells. *Mol. Biotechnol.* **2022**, *64*, 560–574. [CrossRef] [PubMed]
6. Zhong, L.; Tan, W.; Yang, Q.; Zou, Z.; Zhou, R.; Huang, Y.; Qiu, Z.; Zheng, K.; Huang, Z. PRRX1 promotes colorectal cancer stemness and chemoresistance via the JAK2/STAT3 axis by targeting IL-6. *J. Gastrointest. Oncol.* **2022**, *13*, 2989–3008. [CrossRef]
7. Yan, Q.; Fang, X.; Li, C.; Lan, P.; Guan, X. Oncofetal proteins and cancer stem cells. *Essays Biochem.* **2022**, *66*, 423–433. [CrossRef]
8. Pandian, J.; Panneerpandian, P.; Sekar, B.T.; Selvarasu, K.; Ganesan, K. OCT4-mediated transcription confers oncogenic advantage for a subset of gastric tumors with poor clinical outcome. *Funct. Integr. Genom.* **2022**, *22*, 1345–1360. [CrossRef]
9. Ibrahim, D.A.; Elsebai, E.A.; Fayed, A.; Abdelrahman, A.E. Prognostic value of NOTCH1 and OCT4 in gastric carcinoma. *Indian J. Pathol. Microbiol.* **2022**, *65*, 328–335. [CrossRef]
10. Basati, G.; Mohammadpour, H.; Emami-Razavi, A. Association of High Expression Levels of SOX2, NANOG, and OCT4 in Gastric Cancer Tumor Tissues with Progression and Poor Prognosis. *J. Gastrointest. Cancer* **2020**, *51*, 41–47. [CrossRef]
11. Khoshchehreh, R.; Totonchi, M.; Ramirez, J.C.; Torres, R.; Baharvand, H.; Aicher, A.; Ebrahimi, M.; Heeschen, C. Epigenetic reprogramming of primary pancreatic cancer cells counteracts their in vivo tumourigenicity. *Oncogene* **2019**, *38*, 6226–6239. [CrossRef] [PubMed]
12. Jin, X.; Li, Y.; Guo, Y.; Jia, Y.; Qu, H.; Lu, Y.; Song, P.; Zhang, X.; Shao, Y.; Qi, D.; et al. ERα is required for suppressing OCT4-induced proliferation of breast cancer cells via DNMT1/ISL1/ERK axis. *Cell Prolif.* **2019**, *52*, e12612. [CrossRef] [PubMed]
13. Siddiqui, Z.; Srivastava, A.N.; Sankhwar, S.N.; Zaidi, N.; Fatima, N.; Singh, S.; Yusuf, M. Oct-4: A prognostic biomarker of urinary bladder cancer in North India. *Ther. Adv. Urol.* **2019**, *11*, 1756287219875576. [CrossRef] [PubMed]
14. Robinson, M.; Gilbert, S.F.; Waters, J.A.; Lujano-Olazaba, O.; Lara, J.; Alexander, L.J.; Green, S.E.; Burkeen, G.A.; Patrus, O.; Sarwar, Z.; et al. Characterization of SOX2, OCT4 and NANOG in Ovarian Cancer Tumor-Initiating Cells. *Cancers* **2021**, *13*, 262. [CrossRef]
15. Vaddi, P.K.; Stamnes, M.A.; Cao, H.; Chen, S. Elimination of SOX2/OCT4-Associated Prostate Cancer Stem Cells Blocks Tumor Development and Enhances Therapeutic Response. *Cancers* **2019**, *11*, 1331. [CrossRef]
16. Lai, S.C.; Su, Y.T.; Chi, C.C.; Kuo, Y.C.; Lee, K.F.; Wu, Y.C.; Lan, P.C.; Yang, M.H.; Chang, T.S.; Huang, Y.H. DNMT3b/OCT4 expression confers sorafenib resistance and poor prognosis of hepatocellular carcinoma through IL-6/STAT3 regulation. *J. Exp. Clin. Cancer Res.* **2019**, *38*, 474. [CrossRef]
17. Marques, V.; Ourô, S.; Afonso, M.B.; Rodrigues, C.M.P. Modulation of rectal cancer stemness, patient outcome and therapy response by adipokines. *J. Physiol. Biochem.* **2023**, *79*, 261–272. [CrossRef]
18. Shao, M.; Bi, T.; Ding, W.; Yu, C.; Jiang, C.; Yang, Y.; Sun, X.; Yang, M. OCT4 Potentiates Radio-Resistance and Migration Activity of Rectal Cancer Cells by Improving Epithelial-Mesenchymal Transition in a ZEB1 Dependent Manner. *Biomed. Res. Int.* **2018**, *2018*, 3424956. [CrossRef]
19. You, L.; Guo, X.; Huang, Y. Correlation of Cancer Stem-Cell Markers OCT4, SOX2, and NANOG with Clinicopathological Features and Prognosis in Operative Patients with Rectal Cancer. *Yonsei Med. J.* **2018**, *59*, 35–42. [CrossRef] [PubMed]
20. Johari, B.; Rezaeejam, H.; Moradi, M.; Taghipour, Z.; Saltanatpour, Z.; Mortazavi, Y.; Nasehi, L. Increasing the colon cancer cells sensitivity toward radiation therapy via application of Oct4-Sox2 complex decoy oligodeoxynucleotides. *Mol. Biol. Rep.* **2020**, *47*, 6793–6805. [CrossRef]
21. Roudi, R.; Barodabi, M.; Madjd, Z.; Roviello, G.; Corona, S.P.; Panahi, M. Expression patterns and clinical significance of the potential cancer stem cell markers OCT4 and NANOG in colorectal cancer patients. *Mol. Cell Oncol.* **2020**, *7*, e1788366. [CrossRef]
22. Fujino, S.; Miyoshi, N. Oct4 Gene Expression in Primary Colorectal Cancer Promotes Liver Metastasis. *Stem Cells Int.* **2019**, *2019*, 7896524. [CrossRef] [PubMed]

23. American Joint Committee on Cancer. Colon and Rectum. In *AJCC Cancer Staging Manual*, 7th ed.; Edge, S.B., Byrd, D.R., Compton, C.C., Fritz, A.G., Greene, F.L., Trotti, A., Eds.; Springer: New York, NY, USA, 2010; pp. 143–164. ISBN 978-0-387-88440-0.
24. Kruger, N.J. The Bradford Method for Protein Quantitation. In *The Protein Protocols Handbook*, 3rd ed.; Walker, J.M., Ed.; Humana Press: Totowa, NJ, USA, 2009; pp. 17–24, ISBN 978-1-58829-880-5.
25. Sambrook, J.; Fritsch, E.; Maniatis, T. *Molecular Cloning: A Laboratory Manual, 2nd. ed.*; Cold Spring Harbor Laboratory Press: Cold Spring Harbor, NY, USA, 1989; ISBN 0-87969-309-6.
26. Moreno-Londoño, A.P.; Castañeda-Patlán, M.C.; Sarabia-Sánchez, M.A.; Macías-Silva, M.; Robles-Flores, M. Canonical Wnt Pathway Is Involved in Chemoresistance and Cell Cycle Arrest Induction in Colon Cancer Cell Line Spheroids. *Int. J. Mol. Sci.* 2023, *24*, 5252. [CrossRef]
27. Vasefifar, P.; Motafakkerazad, R.; Maleki, L.A.; Najafi, S.; Ghrobaninezhad, F.; Najafzadeh, B.; Alemohammad, H.; Amini, M.; Baghbanzadeh, A.; Baradaran, B. Nanog, as a key cancer stem cell marker in tumor progression. *Gene* 2022, *827*, 146448. [CrossRef] [PubMed]
28. Boman, B.M.; Viswanathan, V.; Facey, C.O.B.; Fields, J.Z.; Stave, J.W. The v8-10 variant isoform of CD44 is selectively expressed in the normal human colonic stem cell niche and frequently is overexpressed in colon carcinomas during tumor development. *Cancer Biol. Ther.* 2023, *24*, 2195363. [CrossRef] [PubMed]
29. Frau, C.; Jamard, C.; Delpouve, G.; Guardia, G.D.A.; Machon, C.; Pilati, C.; Nevé, C.L.; Laurent-Puig, P.; Guitton, J.; Galante, P.A.F.; et al. Deciphering the Role of Intestinal Crypt Cell Populations in Resistance to Chemotherapy. *Cancer Res.* 2021, *81*, 2730–2744. [CrossRef]
30. Pádua, D.; Figueira, P.; Ribeiro, I.; Almeida, R.; Mesquita, P. The Relevance of Transcription Factors in Gastric and Colorectal Cancer Stem Cells Identification and Eradication. *Front Cell Dev. Biol.* 2020, *8*, 442. [CrossRef] [PubMed]
31. Lumsdaine, C.T.; Liu-Smith, F.; Li, X.; Zell, J.A.; Lu, Y. Increased incidence of early onset colorectal adenocarcinoma is accompanied by an increased incidence of rectal neuroendocrine tumors. *Am. J. Cancer Res.* 2020, *10*, 1888–1899.
32. Vergara, E.E.; Núñez, G.A.; Hoyos, J.C.; Lozada-Martínez, I.D.; Suarez, A.; Narvaez-Rojas, A.R. Surgical outcomes and factors associated with postoperative complications of colorectal cancer in a Colombian Caribbean population: Results from a regional referral hospital. *Cancer Rep.* 2023, *6*, e1766. [CrossRef]
33. Vaccaro, C.A.; López-Kostner, F.; Adriana, D.V.; Palmero, E.I.; Rossi, B.M.; Antelo, M.; Solano, A.; Carraro, D.M.; Forones, N.M.; Bohorquez, M.; et al. From colorectal cancer pattern to the characterization of individuals at risk: Picture for genetic research in Latin America. *Int. J. Cancer* 2019, *145*, 318–326. [CrossRef]
34. Mauri, G.; Sartore-Bianchi, A.; Russo, A.G.; Marsoni, S.; Bardelli, A.; Siena, S. Early-onset colorectal cancer in young individuals. *Mol. Oncol.* 2019, *13*, 109–131. [CrossRef]
35. Siegel, R.L.; Wagle, N.S.; Cercek, A.; Smith, R.A.; Jemal, A. Colorectal cancer statistics, 2023. *CA Cancer J. Clin.* 2023, *73*, 233–254. [CrossRef]
36. Musetti, C.; Garau, M.; Alonso, R.; Piñeros, M.; Soerjomataram, I.; Barrios, E. Colorectal Cancer in Young and Older Adults in Uruguay: Changes in Recent Incidence and Mortality Trends. *Int. J. Environ. Res. Public Health* 2021, *18*, 8232. [CrossRef]
37. Vargas-Moranth, R.; Navarro-Lechuga, E. Cancer incidence and mortality in Barranquilla, Colombia. 2008–2012. *Colomb. Med.* 2018, *49*, 55–62. [CrossRef]
38. Shaheen, M.A.; Hegazy, N.A.; Nada, O.H.; Radwan, N.A.; Talaat, S.M. Immunohistochemical expression of stem cell markers CD133 and Oct4 in colorectal adenocarcinoma. *Egypt J. Pathol.* 2014, *34*, 44–51. [CrossRef]
39. Pece, S.; Tosoni, D.; Confalonieri, S.; Mazzarol, G.; Vecchi, M.; Ronzoni, S.; Bernard, L.; Viale, G.; Pelicci, P.G.; di Fiore, P.P. Biological and molecular heterogeneity of breast cancers correlates with their cancer stem cell content. *Cell* 2010, *140*, 62–73. [CrossRef] [PubMed]
40. Brown, R.E.; Ali, Y.D.; Cai, Z. Morphoproteomics Identifies CXCR4 in Undifferentiated Colorectal Cancer: A Case Study with Therapeutic Implications. *Ann. Clin. Lab. Sci.* 2020, *50*, 266–269. [PubMed]
41. Gao, Z.-Y.; Liu, X.-B.; Yang, F.-M.; Liu, L.; Zhao, J.-Z.; Gao, B.; Li, S.-B. Octamer binding transcription factor-4 expression is associated with cervical cancer malignancy and histological differentiation: A systematic review and meta-analysis. *Biosci. Rep.* 2019, *39*, BSR20182328. [CrossRef]
42. Mohamed, S.Y.; Kaf, R.M.; Ahmed, M.M.; Elwan, A.; Ashour, H.R.; Ibrahim, A. The Prognostic Value of Cancer Stem Cell Markers (Notch1, ALDH1, and CD44) in Primary Colorectal Carcinoma. *J. Gastrointest. Cancer* 2019, *50*, 824–837. [CrossRef]
43. Li, H.; Wang, L.; Shi, S.; Xu, Y.; Dai, X.; Li, H.; Wang, J.; Zhang, Q.; Wang, Y.; Sun, S.; et al. The Prognostic and Clinicopathologic Characteristics of OCT4 and Lung Cancer: A Meta-Analysis. *Curr. Mol. Med.* 2019, *19*, 54–75. [CrossRef]
44. Razmi, M.; Ghods, R.; Vafaei, S.; Sahlolbei, M.; Saeednejad-Zanjani, L.; Madjd, Z. Clinical and prognostic significances of cancer stem cell markers in gastric cancer patients: A systematic review and meta-analysis. *Cancer Cell Int.* 2021, *21*, 139. [CrossRef]
45. Zhang, Q.; Han, Z.; Zhu, Y.; Chen, J.; Li, W. The role and specific mechanism of OCT4 in cancer stem cells: A review. *Int. J. Stem Cells* 2020, *13*, 312–325. [CrossRef] [PubMed]
46. Xie, W.; Yu, J.; Yin, Y.; Zhang, X.; Zheng, X.; Wang, X. OCT4 induces EMT and promotes ovarian cancer progression by regulating the PI3K/AKT/mTOR pathway. *Front Oncol.* 2022, *12*, 876257. [CrossRef] [PubMed]

47. Guo, K.; Duan, J.; Lu, J.; Xiao, L.; Han, L.; Zeng, S.; Tang, X.; Li, W.; Huang, L.; Zhang, Y. Tumor necrosis factor-α-inducing protein of Helicobacter pylori promotes epithelial-mesenchymal transition and cancer stem-like cells properties via activation of Wnt/β-catenin signaling pathway in gastric cancer cells. *Pathog. Dis.* **2022**, *80*, ftac025. [CrossRef]
48. Saigusa, S.; Tanaka, K.; Toiyama, Y.; Yokoe, T.; Okugawa, Y.; Ioue, Y.; Miki, C.; Kusunoki, M. Correlation of CD133, OCT4, and SOX2 in rectal cancer and their association with distant recurrence after chemoradiotherapy. *Ann. Surg. Oncol.* **2009**, *16*, 3488–3498. [CrossRef] [PubMed]

Disclaimer/Publisher's Note: The statements, opinions and data contained in all publications are solely those of the individual author(s) and contributor(s) and not of MDPI and/or the editor(s). MDPI and/or the editor(s) disclaim responsibility for any injury to people or property resulting from any ideas, methods, instructions or products referred to in the content.

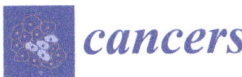

Article

Luciferase Expressing Preclinical Model Systems Representing the Different Molecular Subtypes of Colorectal Cancer

Arne Rotermund [1,†], Martin S. Staege [2,†], Sarah Brandt [1], Jana Luetzkendorf [1], Henrike Lucas [3], Lutz P. Mueller [1] and Thomas Mueller [1,*]

1. Department of Internal Medicine IV, Hematology and Oncology, Medical Faculty, Martin Luther University Halle-Wittenberg, 06120 Halle, Germany; arne.rotermund@student.uni-halle.de (A.R.); sarah.brandt@uk-halle.de (S.B.); jana.luetzkendorf@uk-halle.de (J.L.); lutz.mueller@uk-halle.de (L.P.M.)
2. Department of Surgical and Conservative Pediatrics and Adolescent Medicine, Medical Faculty, Martin Luther University Halle-Wittenberg, 06120 Halle, Germany; martin.staege@medizin.uni-halle.de
3. Institute of Pharmacy, Martin Luther University Halle-Wittenberg, 06120 Halle, Germany; henrike.lucas@pharmazie.uni-halle.de
* Correspondence: thomas.mueller@medizin.uni-halle.de; Tel.: +49-0345-5577211
† These authors contributed equally to this work.

Simple Summary: More insight into the biological diversity of colorectal cancer (CRC) is needed to improve therapeutic outcomes. We aimed at establishing a combined 2D/3D, in vitro/in vivo model system representing the heterogeneity of CRC with regards to the molecular subtypes, allowing bioluminescence imaging-assisted analyses. Comparative characterization of stable luciferase expressing derivatives of well-established CRC cell lines, derived spheroids and subcutaneous xenograft tumors showed that regarding primary tumor characteristics, the 3D-spheroid cultures resembled xenografts more closely than 2D-cultured cells do. Xenograft tumor growth resulted in metastatic spread to the lungs. Furthermore, a bioluminescence-based spheroid cytotoxicity assay was set up in order to be able to perform dose–response relationship studies in analogy to typical monolayer assays. Thus, the model systems can be used in preclinical research applications to study new therapy approaches and represents the biological heterogeneity of CRC.

Abstract: Colorectal cancer (CRC) is a heterogeneous disease. More insight into the biological diversity of CRC is needed to improve therapeutic outcomes. Established CRC cell lines are frequently used and were shown to be representative models of the main subtypes of CRC at the genomic and transcriptomic level. In the present work, we established stable, luciferase expressing derivatives from 10 well-established CRC cell lines, generated spheroids and subcutaneous xenograft tumors in nude mice, and performed comparative characterization of these model systems. Transcriptomic analyses revealed the close relation of cell lines with their derived spheroids and xenograft tumors. The preclinical model systems clustered with patient tumor samples when compared to normal tissue thereby confirming that cell-line-based tumor models retain specific characteristics of primary tumors. Xenografts showed different differentiation patterns and bioluminescence imaging revealed metastatic spread to the lungs. In addition, the models were classified according to the CMS classification system, with further sub-classification according to the recently identified two intrinsic epithelial tumor cell states of CRC, iCMS2 and iCMS3. The combined data showed that regarding primary tumor characteristics, 3D-spheroid cultures resemble xenografts more closely than 2D-cultured cells do. Furthermore, we set up a bioluminescence-based spheroid cytotoxicity assay in order to be able to perform dose–response relationship studies in analogy to typical monolayer assays. Applying the established assay, we studied the efficacy of oxaliplatin. Seven of the ten used cell lines showed a significant reduction in the response to oxaliplatin in the 3D-spheroid model compared to the 2D-monolayer model. Therapy studies in selected xenograft models confirmed the response or lack of response to oxaliplatin treatment. Analyses of differentially expressed genes in these models identified CAV1 as a possible marker of oxaliplatin resistance. In conclusion, we established a combined 2D/3D, in vitro/in vivo model system representing the heterogeneity of CRC, which can be used in preclinical research applications.

Citation: Rotermund, A.; Staege, M.S.; Brandt, S.; Luetzkendorf, J.; Lucas, H.; Mueller, L.P.; Mueller, T. Luciferase Expressing Preclinical Model Systems Representing the Different Molecular Subtypes of Colorectal Cancer. *Cancers* **2023**, *15*, 4122. https://doi.org/10.3390/cancers15164122

Academic Editors: Javier Martinez Useros, Cristina Díaz del Arco, Rodrigo Barderas-Manchado and María Jesús Fernández-Aceñero

Received: 19 June 2023
Revised: 10 August 2023
Accepted: 11 August 2023
Published: 16 August 2023

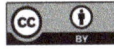

Copyright: © 2023 by the authors. Licensee MDPI, Basel, Switzerland. This article is an open access article distributed under the terms and conditions of the Creative Commons Attribution (CC BY) license (https://creativecommons.org/licenses/by/4.0/).

Keywords: colorectal cancer; preclinical models; bioluminescence imaging; cell lines; spheroids; xenograft tumors; CMS classification

1. Introduction

Cancer cell lines are valuable in vitro model systems that are widely used in basic cancer research and drug discovery [1]. Here, the Cancer Cell Line Encyclopedia has clearly demonstrated that large, annotated cell-line collections may help to enable preclinical stratification patterns for anticancer agents [2–4]. This has been demonstrated again by two recent studies, which investigated important issues of cancer research such as tumor heterogeneity and metastasis [5,6]. Using cell lines, Jin et al. created a first-generation metastasis map (MetMap) that reveals organ-specific patterns of metastasis associated with clinical and genomic features, and demonstrated the utility of this MetMap [5]. In the second study, Kinker et al. described the landscape of heterogeneity within diverse cancer cell lines and identified recurrent patterns of heterogeneity that are shared between tumors and specific cell lines [6]. Thus, cancer cell lines can be useful models with clinical relevance.

Colorectal cancer (CRC) is among the most common cancers and a major cause of cancer mortality [7,8]. CRC is a heterogeneous, clinically diverse disease and is poorly understood biologically. Therefore, more insight into the biological diversity of CRC, especially in relation to its clinical behavior, is needed to improve the therapeutic outcomes. Established CRC cell lines are frequently used and are capable of representing the main subtypes of primary tumors at the genomic level, which validates their utility as tools to investigate colorectal cancer biology and drug responses [9]. Furthermore, several groups have characterized primary CRC tumors based on their gene expression data combined with their genomic features in order to establish biologically distinct molecular subtypes with clinical relevance, which resulted in the emergence of different classification systems [10–15]. Again, CRC cell lines turned out to reflect the differential subtypes among these classification systems and were capable of being used to test specific targeted therapy approaches [16]. Later, the international CRC Subtyping Consortium (CRCSC) was formed with the aim of resolving inconsistencies among the original reported gene expression-based CRC classification systems. This resulted in the establishment of the CMS classification system consisting of four consensus molecular subtypes (CMS), each with distinguishing properties: CMS1 (microsatellite instability immune, 14%), hypermutated, microsatellite unstable and strong immune activation; CMS2 (canonical, 37%), epithelial, marked WNT and MYC signaling activation; CMS3 (metabolic, 13%), epithelial and evident metabolic dysregulation; and CMS4 (mesenchymal, 23%), prominent transforming growth factor-beta activation, stromal invasion and angiogenesis [17]. In addition, there was a fifth group comprising samples with mixed features, labeled as an intermediate group (13%). Besides the biological differences, clear clinical distinctions were evident between the aforementioned groups. Among others, patients with CMS4 tumors displayed worse overall, and relapse-free, survival. The CMS1 population had very poor survival in the situation after relapse, whereas CMS2 patients showed superior survival after relapse [17]. Furthermore, various studies have also reported on different responses to chemotherapy in the different molecular subgroups of the CMS classification.

Gene expression profiles of tumor tissue samples represent the sum of signals derived from the cancer cells and their surrounding tumor microenvironment, the latter of which can impede gene expression analysis, depending on the model used. Moreover, the stromal component in a tumor has been suggested to be crucial for the determination of CMS4 [18,19]. In contrast to these reports, Linnekamp et al. characterized a panel of CRC cell culture models including CRC cell lines, primary cultures and PDX models, and clearly detected CMS4 in all model systems, indicating that CMS4 can be defined as a tumor cell-intrinsic phenotype in addition to the observed accumulation of stromal cells [20]. Moreover, Eide et al. developed a novel CMS classifier, referred to as CMScaller, based on cancer cell-intrinsic and subtype-enriched gene expression markers, thereby providing a solution to the analogous problem of classifying pre-clinical models, which either lack a tumor microenvironment entirely (e.g., cell lines and organoid cultures) or present with a completely different background (e.g., murine xenografts) [21,22]. This is particularly relevant for the classification of CMS1 and CMS4, as interactions between tumor cells and microenvironment play an especially important role in these two subgroups. The CMScaller was shown to perform in primary tumors models and recapitulated the biology of the CMS groups, revealing subtype-dependent drug response profiles when applied to PDX and cell lines [23,24]. Moreover, in a recent study, Joanito et al. performed combined single-cell and bulk transcriptome sequencing and identified two intrinsic epithelial tumor cell states in colorectal tumors, which refined the CMS classification system of colorectal cancer [25].

In the present work, we generated stable, luciferase expressing cell clones from established CRC cell lines, in order to analyze growth, therapy response and metastasis in derived spheroid and nude mouse xenograft models utilizing the endogenous signal. Tumor spheroids are useful in vitro models as they can represent several important aspects of real tumor tissues, e.g., (1) three-dimensional growth with structural organization and physiologically relevant cell–cell and cell–matrix interactions; (2) establishment of tumor microenvironmental characteristics such as nutrient gradients, hypoxia and acidosis; (3) localization-dependent heterogeneous cell growth and differentiation; (4) drug resistance mechanisms [26,27]. Mouse xenograft tumors represent aspects of real tumor tissue even more strongly, since they contain a complete stromal component including vasculature and fibrotic tissue, even though being of murine origin. In addition, a residual immune system consisting of B cells, NK cells, macrophages and dendritic cells is still present in these models, especially in athymic nude mice. In this work, we compared the labeled and cloned CRC cell lines with their derived spheroids and xenograft tumors in terms of gene expression and response to therapy. The aim of the study was to establish a useful preclinical model system, which represents the heterogeneity of CRC, especially in regard to the different subtypes according to the CMS classification system.

2. Materials and Methods

2.1. Cell Lines and Generation of Luciferase Expressing Clones

The colorectal cancer cell lines HT29 (HTB-38), DLD1 (CCL-221), LOVO (CCL-229), SW48 (CCL-231), LS1034 (CRL-2158), SW1463 (CCL-234), COLO205 (CCL-222), LS174T (CL-188), HCT116 (CCL-247) and SW480 (CCL-228) were originally obtained from the ATCC and were authenticated in 2010 at the DSMZ-German Collection of Microorganisms and Cell Cultures GmbH (Braunschweig, Germany). All cell lines were cultivated in RPMI medium (Sigma-Aldrich, Taufkirchen, Germany) containing 10% fetal bovine serum (BioWest, Nuaillé, France) and 1% penicillin/streptomycin (Sigma-Aldrich) at 37 °C/5% CO_2 in a humid atmosphere.

The cDNA of the red-shifted firefly luciferase PLR1 [28], kindly provided by Bruce R. Branchini (Department of Chemistry, Connecticut College, New London, CT, 06320, USA), was cloned into the lentiviral vector system that we previously used [29]. Preparation of the lentiviral particles and the transduction of the used cell lines were performed as previously described [29]. Transduced cell lines were seeded onto 96-well plates to generate single cell clones by means of using limited dilutions. Luciferase (Luc) expressing clones were identified by measuring bioluminescence after supplementation of D-luciferin (Perkin Elmer, Rodgau, Germany) on a Tecan Spark microplate reader (Tecan, Männedorf, Switzerland). Six to ten Luc-positive clones per cell line were picked, expanded and analyzed regarding morphology, growth behavior and drug response in direct comparison to the wild-type cell lines. One clone of each cell line was selected for subsequent experiments. Finally, the newly generated Luc-expressing, cloned cell lines were re-authenticated at the DSMZ in 2020/2021.

2.2. Spheroid Preparation, Growth Kinetics, Drug Treatment

In order to generate single tumor spheroids, tumor cells resuspended in culture medium were seeded onto 96-well plates, which were coated with 0.7% agarose (SeaKem® GTG™ Agarose, Lonza, Basel, Switzerland) before. The cell lines HT29-Luc, DLD1-Luc, LS174T-Luc, LS1034-Luc and SW1463-Luc were able to form compact spheroids within 2 days. For the cell lines LOVO-Luc, SW48-Luc, COLO205-Luc, HCT116-Luc and SW480-Luc, the used culture medium was supplemented with 10 µg/mL collagen I (Ibidi GmbH, Gräfelfing, Germany) in order to support spheroid formation. Compact spheroids were formed within 7 days.

In order to analyze spheroid growth, different amounts of cells (range 150–20,000) were seeded onto agarose-coated 96-well plates. The starting point of the assay (d0) was chosen after the formation of spheroids within two or seven days. On d0, 20 µL D-luciferin solution was added per well and luciferase activity was measured after 15 min incubation time on the Spark microplate reader. Further measurements were performed on d2, d5 and d7. Growth kinetic curves were established by plotting mean values (8 spheroids) over time using GraphPad Prism8. Based on these analyses, a cell line-specific cell amount to be used in our cytotoxicity assays was determined: HT29, DLD1, LS174T, LS1034, SW1463–1500; HCT116, LOVO–300; SW48, SW480–500; COLO205–150.

For the cytotoxicity assay, cells were seeded onto agarose-coated 96-well plates and were treated with serial dilutions of oxaliplatin (Eloxatin, 5 mg/mL, provided from own hospital pharmacy) for seven days after compact spheroids formed. Measurements of luciferase activity were performed as described above. Dose–response curves and calculation of IC_{50} values including standard deviations were carried out using GraphPad Prism8. The IC_{50} values of the groups were then compared using a Welch test.

2.3. RNA Preparation, Microarray Analysis, Molecular Subtyping and Classification

Cell lines were harvested 48 h after seeding and different samples per cell line were pooled. Spheroids were harvested on day 7 (HT29, DLD-1, LS174T, LS1034, SW1463) or day 12 (LOVO, SW48, COLO205, HCT116, SW480) and were pooled. Xenograft tumors (see Section 2.4) were resected from nude mice when they had reached a volume of approximately 1 cm^3. Tumors were sliced in half and, afterwards, one half was fixed in formalin for histological analyses, whereas the other half was immediately processed, performing cell separation using the MACS cell separation technology from Miltenyi (Miltenyi Biotech, Bergisch Gladbach, Germany). Preparation of the tumor mass was performed on a gentleMACS Octo by using the Tumor Dissociation Kit (130-095-929), followed by separation using the Mouse Cell Depletion Kit (130-104-694) and the Death Cell Removal Kit (130-090-101) according to the protocols of the manufacturer. For histological analyses, formalin-fixed samples were embedded in paraffin and then cut to perform hematoxylin/eosin (HE) staining according to standard protocols, as described previously [30].

RNA was extracted using the TRIzol™ Reagent (Thermo Fisher Scientific, Waltham, MA, USA) according to the manufacturer's protocol. For transcriptomic analyses, the Clariom™ D Assay from Applied Biosystems™ (Thermo Fisher Scientific) was used. The processing of the microarrays was performed in the core facility "analyses" of the Center for Medical Basis Research (ZMG) of the Medical Faculty (Martin Luther University Halle-Wittenberg) according to the instructions of the manufacturer. Microarray data will be available from the Gene Expression Omnibus (GEO) database. In addition to our preclinical samples, ten tumor samples and ten normal colon tissue samples from the GEO database (accession number GSE115261 [31]), which was processed using the same microarray, were included in the transcriptomic analyses.

Microarrays were analyzed using the robust multi-array average (RMA) algorithm with the Transcriptome Analysis Console (TAC4.0; Thermo Fisher Scientific). Gene filtering and cluster analysis was performed with TAC4.0. For the genes included in the cluster analysis focusing on cell line-specific genes and differences between tumor and normal samples were filtered for a false discovery rate (FDR) F-test < 0.0001 and a tumor-versus-normal log2 fold change of >5/<−5 (749 probe sets passed these filters). Normal samples were set as the baseline. Genes included in cluster analysis focusing on the different preclinical model systems were filtered for a FDR F-test < 0.01 and 2D cultures were used as baseline. Genes were further filtered for spheroid-versus-2D and xenograft-versus-2D log2 fold changes of >1.5/<−1.5 (152 probe sets) or >2/<−2 (51 probe sets).

The gene expression data were used to classify the samples according to the CMS classification system applying the CMScaller [21]. The classification was performed according to the instructions provided on https://github.com/peterawe/CMScaller (lastly accessed on 10 August 2023). In addition, the datasets were classified using the CRCassigner [14] according to the instructions provided on https://github.com/syspremed/CRCAssigner (lastly accessed on 10 August 2023).

For classification of the intrinsic epithelial tumor cell type, the specific iCMS2 and iCMS3 gene sets provided in the original study [25] were used to calculate scores for iCMS2. Probe sets were mean collapsed to gene names and for all genes, the sample-specific quantile ranks were calculated. Thereafter, two different scores were calculated: For score A, the means of the quantile ranks for the gene sets [25] iCMS2_up (Mq2U), iCMS2_down (Mq2D), iCMS3_up (Mq3U), and iCMS3_down (Mq3D) were calculated for all samples. Score A was calculated as A = (Mq2U/Mq2D) − (Mq3U/Mq3D). In score B, the sums of the quantile ranks for the same gene sets iCMS2_up (Sqi2U), iCMS2_down (Sqi2D), iCMS3_up (Sq3U) and iCMS3_down (Sq3D) were calculated for all samples. The score B was calculated as B = (Sq2U−Sq2D) − (Sq3U−Sq3D). In both scores, higher positive values suggest that the corresponding sample likely belongs to the iCSM2 class. In addition, nearest template prediction [32] was performed using the mentioned gene sets. Based on the calculated distances to the gene classes iCMS2_up (D2U), iCMS2_down (D2D), iCMS3_up (D3U) and iCMS3_down (D3D), the iCMS classes were determined as: (D2U < D2D) and (D3U > D3U) → iCMS2; (D2U > D2D) and (D3U < D3U) → iCMS3; all other constellations → unstable.

Additional datasets from public databases were used for iCMS classification of additional cell lines. From ArrayExpress, the cel files from dataset E-MTAB-2971 were downloaded. In addition, the following the GEO datasets were used: GSM1374426, GSM1374451, GSM1374452, GSM1374456, GSM1374463, GSM1374516, GSM1374517, GSM1374518, GSM1374561, GSM1374562, GSM1374563, GSM1374564, GSM1374627, GSM1374628, GSM1374629, GSM1374630, GSM1374632, GSM1374633, GSM1374759, GSM1374919, GSM1374920, GSM1374925, GSM1374926, GSM1374927, GSM1374928, GSM1374929, GSM1374930, GSM1374933, GSM1374934, GSM1374935, GSM1374937, GSM206450, GSM206455, GSM206459, GSM206463, GSM206467, GSM206501, GSM206517, GSM206519, GSM206524, GSM206547, GSM206548, GSM206552, GSM206553, GSM206554, GSM843481, GSM843482, GSM844580, GSM844713, GSM887141, GSM887274, GSM887277, GSM887278, GSM887303, GSM887479, GSM887632, GSM887644, GSM887667, GSM887668, GSM887674, GSM887675, GSM887677, GSM887679 (GSE57083, GSE8332 [33], GSE34211 [34], GSE36133 [2]).

2.4. Animal Studies, Treatment, Imaging

Generation of subcutaneous xenograft tumors was performed by inoculation of 5 million tumor cells into the right flank of male athymic nude mice (Charles River Laboratories, Sulzfeld, Germany). Monitoring of tumor growth was performed by caliper measurement and volume calculation using the formula $a^2 \times b \times \pi/6$ with 'a' being the short and 'b' the long diameter. For molecular and histological analyses (see Section 2.3), three to four tumors from each cell line model were removed from mice when they had reached a volume of approximately 1 cm^3. To analyze the ability to metastasize, one tumor of each model was allowed to grow to a size of about 2 cm^3. After completing, the lungs were removed, incubated in D-luciferin solution for 10 min and bioluminescence imaging was performed on an IVIS Spectrum (PerkinElmer, Rodgau, Germany).

Selected models were used to analyze the anti-tumor activity of oxaliplatin. For this purpose, mice were divided into two groups ($n = 3$) with similar mean tumor volumes of about 0.150 cm^3 and equal volume distribution at the start of treatment. Treatments comprised weekly intraperitoneal applications of oxaliplatin (8 mg/kg BW) and normal saline (control). Mouse weight and behavior were controlled daily during the course of treatment. The impact of treatment was calculated as the increase in tumor volume after treatment relative to the tumor volume at the start of the treatment on day 0 (mean values ± SD).

3. Results

3.1. Luciferase-Labelled CRC Cell Line Clones form Subcutaneous Xenograft Tumors with Various Differentiation Characteristics and Metastasize to the Lung

We chose ten well-known CRC cell lines, which already have been used in recent classification studies, to establish luciferase-labelled derivatives. The red-shifted firefly luciferase PLR1 [28] was cloned into the vector system that we previously used [29], which contains no further selection marker, enabling the utilization of typical selection markers in subsequent experiments. Single cell cloning was performed in order to achieve homogenous cell populations in regard to the chromosomal locus of the incorporated vector cassette. From several picked clones of each cell line, one was selected based on the criteria luminescence intensity, as well as the morphology, growth behavior and drug response resembling the wild type of the corresponding cell line. The generated luciferase (Luc)-expressing, cloned CRC cell lines were re-authenticated using STR analysis.

All new Luc-labelled derivatives were able to grow as subcutaneous xenograft tumors in nude mice without any differences to the wild-type cell lines. Interestingly, ex vivo bioluminescence imaging revealed metastatic spread to the lungs in each model (Figure 1A). Histological examination of the subcutaneous tumors showed clear differences (Figure 1B). Tumors from LS1034 and SW1463 cells showed well-differentiated structures resembling those of the colonic mucosa, with arranged columnar epithelial cells including goblet cells. LS174T, and to a lesser extent HT29, tumors were characterized by pronounced goblet cell differentiation and displayed only a residual pattern of layered epithelium formation. Tumors from SW48, LOVO, HCT116, SW480 and COLO205 cells showed a completely undifferentiated phenotype although scattered goblet cells could occasionally be observed. In addition, examination of HCT116 and SW480 tumors revealed a high density of small capillary structures. A high content of mitotic figures was a typical feature of COLO205 tumors, which corresponded with their fast growth compared to the other tumor types. DLD1 tumors predominantly displayed an undifferentiated phenotype but in part showed a residual tendency of cellular organization. Together, these analyses showed that the Luc-labelled, cloned cell lines retained the main properties of wild-type cell lines.

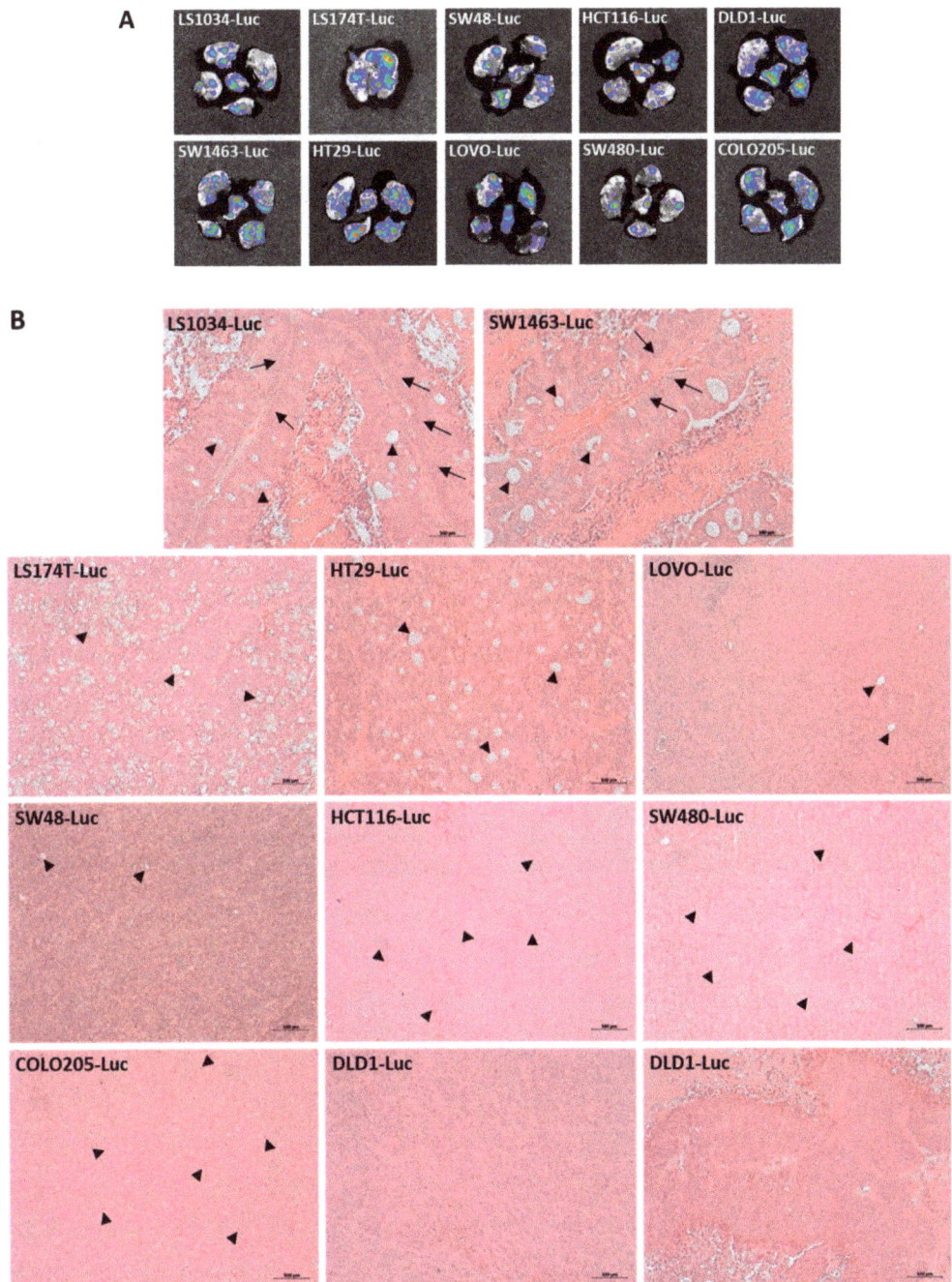

Figure 1. Characteristics of subcutaneous xenograft tumors generated from luciferase expressing CRC cell line clones. (**A**): Lung metastasis analyzed by bioluminescence imaging ex vivo; (**B**): histological examination of tumors after HE staining showing different histological phenotypes. LS1034-Luc and SW1463-Luc: Well differentiated; display of colonic mucosa-like structures with arranged columnar

epithelial cells (arrows), as well as goblet cells (arrowheads). LS174T-Luc and HT29-Luc: Occurrence of pronounced goblet cell differentiation (arrowheads). LOVO-Luc and SW48-Luc: Undifferentiated; scattered goblet cells (arrowheads). HCT116-Luc and SW480-Luc: Undifferentiated; high density of small capillary structures (arrowheads). COLO205-Luc: Undifferentiated; high content of mitotic figures (arrowheads). DLD1-Luc: Predominantly undifferentiated (below middle); residual tendency of cellular organization (below right). (Scale bar: 100 µm). For higher resolution display, see original images (Supplementary File S1).

3.2. Luciferase Expressing Cell Lines as Well as Their Derived Spheroids and Xenograft Tumors Represent Molecular Characteristics of CRC

We performed transcriptomic analyses to characterize the Luc-CRC cell lines, derived spheroids and xenograft tumors. The cell lines LS1034, SW1463, HT29, LS174T and DLD1 were able to form compacted spheroids within one or two days. In contrast, SW48, LOVO, HCT116, SW480 and COLO205 only formed loose aggregates in an equal time span. Medium supplementation with collagen I and a longer incubation time was necessary to achieve the formation of properly compacted spheroids in these models. From xenograft tumors, the human tumor cells were extracted and mouse cells were depleted. Furthermore, ten colorectal tumor samples and ten normal colon tissue samples from publicly available data sources [31] were included for further comparison. First, we performed hierarchical cluster analysis focusing on cell line specific genes and differences between the tumor and the normal tissue samples (Figure 2A, gene set 749 in Supplementary Table S1), revealing a close relation between the cell lines and their derived spheroids and xenograft tumors. In addition, clustering the preclinical model systems together with the tumor samples confirmed that the cell line-based tumor models retain specific characteristics of real tumors when compared to normal tissue. Hierarchical cluster analysis focusing on differences among the preclinical model systems showed that spheroids were located in the main cluster together with cell lines when compared with xenograft tumors (Figure 2B, gene set 152 in Supplementary Table S2). Spheroids of the cell lines SW48, LOVO, HCT116 and COLO205 were more closely related to the cell line group than the others. All of these four cell lines belonged to the group, which were less prone to form spheroids. Although belonging to the same group, the cell line SW480 was able to form spheroids faster when supplemented with collagen I, possibly explaining the clustering together with the other group. Furthermore, to investigate the relation between the three preclinical model systems, we performed a correlation analysis (Pearson) based on the gene set 152 (Supplementary Table S2). This revealed that spheroids resemble xenografts more closely than 2D-cultured cells do in each model, with SW48 as the only exception (Supplementary Table S3).

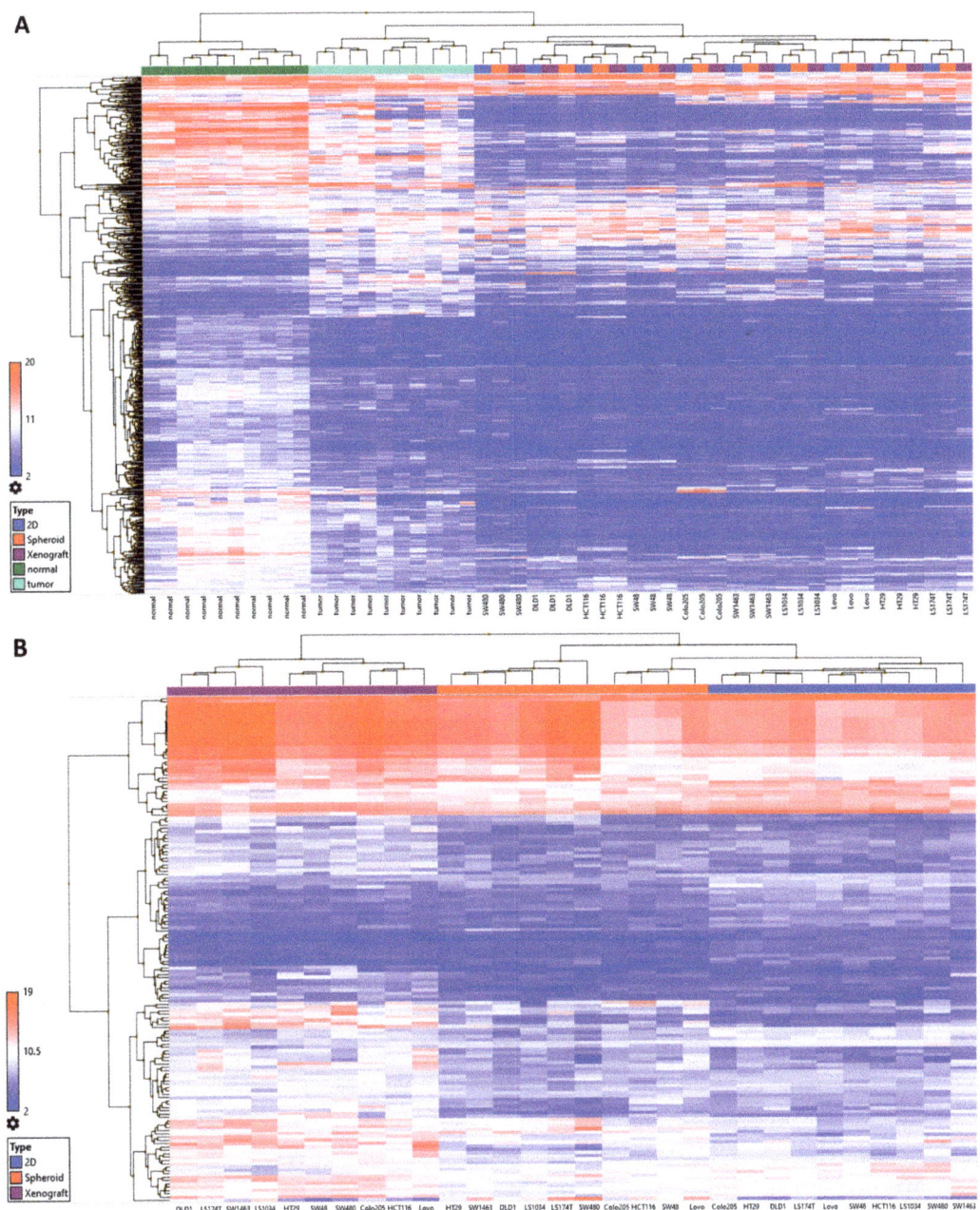

Figure 2. *Cont.*

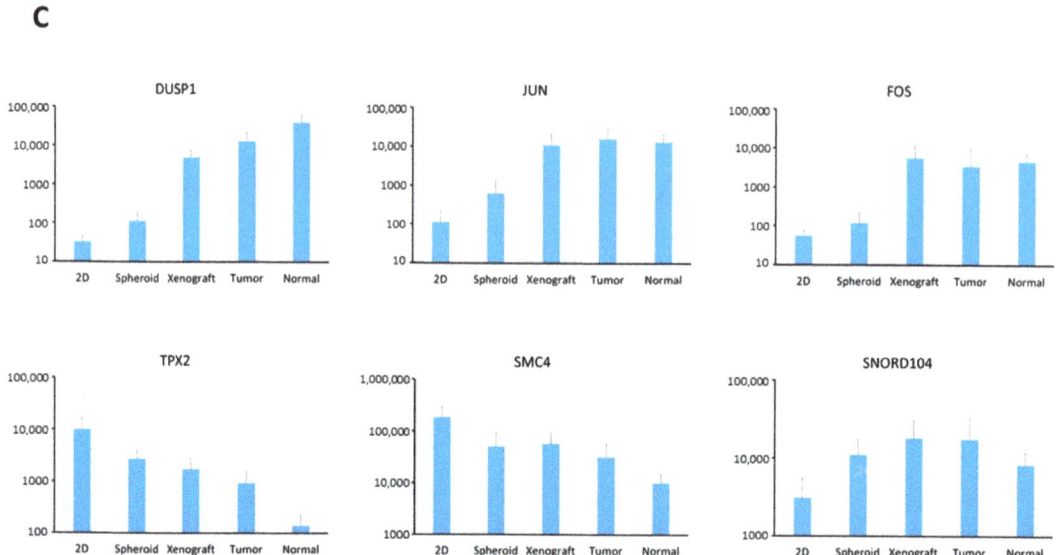

Figure 2. Transcriptomic gene expression and analyses of relationship between cell lines, spheroid and xenograft tumors compared to tumor and normal tissue samples. (**A**): Hierarchical cluster analysis focusing on cell line-specific genes and differences between tumor and normal tissue samples (for parameters see Section 2.3); (**B**): hierarchical cluster analysis focusing on differences among the preclinical model systems (for parameters see Section 2.3); (**C**): examples of genes with model-dependent increasing or decreasing expression pattern compared to tumor and normal tissue samples. Presented are signal intensities. Microarray raw data were analyzed and normalized using the RMA algorithm as indicated in the Materials and Methods section (Section 2.3).

Since spheroid models are described as better reflecting the characteristics of real tumor tissue than cell lines, we questioned whether this phenomenon is associated with a specific pattern of increased or decreased gene expression between the different model systems. Among the 152 genes (Supplementary Table S2) used in the cluster analysis depicted in Figure 2B, 64 genes showed an increasing and 25 genes a decreasing expression pattern. In addition, in three cases, gene expression increased from cell lines to spheroids without further increasing to xenograft tumors, whereas in eighteen cases gene expression decreased without further decreasing in xenograft tumors. Overall, 72% of the 152 genes showed a characteristic pattern indicating that spheroids, more than cell lines, comprise molecular traits of xenograft tumors. Further clustering using a fold-change higher than 2 resulted in a more restricted set of 51 genes, 84% of which showed the described increasing or decreasing expression pattern (Supplementary Table S4). Further analyses in combination with the gene expression data of the tumor and normal tissue samples revealed different, gene-dependent relations between the preclinical models and clinical samples (Supplementary Table S2). For example, the expression of genes such as JUN, FOS and DUSP1 showed an increasing pattern within the model and turned out to be high in both the tumor and normal samples (Figure 2C), suggesting an involvement of these factors in tissue-specific differentiation processes. Decreasing pattern of gene expression within the model associated with lower expression in the tumor and normal samples was found in genes such as TPX2 and SMC4. These genes are involved in cell division processes, thus reflecting the higher proliferation rate of cell lines growing on a monolayer. There were also genes such as SNORD104 whose expression increased from cell lines to tumors, but decreased from tumors to normal tissue, which might point to a tumorigenicity factor. In some cases, gene expression increased within the model, but decreased towards the clinical samples, suggesting the involvement of pure model-specific expression.

3.3. Luciferase Expressing Cell Lines and Their Derived Spheroids and Xenograft Tumors Represent the Main Subtypes of CRC According to the CMS Classification

Next, the CRC models were characterized according to the CMS classification using the CMScaller [21]. In addition, the datasets were analyzed using the CRCassigner, which was developed by Sadanandam et al. as one of the original classification systems, and which uses a cell lineage-related classification [14]. As summarized in Scheme 1, a high concordance between both classification systems could be observed. For example, xenograft tumors of SW48 and LOVO were classified as CMS1 based on the CMScaller and as Inflammatory, which is the corresponding group of the CRCassigner. The concordant CMScaller/CRCassigner classifications of the other xenograft tumors were as follows: LS1034 and SW1463–CMS2/TA (transit amplifying); HT29 and LS174T–CMS3/Goblet-like; HCT116 and SW480–CMS4/Stem-like. Xenograft tumors of COLO205 could not clearly be classified (FDR > 0.2), although there was a clear tendency (lowest distance) to CMS2/TA. DLD1 xenograft tumors were clearly classified as Stem-like by the CRCassigner, which correlated with the closest proximity to CMS4 (lowest distance) obtained by the CMScaller. Interestingly, the clear classification into CMS2/TA and CMS3/Goblet-like correlated well with the specific epithelial differentiation patterns observed in the corresponding xenograft tumors (see Figure 1B). This suggests that the cloned tumor cells still harbor the respective differentiation programs of their origin, which will lead to induction of differentiation processes once they are able to grow as three-dimensional tissue. Moreover, even in those tumors displaying an undifferentiated phenotype, residual signs of cellular differentiation or organization can occasionally be observed.

					CMScaller				CRCassigner				
	d.CMS1	d.CMS2	d.CMS3	d.CMS4	p.value	FDR	prediction (lowest distance)	determination (FDR<0.2)	Inflammatory	Goblet.like	Enterocyte	TA	Stem.like	Subtype	Mixed subtypes
Lovo	0.705	0.763	0.762	0.751	0.546	0.683	CMS1	no label	0.126	-0.073	-0.019	-0.142	0.088	Inflammatory	mixed
Lovo.Sph	0.651	0.703	0.710	0.684	0.001	0.002	CMS1	CMS1	0.065	-0.048	0.013	-0.069	-0.034	Inflammatory	mixed
Lovo.Xeno	0.613	0.734	0.708	0.630	0.001	0.002	CMS1	CMS1	0.130	-0.042	-0.071	-0.155	0.056	Inflammatory	Inflammatory
SW48	0.714	0.790	0.761	0.780	0.868	0.999	CMS1	no label	0.074	-0.053	-0.038	-0.090	0.144	Stem.like	Stem.like
SW48.Sph	0.726	0.779	0.749	0.777	0.999	0.999	CMS1	no label	0.041	-0.037	-0.032	-0.040	0.114	Stem.like	Stem.like
SW48.Xeno	0.614	0.744	0.712	0.687	0.001	0.002	CMS1	CMS1	0.222	-0.035	-0.060	-0.151	0.085	Inflammatory	Inflammatory
LS1034	0.770	0.595	0.710	0.714	0.001	0.002	CMS2	CMS2	-0.314	-0.029	-0.018	0.403	-0.081	TA	TA
LS1034.Sph	0.752	0.606	0.698	0.737	0.001	0.002	CMS2	CMS2	-0.251	0.025	0.060	0.313	-0.163	TA	TA
LS1034.Xeno	0.846	0.664	0.721	0.801	0.130	0.177	CMS2	CMS2	-0.333	0.108	0.080	0.286	-0.102	TA	TA
SW1463	0.729	0.619	0.687	0.739	0.001	0.002	CMS2	CMS2	-0.222	0.112	0.045	0.233	-0.149	TA	TA
SW1463.Sph	0.746	0.605	0.670	0.723	0.001	0.002	CMS2	CMS2	-0.273	0.115	0.057	0.252	-0.141	TA	TA
SW1463.Xeno	0.720	0.605	0.667	0.750	0.001	0.002	CMS2	CMS2	-0.232	0.144	0.043	0.208	-0.187	TA	TA
HT29	0.697	0.761	0.680	0.763	0.072	0.103	CMS3	CMS3	0.051	0.153	0.105	-0.132	-0.104	Goblet.like	Goblet.like
HT29.Sph	0.710	0.726	0.638	0.761	0.001	0.002	CMS3	CMS3	-0.008	0.248	0.141	-0.096	-0.180	Goblet.like	Goblet.like
HT29.Xeno	0.667	0.726	0.650	0.742	0.001	0.002	CMS3	CMS3	0.019	0.248	0.144	-0.143	-0.170	Goblet.like	Goblet.like
LS174T	0.733	0.720	0.666	0.831	0.007	0.010	CMS3	CMS3	-0.099	0.288	0.136	-0.039	-0.252	Goblet.like	Goblet.like
LS174T.Sph	0.679	0.648	0.612	0.723	0.001	0.002	CMS3	CMS3	-0.122	0.319	0.192	-0.030	-0.286	Goblet.like	Goblet.like
LS174T.Xeno	0.730	0.703	0.547	0.803	0.001	0.002	CMS3	CMS3	-0.164	0.482	0.185	-0.068	-0.347	Goblet.like	Goblet.like
HCT116	0.701	0.760	0.759	0.606	0.001	0.002	CMS4	CMS4	0.091	-0.162	-0.028	-0.134	0.293	Stem.like	Stem.like
HCT116.Sph	0.661	0.730	0.736	0.558	0.001	0.002	CMS4	CMS4	0.084	-0.158	-0.053	-0.121	0.266	Stem.like	Stem.like
HCT116.Xeno	0.617	0.720	0.717	0.518	0.001	0.002	CMS4	CMS4	0.178	-0.147	-0.071	-0.169	0.239	Stem.like	Stem.like
SW480	0.692	0.736	0.756	0.576	0.001	0.002	CMS4	CMS4	0.000	-0.128	-0.080	-0.020	0.257	Stem.like	Stem.like
SW480.Sph	0.766	0.759	0.768	0.632	0.153	0.199	CMS4	CMS4	0.030	-0.070	-0.017	-0.096	0.263	Stem.like	Stem.like
SW480.Xeno	0.705	0.691	0.739	0.608	0.001	0.002	CMS4	CMS4	-0.005	-0.036	-0.077	-0.002	0.172	Stem.like	Stem.like
Colo205	0.764	0.730	0.727	0.828	0.966	0.999	CMS3	no label	0.002	0.075	0.004	0.025	-0.083	mixed	mixed
Colo205.Sph	0.691	0.679	0.680	0.755	0.001	0.002	CMS2	CMS2	0.001	0.077	0.018	0.044	-0.147	Goblet.like	mixed
Colo205.Xeno	0.710	0.700	0.726	0.757	0.997	0.999	CMS2	no label	0.011	0.014	-0.024	0.026	-0.011	TA	mixed
DLD1	0.734	0.749	0.768	0.750	0.992	0.999	CMS1	no label	0.022	-0.118	-0.040	0.024	0.113	Stem.like	Stem.like
DLD1.Sph	0.656	0.663	0.680	0.583	0.001	0.002	CMS4	CMS4	0.023	0.036	0.007	-0.017	0.030	Goblet.like	mixed
DLD1.Xeno	0.720	0.742	0.735	0.713	0.999	0.999	CMS4	no label	0.017	-0.055	-0.073	-0.016	0.114	Stem.like	Stem.like

Scheme 1. Molecular classification of cell lines, spheroids and xenograft tumors using the CMScaller [21] and the CRCassigner [14].

Comparing the classification of the xenograft tumors with their corresponding spheroids and cell lines, a consistent classification was observed in each model of CMS2 (LS1034, SW1463), CMS3 (HT29, LS174T) and CMS4 (HCT116, SW480) (Scheme 1). Both cell lines of CMS1 (SW48, LOVO) could not be clearly classified (FDR > 0.2), but they showed the closest proximity to the CMS of the respective xenograft tumor. Notably, in the case of LOVO, the corresponding spheroid was clearly classified into CMS1. Spheroids of COLO205 and DLD1 were assigned to CMS2 and CMS4, respectively, in accordance with the characteristic of their respective xenograft tumors, but their respective cell lines showed the closest proximity to a different CMS, i.e., CMS3 for COLO205 and CMS1 for DLD1. This suggest that both models represent samples of the mixed/intermediate group, which is also supported by the data obtained with the CRCassigner (Scheme 1). Taken together, the established panel of Luc-labelled, cloned cell lines represents the heterogeneity of CRC and their derived spheroids and xenograft tumors are capable of clearly recapitulating the main subtypes of CRC according to the CMS classification.

In a very recent study, two intrinsic epithelial tumor cell states, iCMS2 and iCMS3, were identified in colorectal tumors, which can be used to refine the CMS classification system [25]. In this dual system, iCMS3 comprises the microsatellite unstable (MSI-H) tumors and one-third of the microsatellite-stable (MSS) tumors. Interestingly, the iCMS3 MSS tumors were transcriptomically more similar to MSI-H tumors than to the iCMS2 MSS tumors. In addition, iCMS3 cancers compared to iCMS2 showed worse survival after relapse. Notably, poor prognosis CMS4 tumors were shown to contain either iCMS2 or iCMS3 epithelium, the latter being associated with the worst prognosis of all subgroups [25]. Using the specific gene sets characterizing iCMS2 and iCMS3 provided in the original study, we analyzed our models. We applied two different scores (see Section 2.3 for explanation) in order to accomplish the assignment to either of the two epithelial subtypes (Figure 3). Both of the CMS1 models, LOVO and SW48, could be classified into iCMS3, with concordance reached between both scoring approaches. Thus, they belong to the most representative group of CMS1 (Scheme 2). LS1034 and SW1463 were clearly classified into iCMS2, which is also the common epithelial type of CMS2. The CMS3 model HT29 could not be clearly assigned, since results of both scores differed (Figure 3). While it rather tends to iCMS3, it seems to harbor characteristics of both epithelial subtypes or represents an intermediate type. Most tumors of CMS3 are iCMS3 with MSS (Scheme 2). The other CMS3 model LS174T, which is MSI-H, turned out to be iCMS3 and therefore belonged to the second group of CMS3. SW480 and HCT116 were classified as iCMS2 and iCMS3, respectively, the first therefore representing one of the two large groups of CMS4, whereas the latter belongs to a small group of CMS4 with MSI-H (Scheme 2). Both intermediate models COLO205 and DLD1 turned out to be iCMS3 (Figure 3). Thus, these models clearly differ in their molecular profile. DLD1 represents the iCMS3-MSI type and combines characteristics of CMS4 and CMS1, whereas COLO205 belongs to the iCMS3-MSS type and harbors characteristics of CMS2/CMS3 tumors.

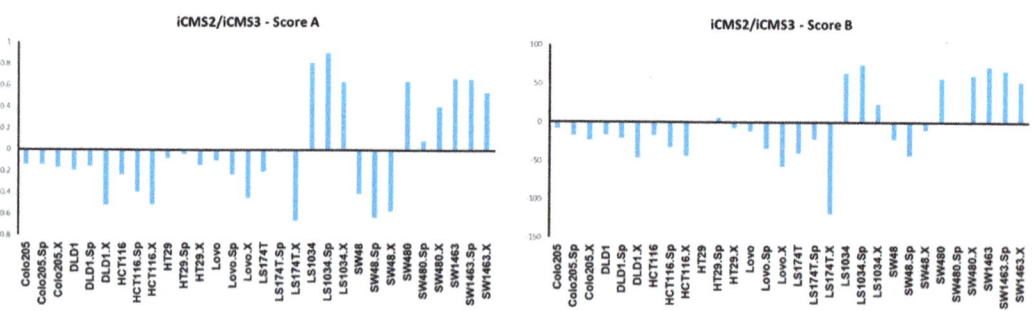

Figure 3. Determination of the intrinsic epithelial subtype iCMS2 vs. iCMS3. (values > 0 means iCMS2 assignment, values < 0 means iCMS3 assignment). Sp: spheroid; X: xenograft tumor.

We noticed that neither of our initially selected models represented the second main group of CMS4 tumors CMS4/iCMS3-MSS (Scheme 2). In order to find cell lines with properties of CMS4/iCMS3-MSS, we analyzed a panel of 13 CRC cell lines, which were classified as CMS4 (w/o MSI-H) in a previous study by Sveen et al. [24], using publicly available data sources. In addition, publicly available datasets from the cell lines used in this study were included for comparison. As shown in Figure 4, there was a high concordance between the luciferase expressing models created in this study and the respective datasets from publicly available data sources regarding the iCMS determination, with COLO205 as one exception. HT29 was confirmed to resemble iCMS3 better than iCMS2. Furthermore, from the 13 CMS4 cell lines, 7 could be assigned to the CMS4/iCMS3-MSS type, whereas the others were classified into iCMS2 (Figure 4). Nearest template prediction [32] was performed in addition to the scoring approach to determine the epithelial subtype, which confirmed the stated results (Supplementary Table S5). Based on these data, the well-established cell lines CaCo2, SW837 and LS123 were chosen and will be included into the panel of this study, in order to achieve and guarantee an adequate representation of the main groups of CMS4 to complete the CRC model (Scheme 2).

	CMS1	CMS2	CMS3	CMS4
iCMS2_MSS	0.2%	40.6% (SW1463, LS1034)	0.9%	14.2% (SW480, CaCo2)
iCMS3_MSS	2.3%	2.4%	11.3% (HT29)	10.1% (SW837, LS123)
iCMS3_MSI	14.0% (LOVO, SW48)	0%	3.0% (LS174T)	1.2% (HCT116)

Scheme 2. Assignment of the cell models applying combined CMS/iCMS classification. The data of the table are from the original study by Joanito et al. [25] showing the percent distribution of subtypes among colorectal cancer, and were complemented with the model names. Red marked cell lines are in preparation for completion of the CRC model.

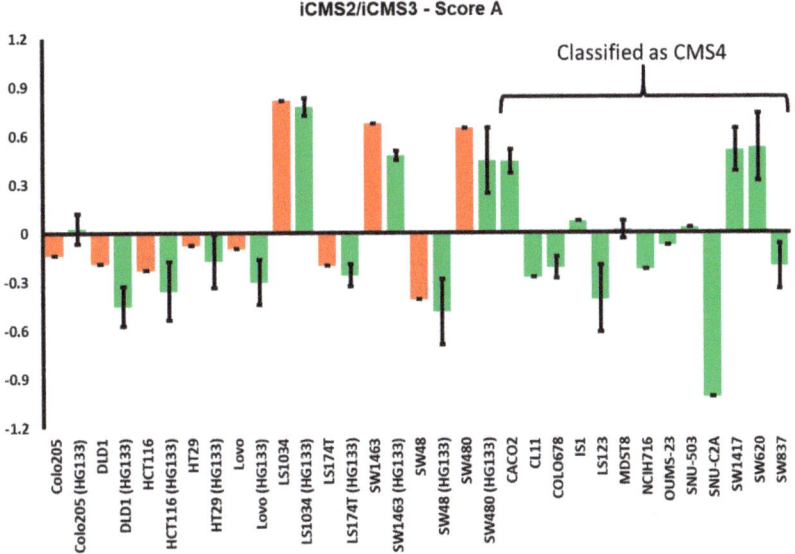

Figure 4. Determination of the intrinsic epithelial subtype iCMS2 vs. iCMS3. (values > 0 means iCMS2 assignment, values < 0 means iCMS3 assignment). Red bars: Cell line models characterized in this study. Green bars: Datasets from public databases (see Section 2.3). Cell lines marked by bracket were classified as CMS4 in a previous study by Sveen et al. [24].

Thus, including the three cell lines in preparation, the completed model comprises thirteen CRC cell lines, with four cell lines clearly representing the iCMS2 epithelial subtype (LS1034, SW1463, SW480, CaCo2), whereas seven cell lines (LOVO, SW48, LS174T, HCT116, DLD1, SW837, LS123) clearly belong to the iCMS3 subtype. The cell lines COLO205 and HT29 seem to represent intermediate types with a similarity to iCMS3. Furthermore, Joanito et al. demonstrated that one of the defining features of iCMS2 was the enrichment in copy number variations (CNV), whereas iCMS3 tumors were diploid or showed infrequent and inconsistent CNV [25]. Data regarding CNV of the cell lines could be found in the study of Berg et al., presented as a percent of the genome affected by copy number aberrations [23]. According to these analyses, CNV is consistently high in the iCMS2 cell lines LS1034, SW1463, SW480 and CaCo2 with 42%, 27%, 38% and 47%, respectively, whereas it is low in the iCMS3 cell lines LOVO, SW48, LS174T, HCT116 and DLD1 with 9%, 10%, 9%, 7% and 8%, respectively. Regarding CNV, COLO205 (45%) and HT29 (43%) clearly show features of iCMS2 confirming their nature as intermediate types harboring characteristics of both epithelial subtypes. Thus, the prevalent iCMS2–iCMS3 dichotomy in CRC as well as the occurrence of intermediate types, as reported by Joanito et al., is reproduced in the cell line models. Interestingly, for three out of the seven cell lines representing the specific CMS4/iCMS3-MSS subgroup of CMS4 tumors (Figure 4) data regarding CNV were available in the study of Berg et al. [23], which revealed a rather high CNV, with 18%, 48% and 30% for C11, COLO678 and SW837, respectively. Together, this shows an inconsistent CNV among iCMS3 cell lines, which is in accordance with the inconsistent CNV among the whole group of iCMS3 tumors, as reported by Joanito et al. [25].

3.4. Establishing a Bioluminescence Based Cytotoxicity Assay for Spheroid Models

The combined data show that tumor spheroids are more suited to be compared to xenograft tumors in regards to characteristics of patient tumors in comparison with the respective cell lines, making them useful models for preclinical drug research. Taking advantage of the endogenous luciferase expression in these models, we set up a bioluminescence-based cytotoxicity assay in order to be able to perform dose–response relationship studies in analogy to typical monolayer assays. In order to determine the optimal assay conditions, we first studied the growth kinetics of each spheroid model in order to prove the expected correlation between cell amount and signal intensity as an important prerequisite. A direct correlation between spheroid mass and signal intensity was confirmed in freshly formed spheroids. However, a near linear growth kinetic in growing and compacted spheroids is highly dependent on the amount of cells seeded at the start of the experiment. The relative decrease in signal intensity in growing spheroids can be explained by their typical characteristics such as the induction of oxygen and nutrient gradients leading to hypoxia, acidosis and heterogeneous cell growth, with proliferating cells at the rim area, and less proliferating/differentiated or even apoptotic/necrotic cells in the core area [35–37]. The characteristic decrease in signal intensity during spheroid growth was observed in each model to a different extent requiring a cell line-specific cell amount to be seeded at the start of the assay (see Section 2.2).

Applying the established assay, we studied the efficacy of oxaliplatin in the spheroid models of the whole panel. Oxaliplatin treatment induced a dose-dependent inhibition of spheroid growth and resulted in a typical dose–response pattern. Next, IC50 values were calculated and compared with existing data obtained from monolayer assays. This revealed clear differences throughout the whole panel (Table 1). In general, seven of the ten used cell lines showed a significantly reduced response to oxaliplatin, and thus a significant increase in IC50 values, when comparing the monolayer model with the spheroid model. This effect is of particular relevance considering that the spheroid assay comprises a prolonged drug treatment of 7 days compared to the monolayer assay (4 days). The alterations in IC50 values also resulted in a different sensitivity pattern within the panel. For example, on the monolayer level, SW1463, LS174T, LOVO and SW48 cells represented the most sensitive cell lines. However, the latter two turned out to be less sensitive in our assay on the spheroid level (LOVO: 0.13 -> 0.37; SW48: 0.08 -> 0.49), whereas the first two remained the most sensitive towards oxaliplatin treatment, indicated by their comparably low IC50 values (Table 1; SW1463: 0.09 -> 0.10; LS174T: 0.11 -> 0.18). The differential gain in resistance cannot be simply explained by the differential spheroid morphology, so that, for example, higher compactness leads to hindered drug penetration. For instance, COLO205 has the greatest increase in IC50 value in the 3D spheroid model, but forms the least compacted spheroids, whereas the spheroids of sensitive SW1463 and LS174T are very dense and compact. This suggests that the differential oxaliplatin sensitivity is instead determined by molecular mechanisms.

Table 1. Oxaliplatin specific IC50 values (µM) ± SD obtained from cytotoxicity assays performed in the monolayer- and the spheroid models and analysis of differences. (Monolayer data are from own previous studies [38]). (*: $p \leq 0.05$, **: $p \leq 0.01$, ***: $p \leq 0.001$, ns: not significant).

Cell Line	Mean Monolayer	SD Monolayer	Mean Spheroid	SD Spheroid	p-Value	Significance
LOVO	0.13	0.02	0.37	0.09	0.0009	***
SW48	0.08	0.00	0.49	0.12	0.0005	***
LS1034	0.30	0.05	0.37	0.14	0.3537	ns
SW1463	0.09	0.04	0.10	0.03	0.7680	ns
HT29	0.26	0.04	2.12	0.97	0.0053	**
LS174T	0.11	0.04	0.18	0.04	0.0778	ns
HCT116	0.24	0.01	1.39	0.33	0.0003	***
SW480	0.43	0.12	2.40	0.95	0.0035	**
COLO205	0.27	0.12	12.44	6.77	0.0159	*
DLD1	2.02	0.36	4.10	0.84	0.0012	**

3.5. Analyzing Response to Oxaliplatin in Nude Mice Xenograft Tumors

We next questioned to what extent the different in vitro sensitivity of spheroids, represented by their specific IC50 value, can predict a specific response towards oxaliplatin treatment in vivo. We therefore analyzed the impact of an oxaliplatin therapy in selected xenograft models (Figure 5). Clear response to oxaliplatin resulting in a substantial tumor growth inhibition over time could only be observed in the SW1463 model. A reduced yet still moderate overall tumor growth inhibition was achieved in the LS174T model. Tumors of the models LOVO, SW48 and HCT116 were completely resistant to oxaliplatin treatment. These results confirmed the lack of oxaliplatin sensitivity of LOVO and SW48 models, which was assumed based on the analyses in the spheroid model. Together, the presented findings suggest that IC50 values above 0.2 µM in the spheroid assay may predict a lack of response to oxaliplatin treatment in the xenograft model. The only selective activity of oxaliplatin within the model reflects the low overall therapeutic activity of this drug as a single agent in CRC.

3.6. Identification of CAV1 as a Putative Marker of Oxaliplatin Resistance

Based on the proven oxaliplatin resistance, we performed analyses of differentially expressed genes comparing the xenograft tumors of SW1463 and LS174T with those of LOVO, SW48 and HCT116 in order to find targets associated with the differential oxaliplatin sensitivity. CAV1 (caveolin 1) was identified as the top-ranked gene with a 400-fold increased expression in resistant vs. sensitive xenograft tumors, (Supplementary Table S6). Furthermore, CAV1 turned out to be the top-ranked gene (375-fold) when performing the same analyses using the spheroid models. In the 2D models, CAV1 was the second listed gene with a 280-fold increased expression in resistant cells. This suggests that a possible CAV1-associated mechanism of oxaliplatin resistance is based on cell intrinsic characteristics in one part, but is further supported under 3D growth conditions. Interestingly, CAV1 has already been linked with drug resistance in general [39] as well as specifically in CRC [40–42]. Therefore, further analyses to explore the role of CAV1 in CRC especially with regard to oxaliplatin-containing chemotherapy are worth performing.

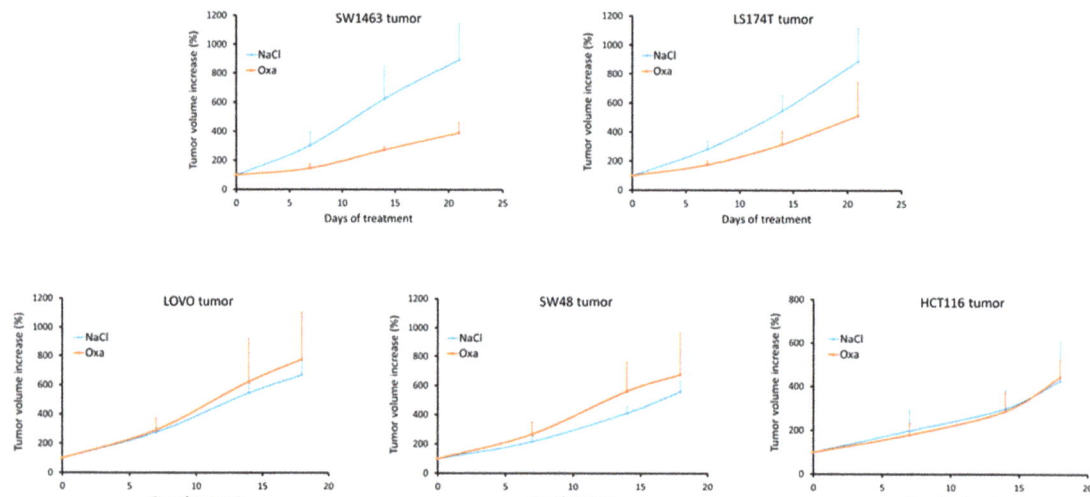

Figure 5. Antitumor activity of oxaliplatin in nude mice xenograft tumors of SW1436, LS174T, LOVO, SW48 and HCT116. Mice were treated with NaCl (control) or oxaliplatin (8 mg/kg BW) on days 0, 7 and 14. The tumor volume increase relative to the start of treatment on day 0 is shown, as mean values ± SD (n = 4, LS174T, LOVO, HCT116; n = 3, SW1463, SW48).

4. Discussion

Cancer is among the world's greatest health problems and one of the leading causes of death worldwide [7]. Since cancer itself is a very heterogeneous and still often poorly understood disease, both from a clinical and a biological perspective, more research is necessary to improve the prevention and treatment of this deadly disease. Cancer cell lines are important and useful tools used especially in preclinical cancer research and drug discovery due to their availability and comparability amongst others [1]. Due to the heterogeneity of cancer and many new discoveries in the area of targeted medicine, the emphasis on treatment stratification is as high as ever before. Therefore, preclinical research needs to establish models, which are able to reproduce the distinct molecular patterns of in vivo tumors in vitro based on standardized cancer cell lines. Promising research was conducted on this topic in recent years, showing the potential of cancer cell line models [5,6].

As CRC is both a leading cause of cancer mortality as well as a very diverse and poorly understood disease, establishing an aforementioned model is of utmost importance, in order to improve preclinical research with the aim of improving therapeutic options. Previous research has already suggested that CRC cell lines have the potential to be used as representative models [9]. The CMS classification established a consistent CRC classification system, dividing CRC into several subgroups with different patterns and properties [17]. Several studies have demonstrated significant differences concerning outcome and efficacy of chemo- and targeted drug therapy connected to the different molecular subtypes [24,43–48]. Interestingly, the molecular stratification of CRC is far from finished as recent work has described the existence of two intrinsic epithelial tumor cell states, iCMS2 and iCMS3, in colorectal tumors, therefore further refining the CMS classification [25]. The so-called IMF-classification was introduced, which is based on the discovered dichotomy of malignant epithelial cells, as well as the microsatellite status and the occurrence of fibrosis inside the tumor tissue [25].

Our panel of luciferase-labeled, cloned CRC cell lines was able to robustly recapitulate the main subtypes of CRC based on the CMS classification in the majority of cases, both in the spheroid as well as in the mouse xenograft model and to lesser extent in the monolayer model. The results for the cell lines were in accordance to the results obtained for the wild-type cell lines in previous reports [23,24]. Further characterization of the models applying combined CMS/iCMS classification including MSS/MSI status revealed the lack of representation of the specific CMS4/iCMS3-MSS subgroup of CMS4 tumors, requiring the complementation with further cell lines. Thus, including the three cell lines in preparation, the completed model comprises thirteen CRC cell lines, which represent the main subtypes of the confined CMS classification integrating the iCMS2–iCMS3 dichotomy (Scheme 2), but also different intermediate types. Therefore, the heterogeneity of CRC is reproduced in the cell line-derived models.

The combined data showed that 3D-spheroid cultures resemble xenografts more closely than 2D-cultured cells do regarding primary tumor characteristics, which can be expected. While unrestrained proliferation is the main task for cancer cells in monolayer models, three-dimensional growth now requires cell–cell interactions and the establishment of a tumor microarchitecture [49]. This notion is supported by our finding that two genes, TPX2 and SMC4, both essential proteins involved in mitosis and cell division, are among the genes which are downregulated in the xenograft and spheroid model, when compared to the 2D monolayer model, whereas JUN, FOS and DUSP1, genes with a role in differentiation processes, were among the most upregulated genes [50,51]. JUN and FOS are part of the transcription factor AP-1, which plays an important role in cell growth and the differentiation and overexpression of these two proteins leads to an increased expression of other oncogenes in several cancer entities [52–54]. DUSP1 on the other hand plays a role in carcinogenesis, tumor progression and response to anti-cancer treatment, as expression of DUSP1 is essential for the resistance of lung cancer cell lines to cisplatin treatment [55,56]. In addition, small nucleolar RNA SNORD104 was identified as a marker whose expression increased from cell lines to tumors, but decreased from tumors to normal tissue, which might point to a tumorigenicity factor in CRC. Interestingly, in a recent report, the overexpression of SNORD104 was shown to promote endometrial cancer growth in preclinical models in vivo and in vitro [57]. Furthermore, SNORD104 was among a marker panel identified as a novel snoRNA expression signature associated with overall survival in patients with lung adenocarcinoma [58]. Therefore, further investigation to explore the role of SNORD104 in CRC is worth performing.

Tumor spheroids are useful in vitro models and are also an easier, cheaper and faster way to create a three-dimensional preclinical model compared to mouse xenograft tumors [26,27]. Recent studies conducted on spheroids also showed the ability of this three-dimensional model to improve preclinical research in the fields of drug discovery, drug penetration, tumor metabolism and tumor migration, among others [59–62]. Furthermore, recent research by Koch et al. showed differences in the chemo- and radioresistance of four established CRC cell lines between a two-dimensional monolayer and a three-dimensional spheroid model [63]. This is in accordance with our observation regarding the different sensitivity to oxaliplatin. Thus, the establishment of a three-dimensional structure and the associated mechanisms may play a role in the development of chemotherapeutic resistance, a common problem for CRC patients, as CRC is capable of a vast number of mechanisms to achieve chemotherapeutic resistance leading to a worse outcome for patients [64]. However, the spheroid model, of course, has limitations when compared to an in vivo tumor, as the first grows in artificial medium and completely lacks the possibility of an interaction between tumor cells and cells of the tumor stroma or the immune system. Mouse xenograft tumor models contain stromal components and a residual immune system, albeit of murine origin, is present even in athymic mice making it an even more realistic clinical model. Nevertheless, our in vitro spheroid model was able to predict a lack of response to oxaliplatin treatment in vivo. CAV1 was identified as a possible marker for oxaliplatin resistance based on analyses in xenograft tumors, which could be completely reproduced in the spheroid models further confirming the usefulness of the in vitro 3D model.

Analysis of the differential oxaliplatin sensitivity with respect to the molecular subtypes represented by the models revealed some interesting clues. For example, a subset of patients with CMS2 featured tumors benefited from oxaliplatin containing chemotherapy regimen compared to other subtypes in the adjuvant setting [48]. Accordingly, only one of our two CMS2 models (SW1463) turned out to be sensitive to oxaliplatin treatment. Furthermore, meta analyses of results of further clinical studies, summarized in Ten Hoorn et al. [46], revealed an overall inferior effect of oxaliplatin-containing therapy compared to irinotecan-based therapy in all other groups than CMS2 in the metastatic setting, with a clear superior effect of the latter in CMS4 tumors. Regarding the iCMS2-iCMS3 dichotomy, a difference in sensitivity to the single drugs, 5-fluorouracil, SN38 and oxaliplatin, in representative models was found to be not significant [25]. Accordingly, among our two oxaliplatin-sensitive models, one was iCMS2 (SW1463) and one iCMS3 (LS174T). In addition, Joanito et al. evaluated two sets of genes whose expression was correlated with drug response [25]. Interestingly, gene sets positively correlated with drug sensitivity to FOLFOX regimen were upregulated in iCMS2 cells and genes correlated with drug resistance were downregulated, whereas iCMS3 cells showed patterns of up- and downregulation suggesting responsiveness to FOLFIRI [25]. This is in accordance with the observations mentioned above, since almost all CMS2 tumors are composed of iCMS2 epithelium, whereas almost all CMS1, almost all CMS3 and half of CMS4 tumors harbor iCMS3 epithelium (see Scheme 2). Together, this confirms the predictive value of specific subtyping of CRC.

5. Conclusions

With our work we aimed to establish a combined 2D/3D, in vitro/in vivo model system capable of representing the heterogeneity of CRC with regards to the molecular subtypes, and allowing bioluminescence imaging-assisted analyses. Our work has also shown that spheroid models do exhibit a higher similarity towards xenograft tumors compared to monolayer models both in terms of expression patterns as well as in terms of response to drug treatment due to the establishment of a three-dimensional structure and the associated mechanisms. Although spheroids do not completely resemble the heterogeneity found inside xenograft and human tumor samples, they are very solid models, especially considering their easy manageability and availability in comparison to xenograft models, with a stronger validity when, for example, performing drug screening studies.

Supplementary Materials: The following supporting information can be downloaded at: https://www.mdpi.com/article/10.3390/cancers15164122/s1, Supplementary File S1: HE stains-original images; Supplementary Table S1: cluster cell line plus tumors vs. normal_749 genes; Supplementary Table S2: model_152 genes_with tumors and normal; Supplementary Table S3: Pearson correlation_2D-Sph-Xeno; Supplementary Table S4: model_51 genes_with tumors and normal; Supplementary Table S5: iCMS determination by NTP; Supplementary Table S6: DEG analyses_Oxa res. vs. sens._2D-Sph-Xeno.

Author Contributions: Conceptualization, T.M.; investigation, A.R., M.S.S., S.B., J.L., H.L. and T.M.; formal analysis, A.R. and M.S.S.; writing—original draft preparation, A.R., M.S.S. and T.M.; writing—review and editing, L.P.M. and T.M. All authors have read and agreed to the published version of the manuscript.

Funding: This research received no external funding.

Institutional Review Board Statement: The animal investigations in this study were approved by the Laboratory Animal Care Committee of Sachsen-Anhalt, Germany, and were performed according to local guidelines (approval codes: 203.h-42502-2-1250 MLU and -1384 MLU).

Informed Consent Statement: Not applicable.

Data Availability Statement: The datasets used and/or analyzed in the current study are available from the corresponding author upon reasonable request.

Acknowledgments: We thank Franziska Reipsch for her excellent technical assistance.

Conflicts of Interest: The authors declare no conflict of interest.

References

1. Mirabelli, P.; Coppola, L.; Salvatore, M. Cancer Cell Lines Are Useful Model Systems for Medical Research. *Cancers* **2019**, *11*, 1098. [CrossRef]
2. Barretina, J.; Caponigro, G.; Stransky, N.; Venkatesan, K.; Margolin, A.A.; Kim, S.; Wilson, C.J.; Lehar, J.; Kryukov, G.V.; Sonkin, D.; et al. The Cancer Cell Line Encyclopedia enables predictive modelling of anticancer drug sensitivity. *Nature* **2012**, *483*, 603–607. [CrossRef]
3. Ghandi, M.; Huang, F.W.; Jane-Valbuena, J.; Kryukov, G.V.; Lo, C.C.; McDonald, E.R., 3rd; Barretina, J.; Gelfand, E.T.; Bielski, C.M.; Li, H.; et al. Next-generation characterization of the Cancer Cell Line Encyclopedia. *Nature* **2019**, *569*, 503–508. [CrossRef]
4. Li, H.; Ning, S.; Ghandi, M.; Kryukov, G.V.; Gopal, S.; Deik, A.; Souza, A.; Pierce, K.; Keskula, P.; Hernandez, D.; et al. The landscape of cancer cell line metabolism. *Nat. Med.* **2019**, *25*, 850–860. [CrossRef] [PubMed]
5. Jin, X.; Demere, Z.; Nair, K.; Ali, A.; Ferraro, G.B.; Natoli, T.; Deik, A.; Petronio, L.; Tang, A.A.; Zhu, C.; et al. A metastasis map of human cancer cell lines. *Nature* **2020**, *588*, 331–336. [CrossRef]
6. Kinker, G.S.; Greenwald, A.C.; Tal, R.; Orlova, Z.; Cuoco, M.S.; McFarland, J.M.; Warren, A.; Rodman, C.; Roth, J.A.; Bender, S.A.; et al. Pan-cancer single-cell RNA-seq identifies recurring programs of cellular heterogeneity. *Nat. Genet.* **2020**, *52*, 1208–1218. [CrossRef]
7. Ferlay, J.; Soerjomataram, I.; Dikshit, R.; Eser, S.; Mathers, C.; Rebelo, M.; Parkin, D.M.; Forman, D.; Bray, F. Cancer incidence and mortality worldwide: Sources, methods and major patterns in GLOBOCAN 2012. *Int. J. Cancer* **2015**, *136*, E359–E386. [CrossRef] [PubMed]
8. Ferlay, J.; Steliarova-Foucher, E.; Lortet-Tieulent, J.; Rosso, S.; Coebergh, J.W.; Comber, H.; Forman, D.; Bray, F. Cancer incidence and mortality patterns in Europe: Estimates for 40 countries in 2012. *Eur. J. Cancer* **2013**, *49*, 1374–1403. [CrossRef]
9. Mouradov, D.; Sloggett, C.; Jorissen, R.N.; Love, C.G.; Li, S.; Burgess, A.W.; Arango, D.; Strausberg, R.L.; Buchanan, D.; Wormald, S.; et al. Colorectal cancer cell lines are representative models of the main molecular subtypes of primary cancer. *Cancer Res.* **2014**, *74*, 3238–3247. [CrossRef] [PubMed]
10. Budinska, E.; Popovici, V.; Tejpar, S.; D'Ario, G.; Lapique, N.; Sikora, K.O.; Di Narzo, A.F.; Yan, P.; Hodgson, J.G.; Weinrich, S.; et al. Gene expression patterns unveil a new level of molecular heterogeneity in colorectal cancer. *J. Pathol.* **2013**, *231*, 63–76. [CrossRef]
11. De Sousa, E.M.F.; Wang, X.; Jansen, M.; Fessler, E.; Trinh, A.; de Rooij, L.P.; de Jong, J.H.; de Boer, O.J.; van Leersum, R.; Bijlsma, M.F.; et al. Poor-prognosis colon cancer is defined by a molecularly distinct subtype and develops from serrated precursor lesions. *Nat. Med.* **2013**, *19*, 614–618. [CrossRef]
12. Marisa, L.; de Reynies, A.; Duval, A.; Selves, J.; Gaub, M.P.; Vescovo, L.; Etienne-Grimaldi, M.C.; Schiappa, R.; Guenot, D.; Ayadi, M.; et al. Gene expression classification of colon cancer into molecular subtypes: Characterization, validation, and prognostic value. *PLoS Med.* **2013**, *10*, e1001453. [CrossRef]
13. Roepman, P.; Schlicker, A.; Tabernero, J.; Majewski, I.; Tian, S.; Moreno, V.; Snel, M.H.; Chresta, C.M.; Rosenberg, R.; Nitsche, U.; et al. Colorectal cancer intrinsic subtypes predict chemotherapy benefit, deficient mismatch repair and epithelial-to-mesenchymal transition. *Int. J. Cancer* **2014**, *134*, 552–562. [CrossRef] [PubMed]
14. Sadanandam, A.; Lyssiotis, C.A.; Homicsko, K.; Collisson, E.A.; Gibb, W.J.; Wullschleger, S.; Ostos, L.C.; Lannon, W.A.; Grotzinger, C.; Del Rio, M.; et al. A colorectal cancer classification system that associates cellular phenotype and responses to therapy. *Nat. Med.* **2013**, *19*, 619–625. [CrossRef] [PubMed]
15. Schlicker, A.; Beran, G.; Chresta, C.M.; McWalter, G.; Pritchard, S.; Weston, S.; Runswick, S.; Davenport, S.; Heathcote, K.; Castro, D.A.; et al. Subtypes of primary colorectal tumors correlate with response to targeted treatment in colorectal cell lines. *BMC Med. Genom.* **2012**, *5*, 66. [CrossRef] [PubMed]
16. Medico, E.; Russo, M.; Picco, G.; Cancelliere, C.; Valtorta, E.; Corti, G.; Buscarino, M.; Isella, C.; Lamba, S.; Martinoglio, B.; et al. The molecular landscape of colorectal cancer cell lines unveils clinically actionable kinase targets. *Nat. Commun.* **2015**, *6*, 7002. [CrossRef]
17. Guinney, J.; Dienstmann, R.; Wang, X.; de Reynies, A.; Schlicker, A.; Soneson, C.; Marisa, L.; Roepman, P.; Nyamundanda, G.; Angelino, P.; et al. The consensus molecular subtypes of colorectal cancer. *Nat. Med.* **2015**, *21*, 1350–1356. [CrossRef]
18. Calon, A.; Lonardo, E.; Berenguer-Llergo, A.; Espinet, E.; Hernando-Momblona, X.; Iglesias, M.; Sevillano, M.; Palomo-Ponce, S.; Tauriello, D.V.; Byrom, D.; et al. Stromal gene expression defines poor-prognosis subtypes in colorectal cancer. *Nat. Genet.* **2015**, *47*, 320–329. [CrossRef]
19. Isella, C.; Terrasi, A.; Bellomo, S.E.; Petti, C.; Galatola, G.; Muratore, A.; Mellano, A.; Senetta, R.; Cassenti, A.; Sonetto, C.; et al. Stromal contribution to the colorectal cancer transcriptome. *Nat. Genet.* **2015**, *47*, 312–319. [CrossRef]
20. Linnekamp, J.F.; Hooff, S.R.V.; Prasetyanti, P.R.; Kandimalla, R.; Buikhuisen, J.Y.; Fessler, E.; Ramesh, P.; Lee, K.; Bochove, G.G.W.; de Jong, J.H.; et al. Consensus molecular subtypes of colorectal cancer are recapitulated in in vitro and in vivo models. *Cell Death Differ.* **2018**, *25*, 616–633. [CrossRef]

21. Eide, P.W.; Bruun, J.; Lothe, R.A.; Sveen, A. CMScaller: An R package for consensus molecular subtyping of colorectal cancer pre-clinical models. *Sci. Rep.* **2017**, *7*, 16618. [CrossRef] [PubMed]
22. Eide, P.W.; Moosavi, S.H.; Eilertsen, I.A.; Brunsell, T.H.; Langerud, J.; Berg, K.C.G.; Rosok, B.I.; Bjornbeth, B.A.; Nesbakken, A.; Lothe, R.A.; et al. Metastatic heterogeneity of the consensus molecular subtypes of colorectal cancer. *NPJ Genom. Med.* **2021**, *6*, 59. [CrossRef] [PubMed]
23. Berg, K.C.G.; Eide, P.W.; Eilertsen, I.A.; Johannessen, B.; Bruun, J.; Danielsen, S.A.; Bjornslett, M.; Meza-Zepeda, L.A.; Eknaes, M.; Lind, G.E.; et al. Multi-omics of 34 colorectal cancer cell lines—A resource for biomedical studies. *Mol. Cancer* **2017**, *16*, 116. [CrossRef]
24. Sveen, A.; Bruun, J.; Eide, P.W.; Eilertsen, I.A.; Ramirez, L.; Murumagi, A.; Arjama, M.; Danielsen, S.A.; Kryeziu, K.; Elez, E.; et al. Colorectal Cancer Consensus Molecular Subtypes Translated to Preclinical Models Uncover Potentially Targetable Cancer Cell Dependencies. *Clin. Cancer Res.* **2018**, *24*, 794–806. [CrossRef]
25. Joanito, I.; Wirapati, P.; Zhao, N.; Nawaz, Z.; Yeo, G.; Lee, F.; Eng, C.L.P.; Macalinao, D.C.; Kahraman, M.; Srinivasan, H.; et al. Single-cell and bulk transcriptome sequencing identifies two epithelial tumor cell states and refines the consensus molecular classification of colorectal cancer. *Nat. Genet.* **2022**, *54*, 963–975. [CrossRef]
26. Costa, E.C.; Moreira, A.F.; de Melo-Diogo, D.; Gaspar, V.M.; Carvalho, M.P.; Correia, I.J. 3D tumor spheroids: An overview on the tools and techniques used for their analysis. *Biotechnol. Adv.* **2016**, *34*, 1427–1441. [CrossRef] [PubMed]
27. Nunes, A.S.; Barros, A.S.; Costa, E.C.; Moreira, A.F.; Correia, I.J. 3D tumor spheroids as in vitro models to mimic in vivo human solid tumors resistance to therapeutic drugs. *Biotechnol. Bioeng.* **2019**, *116*, 206–226. [CrossRef]
28. Branchini, B.R.; Southworth, T.L.; Fontaine, D.M.; Kohrt, D.; Florentine, C.M.; Grossel, M.J. A Firefly Luciferase Dual Color Bioluminescence Reporter Assay Using Two Substrates To Simultaneously Monitor Two Gene Expression Events. *Sci. Rep.* **2018**, *8*, 5990. [CrossRef]
29. Luetzkendorf, J.; Mueller, L.P.; Mueller, T.; Caysa, H.; Nerger, K.; Schmoll, H.J. Growth inhibition of colorectal carcinoma by lentiviral TRAIL-transgenic human mesenchymal stem cells requires their substantial intratumoral presence. *J. Cell Mol. Med.* **2010**, *14*, 2292–2304. [CrossRef]
30. Mueller, T.; Pfankuchen, D.B.; Wantoch von Rekowski, K.; Schlesinger, M.; Reipsch, F.; Bendas, G. The Impact of the Low Molecular Weight Heparin Tinzaparin on the Sensitization of Cisplatin-Resistant Ovarian Cancers-Preclinical In Vivo Evaluation in Xenograft Tumor Models. *Molecules* **2017**, *22*, 728. [CrossRef]
31. Zhang, B.; Babu, K.R.; Lim, C.Y.; Kwok, Z.H.; Li, J.; Zhou, S.; Yang, H.; Tay, Y. A comprehensive expression landscape of RNA-binding proteins (RBPs) across 16 human cancer types. *RNA Biol.* **2020**, *17*, 211–226. [CrossRef] [PubMed]
32. Hoshida, Y. Nearest template prediction: A single-sample-based flexible class prediction with confidence assessment. *PLoS ONE* **2010**, *5*, e15543. [CrossRef]
33. Wagner, K.W.; Punnoose, E.A.; Januario, T.; Lawrence, D.A.; Pitti, R.M.; Lancaster, K.; Lee, D.; von Goetz, M.; Yee, S.F.; Totpal, K.; et al. Death-receptor O-glycosylation controls tumor-cell sensitivity to the proapoptotic ligand Apo2L/TRAIL. *Nat. Med.* **2007**, *13*, 1070–1077. [CrossRef]
34. Hook, K.E.; Garza, S.J.; Lira, M.E.; Ching, K.A.; Lee, N.V.; Cao, J.; Yuan, J.; Ye, J.; Ozeck, M.; Shi, S.T.; et al. An integrated genomic approach to identify predictive biomarkers of response to the aurora kinase inhibitor PF-03814735. *Mol. Cancer Ther.* **2012**, *11*, 710–719. [CrossRef]
35. Bull, J.A.; Mech, F.; Quaiser, T.; Waters, S.L.; Byrne, H.M. Mathematical modelling reveals cellular dynamics within tumour spheroids. *PLoS Comput. Biol.* **2020**, *16*, e1007961. [CrossRef]
36. Mukomoto, R.; Nashimoto, Y.; Terai, T.; Imaizumi, T.; Hiramoto, K.; Ino, K.; Yokokawa, R.; Miura, T.; Shiku, H. Oxygen consumption rate of tumour spheroids during necrotic-like core formation. *Analyst* **2020**, *145*, 6342–6348. [CrossRef]
37. Tindall, M.J.; Dyson, L.; Smallbone, K.; Maini, P.K. Modelling acidosis and the cell cycle in multicellular tumour spheroids. *J. Theor. Biol.* **2012**, *298*, 107–115. [CrossRef]
38. Reipsch, F.; Biersack, B.; Lucas, H.; Schobert, R.; Mueller, T. Imidazole Analogs of Vascular-Disrupting Combretastatin A-4 with Pleiotropic Efficacy against Resistant Colorectal Cancer Models. *Int. J. Mol. Sci.* **2021**, *22*, 13082. [CrossRef]
39. Ketteler, J.; Klein, D. Caveolin-1, cancer and therapy resistance. *Int. J. Cancer* **2018**, *143*, 2092–2104. [CrossRef] [PubMed]
40. Li, Z.; Wang, N.; Huang, C.; Bao, Y.; Jiang, Y.; Zhu, G. Downregulation of caveolin-1 increases the sensitivity of drug-resistant colorectal cancer HCT116 cells to 5-fluorouracil. *Oncol. Lett.* **2017**, *13*, 483–487. [CrossRef]
41. Luo, F.; Li, J.; Liu, J.; Liu, K. Stabilizing and upregulating Axin with tankyrase inhibitor reverses 5-fluorouracil chemoresistance and proliferation by targeting the WNT/caveolin-1 axis in colorectal cancer cells. *Cancer Gen. Ther.* **2022**, *29*, 1707–1719. [CrossRef]
42. Rodel, F.; Capalbo, G.; Rodel, C.; Weiss, C. Caveolin-1 as a prognostic marker for local control after preoperative chemoradiation therapy in rectal cancer. *Int. J. Radiat. Oncol. Biol. Phys.* **2009**, *73*, 846–852. [CrossRef]
43. Okita, A.; Takahashi, S.; Ouchi, K.; Inoue, M.; Watanabe, M.; Endo, M.; Honda, H.; Yamada, Y.; Ishioka, C. Consensus molecular subtypes classification of colorectal cancer as a predictive factor for chemotherapeutic efficacy against metastatic colorectal cancer. *Oncotarget* **2018**, *9*, 18698–18711. [CrossRef] [PubMed]
44. Stintzing, S.; Wirapati, P.; Lenz, H.J.; Neureiter, D.; Fischer von Weikersthal, L.; Decker, T.; Kiani, A.; Kaiser, F.; Al-Batran, S.; Heintges, T.; et al. Consensus molecular subgroups (CMS) of colorectal cancer (CRC) and first-line efficacy of FOLFIRI plus cetuximab or bevacizumab in the FIRE3 (AIO KRK-0306) trial. *Ann. Oncol.* **2019**, *30*, 1796–1803. [CrossRef]

45. Lenz, H.J.; Ou, F.S.; Venook, A.P.; Hochster, H.S.; Niedzwiecki, D.; Goldberg, R.M.; Mayer, R.J.; Bertagnolli, M.M.; Blanke, C.D.; Zemla, T.; et al. Impact of Consensus Molecular Subtype on Survival in Patients With Metastatic Colorectal Cancer: Results From CALGB/SWOG 80405 (Alliance). *J. Clin. Oncol.* **2019**, *37*, 1876–1885. [CrossRef] [PubMed]
46. Ten Hoorn, S.; de Back, T.R.; Sommeijer, D.W.; Vermeulen, L. Clinical Value of Consensus Molecular Subtypes in Colorectal Cancer: A Systematic Review and Meta-Analysis. *J. Natl. Cancer Inst.* **2021**, *114*, 503–516. [CrossRef]
47. Del Rio, M.; Mollevi, C.; Bibeau, F.; Vie, N.; Selves, J.; Emile, J.F.; Roger, P.; Gongora, C.; Robert, J.; Tubiana-Mathieu, N.; et al. Molecular subtypes of metastatic colorectal cancer are associated with patient response to irinotecan-based therapies. *Eur. J. Cancer* **2017**, *76*, 68–75. [CrossRef] [PubMed]
48. Song, N.; Pogue-Geile, K.L.; Gavin, P.G.; Yothers, G.; Kim, S.R.; Johnson, N.L.; Lipchik, C.; Allegra, C.J.; Petrelli, N.J.; O'Connell, M.J.; et al. Clinical Outcome From Oxaliplatin Treatment in Stage II/III Colon Cancer According to Intrinsic Subtypes: Secondary Analysis of NSABP C-07/NRG Oncology Randomized Clinical Trial. *JAMA Oncol.* **2016**, *2*, 1162–1169. [CrossRef]
49. Zanoni, M.; Piccinini, F.; Arienti, C.; Zamagni, A.; Santi, S.; Polico, R.; Bevilacqua, A.; Tesei, A. 3D tumor spheroid models for in vitro therapeutic screening: A systematic approach to enhance the biological relevance of data obtained. *Sci. Rep.* **2016**, *6*, 19103. [CrossRef]
50. Losada, A.; Hirano, T. Dynamic molecular linkers of the genome: The first decade of SMC proteins. *Genes Dev.* **2005**, *19*, 1269–1287. [CrossRef]
51. Neumayer, G.; Belzil, C.; Gruss, O.J.; Nguyen, M.D. TPX2: Of spindle assembly, DNA damage response, and cancer. *Cell Mol. Life Sci.* **2014**, *71*, 3027–3047. [CrossRef]
52. Manios, K.; Tsiambas, E.; Stavrakis, I.; Stamatelopoulos, A.; Kavantzas, N.; Agrogiannis, G.; Lazaris, A.C. c-Fos/c-Jun transcription factors in non-small cell lung carcinoma. *J. BUON* **2020**, *25*, 2141–2143.
53. Shaulian, E.; Karin, M. AP-1 as a regulator of cell life and death. *Nat. Cell Biol.* **2002**, *4*, E131–E136. [CrossRef] [PubMed]
54. Tsiambas, E.; Mastronikolis, N.; Fotiades, P.P.; Kyrodimos, E.; Chrysovergis, A.; Papanikolaou, V.; Mastronikolis, S.; Peschos, D.; Roukas, D.; Ragos, V. c-Jun/c-Fos complex in laryngeal squamous cell carcinoma. *J. BUON* **2020**, *25*, 618–620. [PubMed]
55. Shen, J.; Zhang, Y.; Yu, H.; Shen, B.; Liang, Y.; Jin, R.; Liu, X.; Shi, L.; Cai, X. Role of DUSP1/MKP1 in tumorigenesis, tumor progression and therapy. *Cancer Med.* **2016**, *5*, 2061–2068. [CrossRef]
56. Wang, Z.; Xu, J.; Zhou, J.Y.; Liu, Y.; Wu, G.S. Mitogen-activated protein kinase phosphatase-1 is required for cisplatin resistance. *Cancer Res.* **2006**, *66*, 8870–8877. [CrossRef]
57. Lu, B.; Chen, X.; Liu, X.; Chen, J.; Qin, H.; Chen, S.; Zhao, Y. C/D box small nucleolar RNA SNORD104 promotes endometrial cancer by regulating the 2′-O-methylation of PARP1. *J. Transl. Med.* **2022**, *20*, 618. [CrossRef] [PubMed]
58. Zhang, L.; Xin, M.; Wang, P. Identification of a novel snoRNA expression signature associated with overall survival in patients with lung adenocarcinoma: A comprehensive analysis based on RNA sequencing dataset. *Math. Biosci. Eng.* **2021**, *18*, 7837–7860. [CrossRef]
59. LaBonia, G.J.; Lockwood, S.Y.; Heller, A.A.; Spence, D.M.; Hummon, A.B. Drug penetration and metabolism in 3D cell cultures treated in a 3D printed fluidic device: Assessment of irinotecan via MALDI imaging mass spectrometry. *Proteomics* **2016**, *16*, 1814–1821. [CrossRef]
60. Lv, D.; Hu, Z.; Lu, L.; Lu, H.; Xu, X. Three-dimensional cell culture: A powerful tool in tumor research and drug discovery. *Oncol. Lett.* **2017**, *14*, 6999–7010. [CrossRef]
61. Ramgolam, K.; Lauriol, J.; Lalou, C.; Lauden, L.; Michel, L.; de la Grange, P.; Khatib, A.M.; Aoudjit, F.; Charron, D.; Alcaide-Loridan, C.; et al. Melanoma spheroids grown under neural crest cell conditions are highly plastic migratory/invasive tumor cells endowed with immunomodulator function. *PLoS ONE* **2011**, *6*, e18784. [CrossRef] [PubMed]
62. Sant, S.; Johnston, P.A. The production of 3D tumor spheroids for cancer drug discovery. *Drug Discov. Today Technol.* **2017**, *23*, 27–36. [CrossRef] [PubMed]
63. Koch, J.; Monch, D.; Maass, A.; Gromoll, C.; Hehr, T.; Leibold, T.; Schlitt, H.J.; Dahlke, M.H.; Renner, P. Three dimensional cultivation increases chemo- and radioresistance of colorectal cancer cell lines. *PLoS ONE* **2021**, *16*, e0244513. [CrossRef] [PubMed]
64. Hammond, W.A.; Swaika, A.; Mody, K. Pharmacologic resistance in colorectal cancer: A review. *Ther. Adv. Med. Oncol.* **2016**, *8*, 57–84. [CrossRef] [PubMed]

Disclaimer/Publisher's Note: The statements, opinions and data contained in all publications are solely those of the individual author(s) and contributor(s) and not of MDPI and/or the editor(s). MDPI and/or the editor(s) disclaim responsibility for any injury to people or property resulting from any ideas, methods, instructions or products referred to in the content.

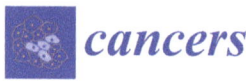

Article

Molecular Classification of Colorectal Cancer by microRNA Profiling: Correlation with the Consensus Molecular Subtypes (CMS) and Validation of miR-30b Targets

Mateo Paz-Cabezas [1,†], Tania Calvo-López [1,†], Alejandro Romera-Lopez [1], Daniel Tabas-Madrid [2], Jesus Ogando [2], María-Jesús Fernández-Aceñero [3], Javier Sastre [1], Alberto Pascual-Montano [2], Santos Mañes [2], Eduardo Díaz-Rubio [1] and Beatriz Perez-Villamil [1,*]

[1] Genomics and Microarrays Laboratory, Medical Oncology Department, Instituto de Investigación Sanitaria San Carlos (IdiSSC), Hospital Clinico San Carlos, 28040 Madrid, Spain
[2] Immunology and Oncology Department, Centro Nacional de Biotecnología (CSIC), 28049 Madrid, Spain
[3] Surgical Pathology, Instituto de Investigación Sanitaria San Carlos (IdiSSC), Hospital Clinico San Carlos, 28040 Madrid, Spain
* Correspondence: beatriz.perezvillamil@salud.madrid.org; Tel.: +34-91-330-3348
† These authors contributed equally to this work.

Citation: Paz-Cabezas, M.; Calvo-López, T.; Romera-Lopez, A.; Tabas-Madrid, D.; Ogando, J.; Fernández-Aceñero, M.-J.; Sastre, J.; Pascual-Montano, A.; Mañes, S.; Díaz-Rubio, E.; et al. Molecular Classification of Colorectal Cancer by microRNA Profiling: Correlation with the Consensus Molecular Subtypes (CMS) and Validation of miR-30b Targets. *Cancers* 2022, 14, 5175. https://doi.org/10.3390/cancers14215175

Academic Editor: Luis Franco

Received: 27 September 2022
Accepted: 19 October 2022
Published: 22 October 2022

Publisher's Note: MDPI stays neutral with regard to jurisdictional claims in published maps and institutional affiliations.

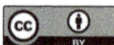

Copyright: © 2022 by the authors. Licensee MDPI, Basel, Switzerland. This article is an open access article distributed under the terms and conditions of the Creative Commons Attribution (CC BY) license (https://creativecommons.org/licenses/by/4.0/).

Simple Summary: Colorectal cancer is one of the most significant causes of cancer mortality worldwide. Patients stratification is central to improve clinical practice and the Consensus Molecular Subtypes (CMS) have been validated as a useful tool to predict both prognosis and treatment response. This is the first study describing that microRNA profiling can define colorectal cancer CMS subtypes as well as mRNA profiling. MicroRNAs small size facilitates its analysis in serum facilitating a real-time analysis of the disease course. Three microRNA subtypes are identified: miR-LS is associated with the low-stroma/CMS2-subtype; miR-MI with the mucinous-MSI/CMS1-subtype and miR-HS with the high-stroma/CMS4-subtype. MicroRNA novel subtypes and association to the CMS classification were externally validated using TGCA data. Analyzing both mRNAs and miRs in the same population enabled identification of miR target genes and altered biological pathways. A miR-mRNA interaction screening and regulatory network selected major miR targets and was functionally validated for the miR30b/SCL6A4 pair.

Abstract: Colorectal cancer consensus molecular subtypes (CMSs) are widely accepted and constitutes the basis for patient stratification to improve clinical practice. We aimed to find whether miRNAs could reproduce molecular subtypes, and to identify miRNA targets associated to the High-stroma/CMS4 subtype. The expression of 939 miRNAs was analyzed in tumors classified in CMS. TALASSO was used to find gene-miRNA interactions. A miR-mRNA regulatory network was constructed using Cytoscape. Candidate gene-miR interactions were validated in 293T cells. Hierarchical-Clustering identified three miRNA tumor subtypes (miR-LS; miR-MI; and miR-HS) which were significantly associated ($p < 0.001$) to the reported mRNA subtypes. miR-LS correlated with the low-stroma/CMS2; miR-MI with the mucinous-MSI/CMS1 and miR-HS with high-stroma/CMS4. MicroRNA tumor subtypes and association to CMSs were validated with TCGA datasets. TALASSO identified 1462 interactions ($p < 0.05$) out of 21,615 found between 176 miRs and 788 genes. Based on the regulatory network, 88 miR-mRNA interactions were selected as candidates. This network was functionally validated for the pair miR-30b/SLC6A6. We found that miR-30b overexpression silenced 3′-UTR-SLC6A6-driven luciferase expression in 293T-cells; mutation of the target sequence in the 3′-UTR-SLC6A6 prevented the miR-30b inhibitory effect. In conclusion CRC subtype classification using a miR-signature might facilitate a real-time analysis of the disease course and treatment response.

Keywords: colorectal cancer; microRNAs; microarray gene-expression profiling; molecular classification; prognostic factors

1. Introduction

Colorectal cancer (CRC) represents a major health problem being the third most frequent cancer and the second cause of cancer death worldwide [1]. CRC is traditionally classified according to clinical and morphological characteristics in TNM stages (American Joint Committee on Cancer). However, the phenotypic diversity of this disease and its clinical behavior are insufficiently explained by the simple histological grade classification and clinical factors in current use. Our group identified four tumor subtypes by transcriptional profiling [2] that largely overlaps in both, subtype distribution and clinic-biological interpretation with the four Consensus Molecular Subtypes (CMS) [3]. Recently relevant reports have confirmed the prognostic and predictive value of CMS subtypes in phase III clinical trials [4–6] supporting the use of the CMS classification as a useful tool for patient management. MicroRNAs (miRs) are noncoding small RNAs that regulate gene activity post-transcriptionally. In cancer, they can function as oncogenes or as tumor suppressors, and miR signatures can serve as promising biomarkers [7,8]. Previous attempts to associate miRs and CRC subtypes have identified members of the miR-200 family downregulated in the mesenchymal/CMS4 subtype [9,10]. However, no other associations between specific miRs and the other three tumor subtypes have been described. In this context, using unsupervised hierarchical clustering analysis, we have analyzed miR expression patterns in the CRC samples used in our previous molecular subtyping study [2] to investigate if miRs allowed CRC tumors classification as well as mRNAs. Since one miR can regulate multiple mRNAs, analyzing both mRNAs and miRs in the same population is an excellent strategy to determine miR target genes and identify altered biological pathways and regulatory networks. In this study we report the identification of three miR molecular subtypes that associate to the described CMSs. This can be an important advance, since it would allow the search of the relevant miRs in serum/plasma of patients and their classification, as other authors have reported for pancreatic adenocarcinoma [11], without the need to obtain biopsies or fragments of the tumor, facilitating real-time analysis of the course of the disease and of the response to the treatment. A just released report, develops a miR classifier using supervised analysis to predict four miR subtypes assigned from the four mRNA CMS subtypes [12]. Using in silico machine learning the study of Adam et al. [12] converts the four mRNA-CMS subtypes to four miR-subtypes. This procedure is different than ours. We used unsupervised analysis that does not constrain any subtype number or class.

2. Materials and Methods

2.1. Patients and RNA

For this study we have analyzed the same CRC patients' cohort used for our previous study, including RNA samples [2]. Tumor samples were taken from the Biobank of the Hospital Clinico San Carlos. The study was conducted according to the guidelines of the Declaration of Helsinki, and approved by the Institutional Review Board and Ethics Committee of Hospital Clinico San Carlos. RNA was extracted from fresh frozen tumor samples using TRIZOL and the homogenizer Ultraturrax T8-S8N-5G. RNA quality was measured with Agilent Bioanalyzer 2100. Only tumors with an RNA Integrity Number (RIN) ≥ 6.5 were included in the analysis.

2.2. MicroRNA Expression Analysis and Tumor Classification

Agilent miR 21827 microarrays were used to analyze the expression of 939 miRs in 97 CRC tumor samples and 19 normal colon samples. Fluorescence was measured and quantile-normalized using Agilent scanner, Feature Extraction and GeneSpring software. 176 miRs were present in 90% of the samples and therefore considered for the following data analysis. Expression data was median centered and Average-linkage-hierarchical clustering (centered Pearson correlation) was carried out to perform unsupervised tumor classification considering the 176 expressed miRs in the 88 tumor samples from our previous study [2] (complete data set was submitted to ArrayExpress (E-MTAB-9288)). Then, Differential expression between miR subtypes was analyzed using one-way ANOVA, Student

Newman-Keuls (SNK) post hoc test and Benjamini-Hochberg multiple test correction. miRs were considered as differentially expressed only if global $p < 0.05$ and fold change > 1.5 considering any of the pairwise subtype comparison.

2.3. Identification of miRs Targets and Correlation with mRNA Expression

TALASSO software [13] was used to find miR-mRNA interactions between the 1722 genes selected from our previous study [2] and the 176 expressed miRs. In order to predict miR-target interactions, TALASSO analyzes miRs expression changes and down-regulation of their putative targets. As criteria to select the most relevant miR-transcript interactions, a class comparison analysis was carried out to find differentially expressed genes between groups.

Unpaired Student-t-test with Benjamini-Hochberg multiple correction was carried out between normal colon tissue and tumors from the low-stroma, high-stroma and Mucinous-MSI subtypes. Selected genes were considered as differentially expressed at $p < 0.05$ and >1.5-fold expression. Then, miRNA-mRNA predicted interactions were used to construct a regulatory network using Cytoscape software v3.6.1 [14]. Only the largest connected component was considered for each network. Centrality measures were determined using NetworkAnalyzer and CentiScaPe 2.2. Clusters with higher interconnections were unveiled using ClusterViz and EAGLE algorithm with default options (CliqueSize Threshold = 3, ComplexSize Threshold = 2). Two global centrality measurements, radiality and closeness centrality, were considered to rank the most relevant nodes, as they reflect not only the immediate connections of a node (the degree of each node) but the overall structure of the network. Combining two centrality measurers increase the reliability of this kind of approaches to predict the most relevant genes in an interaction network [15]. In our data, those two topological parameters predicted the same upmost central genes, considering that miRNA-mRNA interactions between the 20 upmost central nodes for each subtype were selected as putative candidates, along with the interactions between mRNA and miRNAs involved in the most relevant cluster for each subtype.

Potential microRNA-mRNA interaction candidates were annotated and scored using information from [16] with two different combined validated predicting scores (Weighted Scoring by Precision (WSP) and logistic regression score (LRS)). Previously experimentally validated interactions were determined using four different databases Tarbase (http://www.microrna.gr/tarbase), miRTarBase (http://miRTarBase.mbc.nctu.edu.tw/), miR-Walk (http://mirwalk.umm.uni-heidelberg.de) and miRecords (http://miRecords.umn.edu/miRecords/), and also with significant Pearson correlation p-values from Starbase (http://starbase.sysu.edu.cn/). MicroRNA binding sites were predicted by five different algorithms Pita (https://tools4mirs.org/software/target_prediction/pita/), FindTar (http://bio.sz.tsinghua.edu.cn/findtar/), Miranda (https://www.mirbase.org), rnaHybrid (http://bibiserv.techfak.uni-bielefeld.de/rnahybrid/) and TargetScan (http://genes.mit.edu/targetscan). MicroRNA candidate prioritization was assessed using an automated script, considering that the last accession date, for all databases accession dates, are 21 April 2016. Candidate gene-miR interactions were scored and biologically validated in HEK-293T cell line.

2.4. External Dataset Validation

TCGA data for miRNA and mRNA expression in CRC were downloaded from the repository using TCGA Biolinks [17] package, RNAseq using Illumina HiSeq platform was selected to obtain 285 samples with 20,531 features each. Normalized gene expression data for mRNA was classified in CMS subtypes using CMSclassifier R package 3 according to the nearest CMS criteria. Sample clustering: TCGA raw data for miRNA consisted of 444 samples and 1046 features. Expression data from RNAseq was processed using DESeq2 [18] to obtain normalized counts matrix. Prior to the unsupervised clustering of samples according to miRNA expression, we performed a 3D-PCA visualization to filter out those samples with an outlier expression pattern, following this criterion 5 samples from the initial dataset were excluded. Afterwards, gene features with less than 10 counts in more than 90% of samples were filtered out, resulting in 336 features per sample. Hierarchical clustering on samples was performed using hclust function over log2 transformed normalized expression matrix. Pearson correlation as distance measure and ward linkage as agglomeration method were chosen. In order to create the heatmap visualization, gene features were also classified using the same parameters. Finally, subtype association between miRNA and mRNA classification was addressed using Chi-square test (χ^2).

2.5. MicroRNAs Differentially Expressed between Tumor-Epithelia and Tumor-Stroma

MicroRNAs expression data were downloaded from GSE35602 [19]. Differential expression between the epithelial and stromal components of the tumor was analyzed by T-Test and Benjamini-Hochberg Multiple Correction Test using GeneSpring Dx 14.9 software. Selected miRs were considered as differentially expressed at $p < 0.05$ and >1.5-fold expression between tumor epithelia and tumor stroma.

2.6. Evaluation of miRs-Subtypes Using miRaCL20 Classifier

MicroRNAs expression data (miRNA-Seq) from TCGA-COAD were classified using miRaCl classifier [12] available at Github/rsmadam/CMS-miRaCl. Subtype association between miRNA and mRNA classification was determined using Chi-square test (χ^2).

2.7. Cell Lines, Transformation, Transfection and Luciferase Assay

Human HEK-293T cells were grown in Dulbecco's Modified Eagle Medium (DMEM) supplemented with 10% fetal bovine serum (FBS), penicillin-streptomycin, L-Glutamine and NaPyr in a humidified incubator at 37 °C with 5% of CO_2. HmiR0133-MR03 (hsa-miR-30b), HmiT070741-MT06 (FAP), HmiT017418a-MT06 (SLC6A6-A), HmiT017418b-MT06 (SLC6A6-B) and miR-Control plasmids from GeneCopoeia were used. XL1-Blue bacteria were transformed by thermal shock and DNA was extracted using Genomed kit (JETSTAR). HEK-293T cells were cultured in triplicate in 24-well plates (0.05 × 106 cells/well). They were transfected with miR-30b and miR-Control, using Lipofectamine 2000 (Invitrogen). Cells were selected with puromycin and miR-30b levels was checked by RT-PCR using Hs03303066_pri (TaqManTMPri-miR Assays) oligonucleotide and U6 as control. HEK-293T-miR30b-expressing cells were transfected with SLC6A6-A, SLC6A6-B or FAP plasmids. Vectors of these plasmids include Firefly and Renilla luciferase reporter genes. After 12 and 24 h Firefly and Renilla luciferases activity were measured using Dual Luciferase Assay Kit (Promega Madison, WI, USA) in a Tecan Infinite 200 Luminometer. Luciferase intensity measurement was performed by triplicate per condition and analyzed as described [20].

2.8. Site-Directed Mutagenesis

Predicted miR-30b interaction site at the SLC6A6 3′-UTR (2225-TGTTTAC-2231 nucleotides) was modified using QuikChange site-directed mutagenesis kit (Agilent Technologies, Palo Alto, CA, U.S.A). The oligonucleotide 5′-cctatgagaatctaatgttattacaaagcaggaaa gccgccggcc-3′ (2207 to 2251 nucleotides) was designed using QuikChange Primer Design Tool. G2226T, T2228G and C2231A nucleotides were changed to destabilize the predicted interaction with miR-30b.

2.9. Statistical Analysis

Luciferase analysis results were analyzed using Student's t-test to compare mutated vs control mir-30b. Subtype association was addressed using χ^2 Chi-square test. In order to compare the distribution of qualitative variables between groups Fisher exact test was applied (as all the variables presented less than 5 events in at least one of the categories) and "Mantel-Haenzel Test" for b-catenin linear categories. Mean comparison of quantitative variables between subtypes was performed using Kruskal-Wallis test. Statistical analysis was performed using GraphPad Prism 6 and R software.

3. Results

3.1. Tumor Classification Based on miR Expression Patterns and Association to mRNA Subtypes

MicroRNAs arranged tumor samples in three clusters (Figure 1). There is a significant association ($p < 0.001$) of the three miR subtypes with the four mRNA subtypes identified by us [2] as well as with the CMS subtypes [3] (Table 1). Supplementary Table S1 shows the classification of the 88 tumors from our previous study [2] using the SSP and RF [3]. miR-Cluster-1 contains 27 tumors showing a higher proportion of tumors belonging to the low-stroma-subtype, as well as the lowest proportion of stromal component in the tumors; consequently, we named this subtype miR-LS (miR-Low-Stroma). Additionally, miR-LS show a significant association with CMS2 whether random forest (RF) or single sample predictor (SSP) were used for sample classification. The highest proportion of tumors from the mucinous-MSI-subtype as well as from CMS1 are in miR-cluster-2 which contains 31 tumors; mucinous histology as well as microsatellite instability (MSI) are associated to this cluster, accordingly we term this cluster miR-MI (Mucinous, Instable). Cluster-3 with 30 tumors contains the highest proportion of tumors of the high-stroma-subtype as well as the highest proportion of stroma in the tumors; we term this cluster miR-HS (High Stroma). Like-wise, the highest proportion of tumors classified as CMS4 associate to miR-HS subtype.

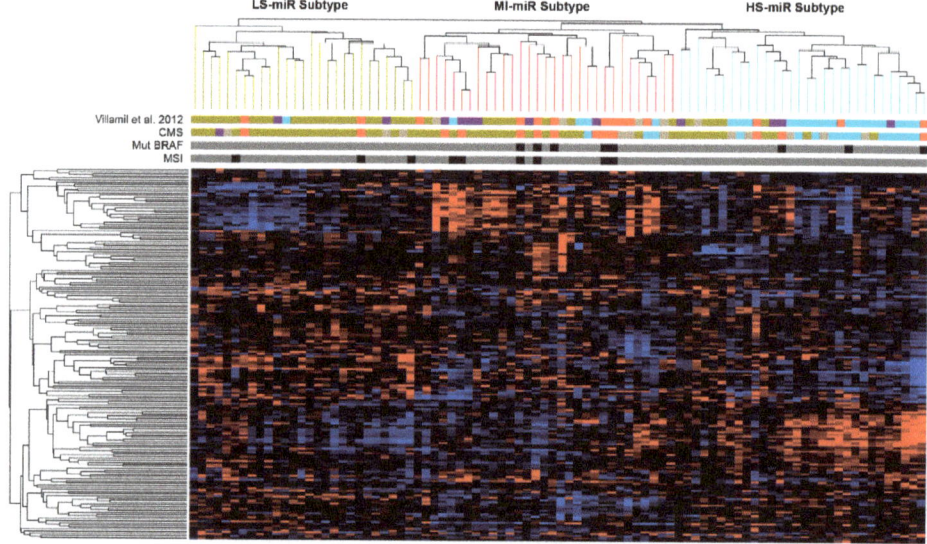

Figure 1. Molecular classification of tumors and miRs. Centered Pearson correlation and average-linkage-hierarchical clustering of the 88 tumor samples and 176 miRs in three miR tumor subtypes (miR-LS pistachio-green lines; miR-MI red lines and miR-HS light blue lines). Villamil et al. subtypes, CMSs, BRAF mutations and MSI are specified below the tree. Low-stroma-subtype/CMS2: pistachio green bar; mucinous-MSI-subtype/CMS1: red bar; high-stroma-subtype/CMS4: light blue; immunoglobulin-related: purple bar; unclassified samples: beige bar. Black bar: BRAF mutated and MSI; grey bar: BRAF wt and MSS. Heatmap intensities: 3.099 (red) to −3.099 (dark blue).

Table 1. Association of miRNA clusters to Villamil et al. subtypes, to CMS and to clinic-biological parameters.

		miR-LS (n = 27)	miR-MI (n = 30)	miR-HS (n = 31)	p Value
Villamil et al., 2012 Subtypes	Low Stroma	22	7	6	
	Immunoglobul	2	6	4	
	High Stroma	1	4	17	0.000 χ^2
	Mucinous-MSI	2	9	3	
	Unclassified	0	4	1	
RF	CMS1	1	7	2	
	CMS2	15	9	10	
	CMS3	4	0	0	0.000 χ^2
	CMS4	0	3	13	
	NA	7	11	6	
SSP	CMS1	2	8	3	
	CMS2	21	16	11	
	CMS3	1	0	0	0.001 χ^2
	CMS4	0	3	12	
	NA	3	3	5	
Microsatellite	MSS	24	24	31	0.036 χ^2
	MSI	3	6	0	
Histologic type	Conventional	26	24	28	0.144 χ^2
	Mucinous	1	6	3	
BRAF	WT	27	25	28	0.091 χ^2
	Mut	0	5	3	
FF Stroma	Range	(5–28)	(5–40)	(8–65)	0.000 ^{KW}
	Median	7.5	13.75	22.5	
FFPE Stroma	Range	(5–20)	(5–40)	(5–60)	0.004 ^{KW}
	Median	10	10	20	

RF: Random Forest, SSP: single sample predictor. FF: Fresh-Frozen, FFPE: Formalin Fixed Paraffin embedded. ^{KW}: Kruskal Wallis, χ^2: Chi-Squared test.

3.2. External Dataset Validation

CRC data from TCGA were classified according to the CMS subtypes, resulting in the following subtype distribution for the 285 samples: CMS1 (59), CMS2 (144), CMS3 (33) and CMS4 (49). Hierarchical clustering of miRNA expression (Supplementary Figure S1) unveiled three different groups according to miR expression with the following correspondence with CMS subtypes determined by mRNA expression (Supplementary Table S2), this association presented a significant correlation ($p < 0.0001$) and was performed in those 228 samples with mRNA and miRNA data.

3.3. Comparison between miR-LS, miR-HS and miR-MI with the miRCL20 Classifier Subtypes

Association between unsupervised miRNA subtypes (miR-LS, miR-HS, miR-MI) and miRaCl20 (CMS subtyping using miRNA data) was addressed in both TCGA data and Agilent CRC miRNA microarray dataset.

CMS distribution in TCGA data according to miRaCl20 supervised classifier resulted in 41 CMS1, 90 CMS2, 22 CMS3, 73 CMS4 and 2 unclassified for the total 228 samples. In the case of the microarray dataset samples were distributed: 23 CMS1, 44 CMS2, 9 CMS3 and 12 CMS4 for the 88 samples.

Association between the three miR subtypes (miR-LS, miR-HS, miR-MI) and miRaCl CMS subtypes (Supplementary Figures S2 and S3) is significant resulting pvalue of Chi-square test (χ^2) was $< 2 \times 10^{-16}$ in both cases, with a wider consensus in high-stroma- and low-stroma- subtypes (CMS4 and CMS2).

3.4. Stromal or Epithelial Localization of the miRs Differentially Expressed between Subtypes

Stroma proportion is associated to miR-subtypes (Table 1) but our study was not designed to distinguish miR expression between the stromal or epithelial components of the tumor. To find the contribution of stroma or epithelia to miR expression we took advantage of the study of Nishida et al. [19] in which miR expression was specifically analyzed using laser microdissection, in tumor stroma and in tumor epithelia. From the 176 miRs selected for tumor classification, 45 miRs were significantly differentially expressed at $p < 0.05$ and FC > 1.5 between tumor epithelia and tumor stroma.

The 176 miRs were also arranged in clusters. Among all, three of them showed the most significant miRs differentially expressed between clusters. Interestingly, two of these clusters contained miRs differentially expressed between tumor-stroma and tumor-epithelia as well (Supplementary Table S3).

MicroRNA-Cluster-A contains miRs that are down-regulated mainly in the miR-LS-subtype and up-regulated in the miR-MI-subtype (Figure 2A). It is worth noting that among the miRs of this cluster are viral miRs such as the human cytomegalovirus-encoded miR, hcmv-miR-UL70-3p and the Kaposi's sarcoma-associated herpesvirus miRs: kshv-miR-K12-3 and kshv-miR-K12-10b. Other relevant miRs of this cluster that have been shown to be involved in CRC progression are miR-572 [21], miR-1246 [22], and miR-494 [23]. This group of miRs does not show particularly a specific stromal or epithelial localization (Supplementary Table S3).

MicroRNA-Cluster-B contains miRs that are particularly inhibited in the miR-HS-subtype (Figure 2B). miR-141; miR-200a; miR-200b; miR-200c and miR-429 are in this cluster and belong to the miR-200 family. Other relevant miRs down-regulated in this cluster are miR-378 and miR-194. The miRs of this cluster are down-regulated in the stroma and up-regulated in the epithelia (Supplementary Table S3).

MicroRNA-Cluster-C contains miRs that are upregulated in the miR-HS-subtype (Figure 2C). Members of the miR-30 family and of the miR-100 family such as miR-100, miR-125 and miR-99 are in microRNA-Cluster-C. Other relevant miRs of this cluster are miR-143 and miR-145. These miRs are up-regulated in the stroma and down-regulated in the epithelia (Supplementary Table S3).

3.5. Identification of miRs Targets, Selection of Relevant Interactions Associated to Subtypes and Altered Pathways

TALASSO software [13] identified 1462 significant ($p < 0.05$) interactions between 176 miRs and 788 genes out of the 21615 putative interactions (Supplementary Table S4). Out of the 788 genes showing significant miR interactions, 166 genes were differentially expressed in Low-stroma/subtype, 158 in High-stroma/subtype and 78 in Mucinous-MSI/subtype.

In order to identify relevant targets in miR-mRNA interaction patterns, three subtype specific network graphs were generated using those predicted interactions with differential expression (Supplementary Figure S4). MicroRNAs and mRNAs were represented as nodes, connected according to the in-silico predicted interactions ($p < 0.05$), topological parameters and selecting criteria for the obtained networks are available in Supplementary Table S5.

A list of 88 mRNA-miR interactions was annotated and ranked (Supplementary Table S6), After discarding those interactions that were already biologically validated and taking in consideration the observed expression profiles between subtypes, network centrality values and annotated scores for each interaction, we decided to focus on studying miR-30b-FAP and miR-30b-SLC6A6 interactions as final candidates for biological validation. Moreover, miR-30b and their targets (FAP and SLC6A6) belong to the most connected cluster in miR-HS interaction network (Figure 3), being the subtype featuring the lowest survival.

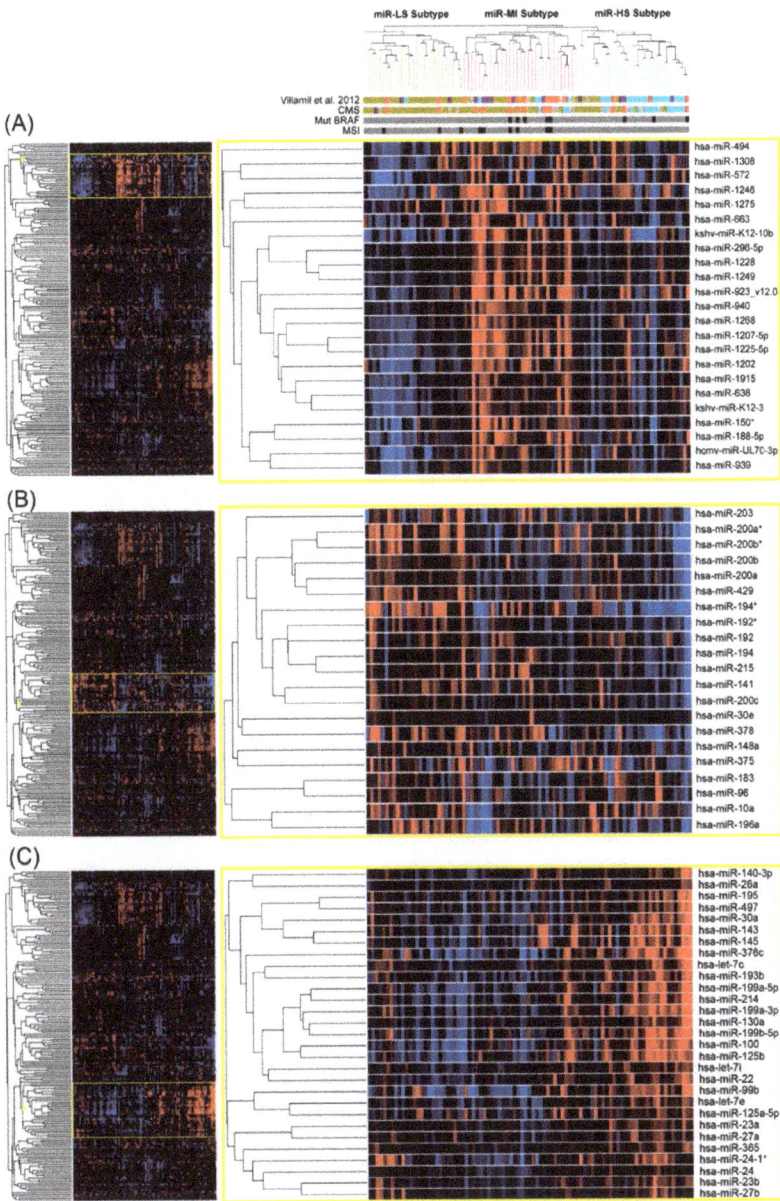

Figure 2. MicroRNAs distribution between Subtypes. (**A**) miRNA-Cluster-A: miRs down-regulated in the miR-LS-subtype and up-regulated in the miR-MI-subtype (23 miRs located in the heatmap between the 7th and the 29th miRs). (**B**) miRNA-Cluster-B: miRs inhibited in the miR-HS-subtype (21 miRs located in the heatmap between the 89th and the 109th miRs). (**C**) miRNA-Cluster-C: miRs upregulated in the miR-HS-subtype (29 miRs located in the heatmap between the 114th and the 142nd miRs). Heatmap intensities: 3.099 (red) to −3.099 (dark blue).

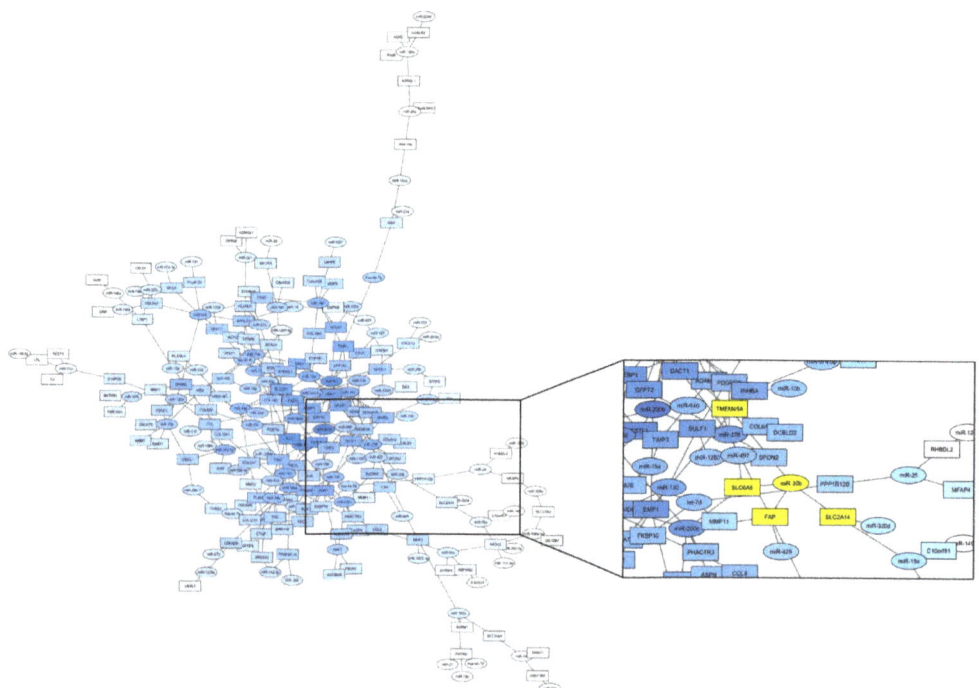

Figure 3. Regulatory Network of the High-Stroma/CMS4-miR-HS-subtype. Nodes reflect mRNAS (squares) and miRNAS (circles), while edges represent a predicted interaction between them. Grey intensity is mapped to each node's closeness centrality value, the lighter nodes being the most marginal nodes. Square details the interactions between miR-30b and their first neighbors (those genes with a predicted interaction) represented as striped squares.

3.6. SCL6A6 Up-Regulated in the High-Stroma/CMS4 Subtype Shows Specific Interaction with miR-30b In Vitro

The genes SLC6A6 and FAP, that are up-regulated in the High-stroma/CMS4 subtype, show in-silico interaction with miR-30b (Figure 3) which is down-regulated in tumors and in the stroma versus the epithelia component of the tumor (Supplementary Table S3). In order to validate in-silico predicted miR-transcript interactions, HEK-293T cells were transfected with a miR-30b expression plasmid and with reporter plasmids containing 3'UTR regions of the genes SLC6A6 and FAP. Since SLC6A6 3'UTR region is too long, two different reporter plasmids were used SLC6A6-A (between 2174 and 4573) carrying the putative miR-30b binding site (2225-TGTTTAC-2231) and SLC6A6-B (from 4353 to 6528 nucleotide). MicroRNA-30b significantly ($p = 0.0038$) decrease luciferase activity of the SLC6A6-A reporter plasmid. No significant differences in luciferase activity were found when the putative binding site in SLC6A6-A is mutated or when plasmid SLC6A6-B lacking miR-30b predicted binding site is used (Figure 4). When using FAP 3'UTR reporter plasmid, no differences were found between miR-30b and miR-Control (not shown). These results indicate that miR-30b binds to SLC6A6 3'UTR region to decrease SLC6A6 3'UTR-driven reporter expression.

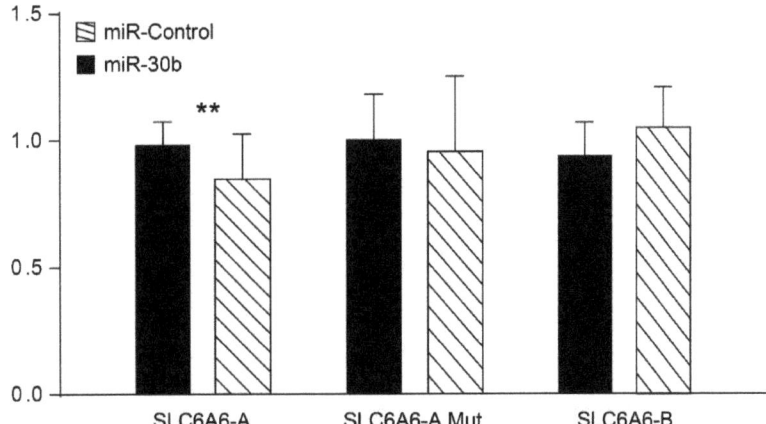

Figure 4. miR-30b target SLC6A6 expression. Luciferase reporter assays of HEK-293 cells transduced with pre-miR-30b or a control miR, and transfected with the 3′-UTR of SLC6A6-A wild-type, SLC6A6-A mutated in the target sequence, or SLC6A6-B lacking the predicted miR-30b binding site. Luciferase activity was normalized to that of control-transfected cells. Data shown as mean ± SEM of triplicates per experiment ($n = 3$). ** $p < 0.005$.

4. Discussion

Tumor molecular classification using unsupervised analysis of gene expression is a powerful tool that has been widely applied to distinguish tumor subgroups with shared biological programs and similar clinical behavior [24]. In contrast, tumor subtyping using unsupervised analysis of miR expression has been barely employed. MicroRNAs are shown to regulate gene expression, and both, miR and mRNA expression patterns are altered in cancer [8]. Since miRs and mRNAs coordinately regulate pathways involved in CRC, our hypothesis was that miR profiling, could also classify CRC in molecular subtypes and that these miR-subtypes, would probably correlate with the described mRNA tumor subtypes [2,3]. In this report we describe the identification of three tumor subtypes based on miR expression patterns that correlates significantly with the four tumor subtypes previously discovered [2,3]. Subtype miR-LS is associated with low-stroma-subtype and CMS2, miR-MI is associated with mucinous-MSI-subtype and CMS1 and miR-HS is associated with high-stroma-subtype and CMS4. Consequently, it is feasible to classify colorectal tumors in the described molecular subtypes by miRs expression profiling. As expected, this correlation is also maintained when the CMS are assigned using miRNA data through miRaCl classifier. Despite of being two strategies for miR classification, they differ in their approach; whereas miRaCl classifier is a supervised method to determine the CMS subtype according to the miR data, our classification does not take any kind of previous assumption to segregate samples. Despite those differences, both classifications have a high correlation in high and low stroma subtypes, supporting the continuous flow of evidence of the role of stroma in the course of the colorectal disease.

This could be an important advance, since it would allow in future the search of these miRs in plasma and the classification of patients without the need to obtain tumor fragments, facilitating real-time analysis of the course of the disease and the response to treatment, as has been described for pancreatic adenocarcinoma [11].

MicroRNA-Cluster-A contains miRs that are up-regulated in the miR-MI-subtype and shows high expression of miRs belonging to the herpesvirus family [25,26]. It has been shown that viral miRs are able to modulate innate immune responses. MSI and CMS1 tumors are characterized by a higher level of tumor-infiltrating lymphocytes and activation of immune evasion pathways. MicroRNA-Cluster-B contains miRs down-regulated in the miR-HS-subtype. These miRs have been shown to be down-regulated in the stroma compared to the epithelia component of the tumor [19] as well. MicroRNA-Cluster-B is mainly composed with members of the miR-200 family. It has been reported that methylation of the miR-200 promoter identifies tumors of the CMS4 [9,10] this agrees with the lower expression of these miRs in the miR-HS-subtype we found in our results. Other relevant miRs down-regulated in this cluster are miR-378 and miR-194. Low levels of miR-378 and miR-194 are implicated in the malignant phenotype of CRC and restoration of their expression inhibits EMT (Epithelial-Mesenchymal Transition) and prevent the migration and invasion of colon cancer cells [27,28].

MicroRNA-Cluster-C contains members of the miR-30 family and of the miR-100 family and are up-regulated in the miR-HS-subtype. Interestingly miRs of this cluster have been reported to be up-regulated in the stroma and down-regulated in the epithelia component of the tumor [19]. Overexpression of miR-100 and miR-125b has been associated with resistance to cetuximab treatment [29]. Other relevant miRs of this cluster are miR-143 and miR-145, these miRs are frequently reduced in colon cancer [30]. We found that when compared with normal colon tissue, tumor miR-143 and miR-145 levels are down regulated around three-fold in clusters miR-LS and miR-MI. However, miR-143 and miR-145 are up-regulated in miR-HS subtype when compared to the other miR clusters but still inhibited with respect to normal colon tissue. An elegant report shows that miR-143 and miR-145 are expressed in the intestinal mesenchyme [31]; this could explain the higher miR-143 and miR-145 in the miR-HS-subtype.

Appropriate integration of miR and mRNA expression profiles is essential to properly understand regulatory pathways and cellular dysfunction in CRC. Elucidating miR targets by bioinformatic analysis permits the identification of a panoply of miR-mRNA possible interactions that need to be ranked. Network analysis is an excellent tool for the selection of the most significant miR-mRNA interactions. Although relevant nodes were found in the three subtypes analyzed (low-stroma, high-stroma and Mucinous-MSI) for in vitro validation we focused on the high-stroma-subtype associated with a poor clinical outcome. The best scores within non-biologically-validated interactions were obtained between miR-30b which is down-regulated in the miR-HS subtype, and FAP or SLC6A6 genes, which are up-regulated in the high-stroma-subtype. High FAP and SLC6A6 levels are associated with worse prognosis in CRC [32,33]. We could not biologically validate miR-30b and FAP interaction; however, miR-30b has been shown to silence SLC6A6 expression. Since higher levels of SLC6A6 are associated with maintenance of stem-cells properties and with chemoresistance [33] restoring miR-30b could be a promising strategy for the treatment of CRC patients of the High-stroma/CMS4 subtype.

5. Conclusions

In summary, we show that miR profiles classify colorectal tumors with a straight correlation with the molecular subtypes identified by transcriptional profiling. miR-LS is associated with low-stroma/CMS2, miR-MI with the mucinous-MSI/CMS1 and miR-HS with high-stroma/CMS4 subtypes. Furthermore, the miR/mRNA network identified in High-stroma/CMS4 subtype was validated for the miR30b/SCL6A4 pair. Considering this, using miRs as a classifier provides a promising scenario, the classification of colorectal cancer patients by miR determination in plasma, allowing the classification of patients avoiding invasive procedures and allowing real-time analysis of the course of the disease and response to treatment by liquid biopsy.

Supplementary Materials: The following supporting information can be downloaded at: https://www.mdpi.com/article/10.3390/cancers14215175/s1, Table S1: Association of Villamil et al. 2012 Subtypes and CMS; Table S2: miR vs CMS subtypes in TCGA; Table S3: miRs differentially expressed between clusters; Table S4: TALASSO Interaction between miRs and target genes; Table S5: Topological parameters of regulatory networks; Table S6: Final interactions; Figure S1: Hierarchical Clustering of miR expression from the TCGA dataset; Figure S2: Association between miR subtypes (miR-LS; miR-MI; miR-HS) and miRaCL20A (miRNA CMS); Figure S3: TCGA: Association between miR subtypes (miR-LS; miR-MI; miR-HS) and miRaclCL20 (CMS); Figure S4: Regulatory networks of miRNA-mRNA interactions in each CRC tumor subtype.

Author Contributions: Conceptualization, S.M., E.D.-R. and B.P.-V.; methodology, T.C.-L., M.P.-C., A.R.-L. and J.O.; software, M.P.-C., D.T.-M. and A.P.-M.; validation, M.P.-C.,T.C.-L. and M.-J.F.-A.; formal analysis, M.P.-C., T.C.-L. and M.-J.F.-A.; investigation, M.P.-C., T.C.-L., J.S. and B.P.-V.; resources, S.M., E.D.-R., J.S. and B.P.-V.; data curation, M.P.-C., D.T.-M. and A.P.-M.; writing, M.P.-C., T.C.-L. and B.P.-V.; writing-review and editing, T.C.-L., M.P.-C. and B.P.-V.; visualization, M.P.-C., T.C.-L. and B.P.-V.; supervision, S.M. and B.P.-V.; project administration, B.P.-V.; funding acquisition, S.M., E.D.-R. and B.P.-V. All authors have read and agreed to the published version of the manuscript.

Funding: This work was partially funded by: IMMUNOTHERCAN Comunidad de Madrid S2017/BMD-3733; Fundacion Mutua Madrileña AP151962014; Bayer Healthcare BPV.M01BAY; Fundacion Rodriguez-Pascual EDRFERP.2013; Fundacion 2000 Merck-Serono F01MSER13. PID2020-116303RB-I00/MCIN/AEI/10.13039/501100011033.

Institutional Review Board Statement: The study was approved by the Institutional Review Board of the Hospital and the Ethical Committee. The study was conducted according to the guidelines of the Declaration of Helsinki, and approved by the Institutional Review Board and Ethics Committee of Hospital Clinico San Carlos. CEIC Hospital Clinico San Carlos n°: 17/241-E-BS.

Informed Consent Statement: The Bank of Tumors follows the rules established by the hospital including the patient consent approved by the Ethical Committee of the Hospital Clinico San Carlos.

Data Availability Statement: ArrayExpress E-MTAB-9288.

Conflicts of Interest: The authors declare no conflict of interest.

References

1. Sung, H.; Ferlay, J.; Siegel, R.L.; Laversanne, M.; Soerjomataram, I.; Jemal, A.; Bray, F. Global cancer statistics 2020: GLOBOCAN estimates of incidence and mortality worldwide for 36 cancers in 185 countries. *CA. Cancer J. Clin.* **2021**, *71*, 209–249. [CrossRef] [PubMed]
2. Perez-Villamil, B.; Romera-Lopez, A.; Hernandez-Prieto, S.; Lopez-Campos, G.; Calles, A.; Lopez-Asenjo, J.; Sanz-Ortega, J.; Fernandez-Perez, C.; Sastre, J.; Alfonso, R.; et al. Colon cancer molecular subtypes identified by expression profiling and associated to stroma, mucinous type and different clinical behaviour. *BMC Cancer* **2012**, *12*, 260. [CrossRef]
3. Guinney, J.; Dienstmann, R.; Wang, X.; de Reyniés, A.; Schlicker, A.; Soneson, C.; Marisa, L.; Roepman, P.; Nyamundanda, G.; Angelino, P.; et al. The consensus molecular subtypes of colorectal cancer. *Nat. Med.* **2015**, *21*, 1350–1356. [CrossRef] [PubMed]
4. Hoorn, S.T.; de Back, T.R.; Sommeijer, D.W.; Vermeulen, L. Clinical Value of Consensus Molecular Subtypes in Colorectal Cancer: A Systematic Review and Meta-Analysis. *J. Natl. Cancer Inst.* **2021**, *144*, 503–516. [CrossRef]
5. Mooi, J.K.; Wirapati, P.; Asher, R.; Lee, C.K.; Savas, P.; Price, T.J.; Townsend, A.; Hardingham, J.; Buchanan, D.; Williams, D.; et al. The prognostic impact of consensus molecular subtypes (CMS) and its predictive effects for bevacizumab benefit in metastatic colorectal cancer: Molecular analysis of the AGITG MAX clinical trial. *Ann. Oncol.* **2018**, *29*, 2240–2246. [CrossRef] [PubMed]
6. Lenz, H.; Ou, F.; Venook, A.P.; Hochster, H.S.; Niedzwiecki, D.; Goldberg, R.M.; Mayer, R.J.; Bertagnolli, M.M.; Blanke, C.D.; Zemla, T.; et al. Impact of consensus molecular subtype on survival in patients with metastatic colorectal cancer: Results from CALGB/SWOG 80405 (Alliance). *J. Clin. Oncol.* **2019**, *37*, 1876–1885. [CrossRef] [PubMed]
7. Al-Akhrass, H.; Christou, N. The clinical assessment of microrna diagnostic, prognostic, and theranostic value in colorectal cancer. *Cancers* **2021**, *13*, 2916. [CrossRef] [PubMed]
8. Rupaimoole, R.; Slack, F.J. MicroRNA therapeutics: Towards a new era for the management of cancer and other diseases. *Nat. Rev. Drug Discov.* **2017**, *16*, 203–221. [CrossRef] [PubMed]
9. Fessler, E.; Jansen, M.; De Sousa E Melo, F.; Zhao, L.; Prasentyanti, P.R.; Rodermond, H.; Kandimalla, R.; Linnekamp, J.F.; Franitza, M.; van Hoof, S.R.; et al. A multidimensional network approach reveals microRNAs as determinants of the mesenchymal colorectal cancer subtype. *Oncogene* **2016**, *35*, 6026–6037. [CrossRef] [PubMed]
10. Cantini, L.; Isella, C.; Petti, C.; Picco, G.; Chiola, S.; Ficarra, E.; Caselle, M.; Medico, E. MicroRNA-mRNA interactions underlying colorectal cancer molecular subtypes. *Nat. Commun.* **2015**, *6*, 8878. [CrossRef] [PubMed]
11. Kandimalla, R.; Shimura, T.; Mallik, S.; Sonohara, F.; Tsai, S.; Evans, D.B.; Kim, S.C.; Baba, H.; Kodera, Y.; Von Hoff, D.; et al. Identification of Serum miRNA Signature and Establishment of a Nomogram for Risk Stratification in Patients with Pancreatic Ductal Adenocarcinoma. *Ann. Surg.* **2022**, *275*, E229–E237. [CrossRef] [PubMed]
12. Adam, R.S.; Poel, D.; Ferreira, L.M.; Spronck, J.M.A.; de Back, T.R.; Torang, A.; Gomez, P.M.B.; ten Hoorn, S.; Markowetz, F.; Wang, X.; et al. Development of a miRNA-based classifier for detection of colorectal cancer molecular subtypes. *Mol. Oncol.* **2022**, *16*, 2693–2709. [CrossRef] [PubMed]

13. Muniategui, A.; Nogales-Cadenas, R.; Vázquez, M.; Aranguren, X.L.; Aguirre, X.; Luttun, A.; Prosper, F.; Pascual-Montano, A.; Rubio, A. Quantification of miRNA-mRNA interactions. *PLoS ONE* **2012**, *7*, e30766. [CrossRef] [PubMed]
14. Shannon, P.; Markiel, A.; Ozier, O.; Baliga, N.S.; Wang, J.T.; Ramage, D.; Amin, N.; Schwikowski, B.; Ideker, T. Cytoscape: A Software Environment for Integrated Models. *Genome Res.* **2003**, *13*, 2498–2504. [CrossRef] [PubMed]
15. Del Rio, G.; Koschützki, D.; Coello, G. How to identify essential genes from molecular networks? *BMC Syst. Biol.* **2009**, *3*, 102. [CrossRef]
16. Tabas-Madrid, D.; Muniategui, A.; Sánchez-Caballero, I.; Martínez-Herrera, D.J.; Sorzano, C.O.S.; Rubio, A.; Pascual-Montano, A. Improving miRNA-mRNA interaction predictions. *BMC Genomics* **2014**, *15* (Suppl. 10), S2. [CrossRef] [PubMed]
17. Colaprico, A.; Silva, T.C.; Olsen, C.; Garofano, L.; Cava, C.; Garolini, D.; Sabedot, T.S.; Malta, T.M.; Pagnotta, S.M.; Castiglioni, I.; et al. TCGAbiolinks: An R/Bioconductor package for integrative analysis of TCGA data. *Nucleic Acids Res.* **2016**, *44*, e71. [CrossRef]
18. Love, M.I.; Huber, W.; Anders, S. Moderated estimation of fold change and dispersion for RNA-seq data with DESeq2. *Genome Biol.* **2014**, *15*, 550. [CrossRef]
19. Nishida, N.; Magahara, M.; Sato, T.; Mimori, K.; Sudo, T.; Tanaka, F.; Shibata, K.; Ishii, H.; Sugihara, K.; Doki, Y.; et al. Microarray analysis of colorectal cancer stromal tissue reveals upregulation of two oncogenic miRNA clusters. *Clin. Cancer Res.* **2012**, *18*, 3054–3070. [CrossRef]
20. Ogando, J.; Tardáguila, M.; Díaz-Alderete, A.; Usategui, A.; Miranda-Ramos, V.; Martínez-Herrera, D.J.; de la Fuente, L.; García-León, M.J.; Moreno, M.C.; Escudero, S.; et al. Notch-regulated MIR-223 targets the aryl hydrocarbon receptor pathway and increases cytokine production in macrophages from rheumatoid arthritis patients. *Sci. Rep.* **2016**, *6*, 20223. [CrossRef]
21. Wang, S.; He, X.; Zhou, R.; Jia, G.; Qiao, Q. STAT3 induces colorectal carcinoma progression through a novel miR-572-MOAP-1 pathway. *Onco. Targets Ther.* **2018**, *11*, 3475–3484. [CrossRef]
22. Wang, S.; Zeng, Y.; Zhou, J.; Nie, S.; Peng, Q.; Gong, J.; Huo, J. MicroRNA-1246 promotes growth and metastasis of colorectal cancer cells involving CCNG2 reduction. *Mol. Med. Rep.* **2016**, *13*, 273–280. [CrossRef]
23. Sun, H.; Chen, X.; Ji, H.; Wu, T.; Lu, H.; Zhang, Y.; Li, H.; Li, Y. MiR-494 is an independent prognostic factor and promotes cell migration and invasion in colorectal cancer by directly targeting PTEN. *Int. J. Oncol.* **2014**, *45*, 2486–2494. [CrossRef] [PubMed]
24. Rhodes, D.R.; Chinnaiyan, A.M. Integrative analysis of the cancer transcriptome. *Nat. Genet.* **2005**, *37*, S31–S37. [CrossRef] [PubMed]
25. Wang, Y.; Lin, Y.; Guo, Y.; Pu, X.; Li, M. Functional dissection of human targets for KSHV-encoded miRNAs using network analysis. *Sci. Rep.* **2017**, *7*, 3159. [CrossRef] [PubMed]
26. Naqvi, A.R.; Shango, J.; Seal, A.; Shukla, D.; Nares, S. Viral miRNAs alter host cell miRNA profiles and modulate innate immune responses. *Front. Immunol.* **2018**, *9*, 433. [CrossRef]
27. Zeng, M.; Zhu, L.; Li, L.; Kang, C. miR-378 suppresses the proliferation, migration and invasion of colon cancer cells by inhibiting SDAD1. *Cell. Mol. Biol. Lett.* **2017**, *22*, 12. [CrossRef]
28. Chang, H.; Ye, X.; Pan, S.; Kuo, T.; Liu, B.C.; Chen, Y.; Huang, T. Overexpression of miR-194 Reverses HMGA2-driven Signatures in Colorectal Cancer. *Theranostics* **2017**, *7*, 3889–3900. [CrossRef] [PubMed]
29. Lu, Y.; Zhao, X.; Liu, Q.; Li, C.; Graves-Deal, R.; Cao, Z.; Singh, B.; Franklin, J.L.; Wang, J.; Hu, H.; et al. LncRNA MIR100HG-derived miR-100 and miR-125b mediate cetuximab resistance via Wnt/β-catenin signaling. *Nat. Med.* **2017**, *23*, 1331–1341. [CrossRef] [PubMed]
30. Michael, M.Z.; O'Connor, S.M.; van Holst Pellekaan, N.G.; Young, G.P.; James, R.J. Reduced Accumulation of Specific MicroRNAs in Colorectal Neoplasia. *Mol. Cancer Res.* **2003**, *1*, 882–891.
31. Chivukula, R.R.; Shi, G.; Acharya, A.; Mills, E.W.; Zeitels, L.R.; Anandam, J.L.; Abdelnaby, A.A.; Balck, G.C.; Mansour, J.C.; Yopp, A.C.; et al. An essential mesenchymal function for miR-143/145 in intestinal epithelial regeneration. *Cell* **2014**, *157*, 1104–1116. [CrossRef] [PubMed]
32. Liu, F.; Qi, L.; Liu, B.; Liu, J.; Zhang, H.; Che, D.; Cao, J.; Shen, J.; Geng, J.; Bi, Y.; et al. Fibroblast activation protein overexpression and clinical implications in solid tumours: A meta-analysis. *PLoS ONE* **2015**, *10*, e0116683. [CrossRef]
33. Yasunaga, M.; Matsumura, Y. Role of SLC6A6 in promoting the survival and multidrug resistance of colorectal cancer. *Sci. Rep.* **2014**, *4*, 4852. [CrossRef] [PubMed]

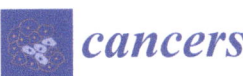

Article

Characteristics of ABCC4 and ABCG2 High Expression Subpopulations in CRC—A New Opportunity to Predict Therapy Response

Jakub Kryczka and Joanna Boncela *

Laboratory of Cell Signaling, Institute of Medical Biology, Polish Academy of Sciences, 93-232 Lodz, Poland; jkryczka@cbm.pan.pl
* Correspondence: jboncela@cbm.pan.pl

Simple Summary: Colorectal cancer (CRC) is one of the most common malignancies worldwide, causing thousands to die each year. Its complex molecular nature leads to significant heterogeneity and variable responses to therapy. ABC proteins, which for many years were regarded as the pillar of the resistance to chemotherapy because they export anticancer drugs from cancer cells, have recently been identified as interesting molecular markers associated with many other physiological functions. We previously reported that during the phenotypic transition, CRC differentially regulates the expression of two transporters, ABCC4 and ABCG2. In cells with a mesenchymal and invasive phenotype, ABCC4 is upregulated, and ABCG2 is downregulated. We have therefore decided to explore this phenomenon by analysing samples from CRC patients with high expression of either ABCC4 or ABCG2 to determine their potential use as markers of therapeutic outcome.

Abstract: Background: Our previous findings proved that ABCC4 and ABCG2 proteins present much more complex roles in colorectal cancer (CRC) than typically cancer-associated functions as drug exporters. Our objective was to evaluate their predictive/diagnostic potential. Methods: CRC patients' transcriptomic data from the Gene Expression Omnibus database (GSE18105, GSE21510 and GSE41568) were discriminated into two subpopulations presenting either high expression levels of ABCC4 (ABCC4 High) or ABCG2 (ABCG2 High). Subpopulations were analysed using various bioinformatical tools and platforms (KEEG, Gene Ontology, FunRich v3.1.3, TIMER2.0 and STRING 12.0). Results: The analysed subpopulations present different gene expression patterns. The protein–protein interaction network of subpopulation-specific genes revealed the top hub proteins in ABCC4 High: RPS27A, SRSF1, DDX3X, BPTF, RBBP7, POLR1B, HNRNPA2B1, PSMD14, NOP58 and EIF2S3 and in ABCG2 High: MAPK3, HIST2H2BE, LMNA, HIST1H2BD, HIST1H2BK, HIST1H2AC, FYN, TLR4, FLNA and HIST1H2AJ. Additionally, our multi-omics analysis proved that the ABCC4 expression correlates with substantially increased tumour-associated macrophage infiltration and sensitivity to FOLFOX treatment. Conclusions: ABCC4 and ABCG2 may be used to distinguish CRC subpopulations that present different molecular and physiological functions. The ABCC4 High subpopulation demonstrates significant EMT reprogramming, RNA metabolism and high response to DNA damage stimuli. The ABCG2 High subpopulation may resist the anti-EGFR therapy, presenting higher proteolytical activity.

Keywords: ABCC4; ABCG2; CRC; immune cell infiltration; metastasis; CRC subpopulations; CRC diagnostic and prognostic biomarkers

Citation: Kryczka, J.; Boncela, J. Characteristics of ABCC4 and ABCG2 High Expression Subpopulations in CRC—A New Opportunity to Predict Therapy Response. *Cancers* 2023, *15*, 5623. https://doi.org/10.3390/cancers15235623

Academic Editors: Rodrigo Barderas-Manchado, Cristina Díaz del Arco, María Jesús Fernández-Aceñero and Javier Martinez Useros

Received: 30 October 2023
Revised: 23 November 2023
Accepted: 25 November 2023
Published: 28 November 2023

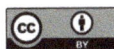

Copyright: © 2023 by the authors. Licensee MDPI, Basel, Switzerland. This article is an open access article distributed under the terms and conditions of the Creative Commons Attribution (CC BY) license (https://creativecommons.org/licenses/by/4.0/).

1. Introduction

Colorectal cancer (CRC) remains one of the most common cancers and the leading cause of cancer-related mortality worldwide [1]. Currently, the most effective treatment for CRC is primary tumour resection with adequate histologic margin, often preceded or followed by adjuvant chemotherapy [2]. However, approximately 25% of patients with CRC will develop distant metastases at the time of initial diagnosis, which is the leading cause of cancer-related mortality. Additionally, up to 50% of patients develop distant metastases as the disease progresses. Predominant sites of CRC metastasis are the liver, lung and peritoneum [3]. CRC is a highly heterogeneous cancer. This results from the cellular plasticity of epithelial-to-mesenchymal transition (EMT) and the different sites of origin. Proximal colon (right-sided) tumours predominantly show flat histology and mutations in the DNA mismatch repair pathway. In contrast, distal colon (left-sided) tumours show polypoid morphology and mutations related to the chromosome instability pathway, such as KRAS, APC, PIK3CA and p53 [4]. The heterogeneity of CRC is a key determinant of their variable response or resistance to therapy. Unfortunately, CRC is one of the most therapy-resistant malignancies, highly unresponsive to immunotherapy and various chemotherapeutic regimens based on a combination of 5-fluorouracil (5FU), oxaliplatin (OxP) and irinotecan (IRI) [2,5–7]. The activity of specific transporters belonging to the ATP-binding cassette (ABC) protein family, such as ABCB1, the ABCC family, and ABCG2, has been closely associated with both acquired and innate chemoresistance due to their ability to export large amounts of various xenobiotics [8,9]. In CRC, the clinical studies focused mainly on ABCG2 and its role in irinotecan response. ABCG2 mRNA expression was found to be lower in tumours than in normal colonic tissue. These data suggest that primary colon cancer cells initially downregulate ABCG2 mRNA expression [10]. Our previous studies show that CRC overexpressing Snail, an EMT-initiating transcription factor, reveals upregulation in ABCC4 and downregulation in ABCG2 protein expression [11,12]. These results may indicate that ABCC4 expression is associated with the acquisition of mesenchymal features by cells, and, in a more general sense, the expression pattern of ABCC4/ABCG2 may be a determinant of phenotypic transition in CRC. We analysed microarray data from the public Gene Expression Omnibus (GEO) database to confirm this observation. We found that ABCC4 was significantly upregulated, whereas ABCG2 was downregulated in primary tumours in comparison to normal colon tissue.

Interestingly, ABC expression profiles constantly change during ongoing EMT and cancer progression. In recent years, an increasing number of studies have shown that loss or inhibition of ABC transporters affects cellular phenotypes closely associated with differentiation, migration/invasion and malignant potential in various cancers. In addition, loss of ABC transporters in both xenograft and transgenic mouse models of cancer can affect tumour initiation and progression. [13–15]. These effects are probably a result of their normal physiological function as exporters of endogenous metabolites and signalling molecules. Thus, ABC transporters play a much more complex role in cancer development than drug efflux [11,16]. To further investigate the importance of ABC proteins and their engagement in different cancer-related processes, in this manuscript, we decided to compare two CRC subgroups presenting high expression levels of two ABC members: ABCC4 and ABCG2.

2. Material and Methods

2.1. Microarray Data Processing and Analysis

Gene expression profiles with accession numbers GSE18105 (https://www.ncbi.nlm.nih.gov/geo/query/acc.cgi?acc=GSE18105, accessed on 4 September 2023), GSE21510 (https://www.ncbi.nlm.nih.gov/geo/query/acc.cgi?acc=GSE21510, accessed on 4 September 2023) GSE41568 (https://www.ncbi.nlm.nih.gov/geo/query/acc.cgi?acc=GSE41568, accessed on 4 September 2023), GSE83129 (https://www.ncbi.nlm.nih.gov/geo/query/acc.cgi?acc=GSE83129, accessed on 4 September 2023) and GSE62080 (https://www.ncbi.nlm.nih.gov/geo/query/acc.cgi?acc=GSE62080, accessed on 4 September 2023) were downloaded from The Gene Expression Omnibus (GEO) database (http://www.ncbi.nlm.nih.gov/geo/) (accessed on 4 September 2023) and analysed similarly to our previous work [16]. All data were processed using the GEO2R online analytical tool (# Version info: R 4.2.2, Biobase 2.58.0, GEOquery 2.66.0, limma 3.54.0) [17]. Linear projections of gene mRNA level were performed using Orange 3.31.1 software as previously presented by us [16]. mRNA levels were calculated and visualised using JASP 0.16.0.0 software (https://jasp-stats.org/, accessed on 4 September 2023), as shown in [18].

2.2. Survival Probability Analysis

The survival rate for patients presenting the high and low expression of chosen differently expressed genes (DEGs) was analysed in CRC patients using TCGA data, the Human Protein Atlas (www.proteinatlas.org, accessed on 4 September 2023) "pathology" section [19,20] and TIMER2.0 platform (http://timer.cistrome.org/, accessed on 4 September 2023) [21]. The presented data used the best expression cut-off suggested by HPA.

2.3. Enrichment Analysis

Functional enrichment software tool FunRich (v3.1.3) (http://www.funrich.org/, accessed on 4 September 2023) supported by the Gene Ontology (GO) (http://geneontology.org/, accessed on 4 September 2023) database was used to compare, analyse and visualise the Biological Process (BP) and Molecular Functions (MF) differences associated to the proteins encoded by differently expressed genes (DEGs) in ABCC4 High- and ABCG2 High-level presenting subfractions of CRC patient samples analogues to our previous work [22].

2.4. Hierarchical Clustering

The top proteins upregulated in both the ABCC4 High and ABCG2 High CRC subgroups were used to create a bidirectional hierarchical clustering heatmap with their respective mRNA levels. The hierarchical clustering method results in a hierarchical dendrogram highlighting similarities and differences between the subjects analysed. The calculation and visualisation were performed using the Orange open source machine learning and data visualisation platform 3.31.1 (https://orangedatamining.com/, accessed on 4 September 2023), as previously described [16,22].

2.5. Protein–Protein Interaction Network

Protein–protein interaction (PPI) networks of top proteins expressed by ABCC4 High and ABCG2 High CRC subgroups were created and visualised using the STRING version 12.0 online platform (https://string-db.org/, accessed on 4 September 2023) and Cytoscape 3.9.1. as presented by us [16,22,23].

2.6. Analysis of Immune Cell Tumour Infiltration

The Tumor Immune Estimation Resource—TIMER2.0 platform (http://timer.cistrome.org/, accessed on 4 September 2023) was used to analyse immune cell infiltration. TIMER2.0 employs immunedeconv—an R package that integrates six state-of-the-art algorithms (TIMER, xCell, MCP-counter, CIBERSORT, EPIC and quanTIseq) to statistically predict tumour infiltration by selected immune cell types using The Cancer Genome Atlas (TCGA) database. Similar to our previous work, the data were analysed and visualised using the xCell algorithm [22].

2.7. Statistics

Statistical evaluation was performed using the normality test (Shapiro–Wilk), followed by the Student's t-test (in the case of normally distributed data) or the Mann–Whitney U test (in the case of non-normally distributed data). Calculations and graphs were performed using Orange data mining 3.31.1 software and JASP 0.16.0.0 software; p values < 0.05 were considered statistically significant for all analyses: * $p < 0.05$; ** $p < 0.005$; *** $p < 0.001$, NS-not statistically significant. Pearson's linear correlation analysis was performed using JASP 0.16.0.0 software with Pearson correlation coefficient presented as colour intensity and numerical values on the correlation matrix. The correlation statistical value was shown as follows: * $p < 0.05$; ** $p < 0.005$; *** $p < 0.001$, no indication—not statistically significant.

3. Results

3.1. Analysis of ABCC4 and ABCG2 Expression Level in CRC

Data containing mRNA levels of approximately 40,000 "hits" detected by microarrays chips in colorectal cancer tumours and normal colon tissue were downloaded from the GEO database (https://www.ncbi.nlm.nih.gov/geo/, accessed on 4 September 2023). Two datasets were analysed: GSE18105 (composed of n = 111) and GSE21510 (composed of n = 148). Expression of ABCC4 and ABCG2 in CRC samples and normal colon tissue was analysed in each dataset independently, as shown in Figure 1A–D. ABCC4 presents significantly higher expression in CRC samples than in normal colon tissue, whereas ABCG2 expression is considerably higher in normal colon tissue than in CRC. Interestingly, the TIMER2.0 platform [24]-based analysis of the TCGA database proves that neither ABCC4 (Figure 1E) nor ABCG2 (Figure 1F) expression level presents any statistically significant association with survival rate. Additionally, further analysis performed with the TIMER2.0 platform and TCGA database proved that expression of the mutated (including any type of mutation) variant of ABCC4 negatively correlates with the expression level of wild type (WT) of ABCC4 (Pearson correlation $p = -0.233$) and positively with ABCG2 (Pearson correlation efficiency $p = 0.666$) (Figure 1G,H).

3.2. Correlation of Immune Cell Infiltration with ABCG2 and ABCC4 Expression Levels in CRC

The tumour microenvironment (TME) is composed of cancer cells, normal cells (tissue of origin), cancer-associated fibroblasts (CAFs) and various immune cells such as CD8 + T cells, natural killer cells (NK cells), regulatory T cells (Treg cells), tumour-associated macrophages (TAM), and Dendritic cells (DC). The cellular components of TME regulate tumour survival and promote metastasis. In recent years, many studies have investigated the role of tumour infiltration by immune cells [25,26]. In the case of CRC, intratumoral infiltration by CD8+ and CD4+ T cells is concerned with a favourable prognostic factor increasing patients' overall survival rate, whereas M2 tumour-associated macrophages (M2-TAMs) infiltration promotes cancer cell proliferation and increases metastatic potential [27–29]. Using the TIMER2.0 platform and gene-signature-based algorithm—xCELL, we analysed the correlation of ABCC4 and ABCG2 mRNA levels with immune cell infiltration (Table 1 and Supplementary Figure S1) [24,30]. Our analysis proves that both ABCC4 and ABCG2 levels present a negative correlation with CD4+ and CD8+ T-cell infiltration but a positive correlation with CAFs infiltration. Interestingly, the mRNA level of mutated ABCC4 shows a high positive correlation with CD4+ (CD4+ Th2 log2FC = 0.565 (Figure 2A) and CD4+ Th1 log2FC = 0.805 (Figure 2B)) and CD8+ (CD8+ central memory log2FC = 1.401 (Figure 2C) and CD8+ naive log2FC = 0.526 (Figure 2D)) T-cell infiltration, with no impact on other immune cells.

3.3. Identification of ABCC4 and ABCG2 High Expression CRC Subsets

Even though ABCG2 presents significantly lower expression in CRC samples than in the normal colon, a small subfraction showing a high mRNA level is observed. Additionally, CRC cells present various ranges of ABCC4 expression. Thus, we decided to identify and analyse differences between CRC subfractions presenting high ABCC4 (ABCC4 H) and high ABCG2 (ABCG2 H) levels. First, we have selected two CRC subgroups for each of the analysed datasets using Orange data mining 3.31.1 software and a VizRank-based algorithm ("linear projection"). The first subgroup presented a high ABCC4 level and low ABCG2 level, whereas the second subgroup presented the opposite expression pattern, as shown in Figure 3A,B [31]. Next, gene expression patterns specific to each subgroup were compared using the online tool GEO2R with an adjustable p value < 0.05 for every dataset (Figure 3C). This analysis provided 867 upregulated genes for the ABCC4 High subgroup and 918 upregulated genes for the ABCG2 subgroup in the GSE18105 dataset and analogously 970 and 1275 for GSE21510 (Figure 3D). Finally, using the Venn Diagram, 704 genes significantly upregulated in the ABCC4 High CRC subgroup and 772 genes upregulated in ABCG2 HIGH CRC subgroups were identified in both datasets, as shown in Figure 3E.

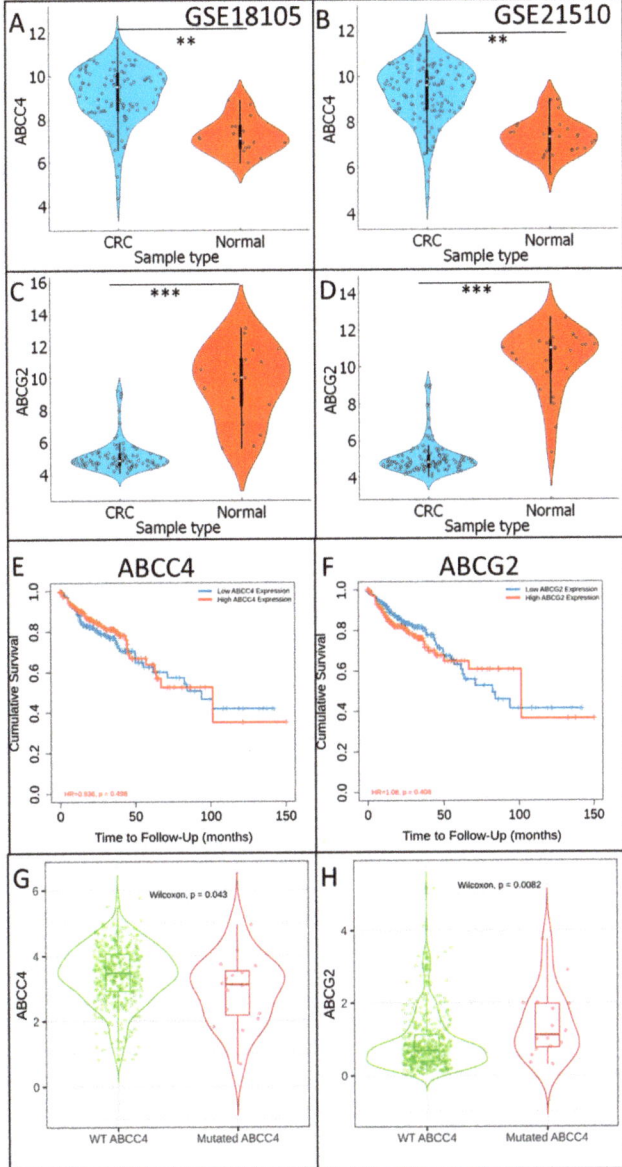

Figure 1. ABCC4 and ABCG2 involvement in CRC progression. ABCC4 and ABCG2 expression levels in "CRC" and noncancerous "Normal" colon tissue were calculated using data from GSE18105 (**A,C**) and GSE21510 (**B,D**) and visualised using Orange data mining 3.31.1 software. A normality test (Shapiro–Wilk) was performed, followed by the Mann–Whitney U test ** $p < 0.005$; *** $p < 0.001$; ABCC4 (**E**) and ABCG2 (**F**) impact on survival rate was analysed using TCGA data and visualised by the TIMER2.0 platform. The correlation of ABCC4 (**G**) and ABCG2 (**H**) wild-type (WT) and mutated variants was calculated using TCGA data and visualised by the TIMER2.0 platform. Wilcoxon test was performed, and the *p*-value is indicated in the figure.

Table 1. Correlation of immune cell infiltration of CRC tumour subfractions presenting high ABCG2 or ABCC4 expression level. Data were obtained using the TIMER2.0 platform and TCGA database.

	Infiltrating Cells	Correlation Rho	p
ABCC4 H			
	CAFs	0.188	1.72×10^{-3}
	Neutrophils	0.226	8.01×10^{-6}
	NK	−0.181	2.54×10^{-3}
	Macrophage	0.326	3.26×10^{-8}
	Macrophage M1	0.358	9.51×10^{-10}
	Macrophage M2	0.304	2.86×10^{-7}
	CD8+ T-cell effector memory	−0.119	4.87×10^{-2}
	CD8+ T-cell-naive	−0.143	1.75×10^{-2}
	CD4+ T cell Th1	−0.207	5.41×10^{-4}
	CD4+ central memory	−0.127	3.50×10^{-2}
ABCG2 H			
	CAFs	0.182	2.48×10^{-3}
	Neutrophils	0.119	4.89×10^{-2}
	Class-switched memory B cells	−0.228	1.35×10^{-4}
	CD8+ T-cell central memory	−0.14	2.04×10^{-2}
	CD4+ T-cell effector memory	−0.153	1.12×10^{-2}
	CD4+ T cell Th2	−0.143	1.75×10^{-2}
	CD4+ T cell non-regulatory	−0.138	2.20×10^{-2}

3.4. Enrichment Analysis of DEGs Unique to ABCC4 High or ABCG2 High CRC Subsets

Genes upregulated in ABCC4 High and ABCG2 High CRC subgroups were analysed using the FunRich platform supported by the Gene Ontology database to verify differences in enrichment of Biological Processes (BP) (Figure 4A) and Molecular Functions (MF) (Figure 4B). The ABCC4 High CRC subgroup presents significantly higher enrichment in processes related to DNA and RNA binding, regulation of gene expression and response to DNA damage. In contrast, the ABCG2 High CRC subgroup demonstrates significant enrichment in positive regulation of apoptotic processes, cell adhesion, extracellular matrix decomposition, actin filament assembly and cell migration.

3.5. Correlation of ABCC4 and ABCG2 Expression Levels with Major Dysregulated Protein Hubs

Having established enriched biological processes, we shifted our focus to major dysregulated protein hubs. Thus, data containing upregulated genes from each subgroup were used to draw a protein–protein interaction (PPI) network via the STRING (ver. 12.0) platform (https://string-db.org/, accessed on 4 September 2023) (supplementary Figure S1). Next, the PPI network was analysed using Cytoscape 3.9.1 (https://cytoscape.org/, accessed on 4 September 2023) to identify the top 10 protein hubs (for each subgroup) with the highest number of direct protein interaction counted as the highest number of drawn "edges" (Table 2), similar to our previous study [16]. This type of analysis provides insight into critical proteins that, by direct interactions, influence various processes and thus potentially can be utilised as molecular targets for future therapies. To further analyse and verify the correctness of chosen protein hubs, a hierarchical clustering analysis of data consisting of mRNA levels of 20 chosen DEGs from all CRC patients (GSE18105 and GSE21510) was performed (Figure 5A). Step by step, this analysis connects most similar subjects, forming clusters (branches) until all clusters are defined. The obtained hierarchical dendrogram proves that protein hubs upregulated in ABCC4 High CRC subgroups cluster together with ABCC4 on one arm (branch). In contrast, protein hubs were observed for the ABCG2 High subgroup on the second arm, together with ABCG2. Additionally, using Orange data mining 3.31.1 software and the FreeViz tool, ABCC4 High and ABCG2 High CRC patients cluster differentiation, using top protein hubs, was visualised (Figure 5B). Next, the Pearson correlation matrix was created to analyse the mutual interaction of genes that encode the chosen top networking protein hub (Figure 5C). Interestingly, selected protein hubs demonstrate a substantial amount of interaction with each other, forming stable clusters presented in Figure 6. The cluster formed for the CRC subgroup characterised by high ABCC4 (Figure 6A) expression enriches biological processes such as GO:0003723—RNA binding and GO:0003676—Nucleic acid binding (according to the Gene Ontology database). Arguably, two of the most important proteins of this cluster are RPS27A and NOP58. RPS27 shows the highest number of edges, directly interacting with 10% of all proteins observed in this group (87 out of 867 proteins), whereas NOP58 presents the highest connectivity inside the cluster. Both proteins play important antiapoptotic roles [32,33]. On the other hand, the ABCG2 High cluster (Figure 6B) presented enrichment in GO:0046982—Protein heterodimerisation activity, GO:0046983—Protein dimerisation activity and GO:0005515—Protein binding.

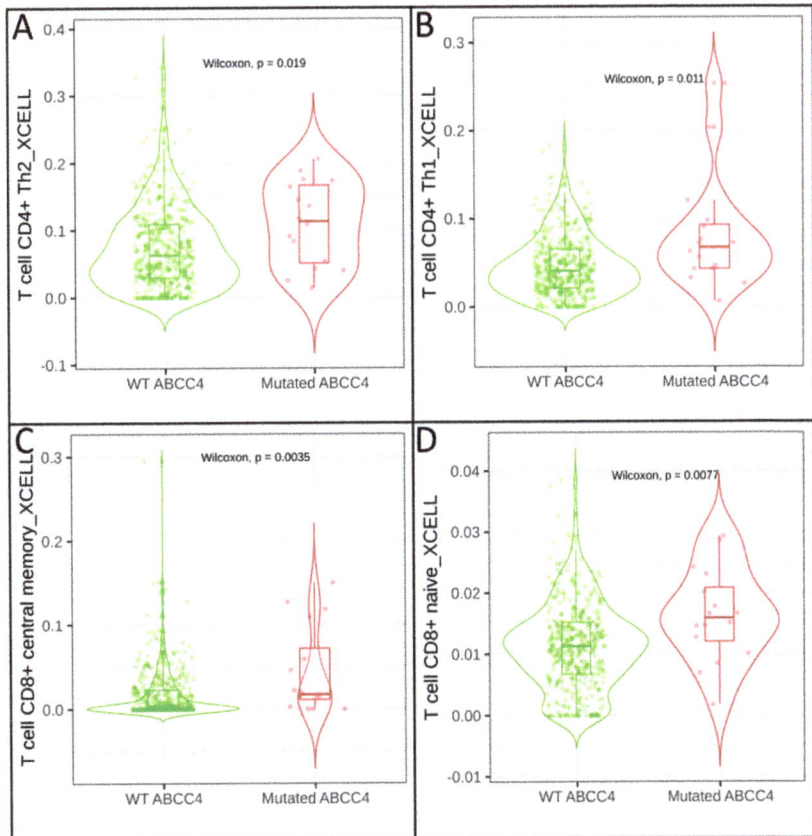

Figure 2. Correlation of mutated *ABCC4* gene expression and immune cell infiltration of CRC. ABCC4 presents a high positive correlation with CD4+ Th2 log2FC = 0.565 (**A**) and CD4+ Th1 log2FC = 0.805 (**B**), CD8+ central memory log2FC = 1.401 (**C**) and CD8+ naive log2FC = 0.526 (**D**) T-cell infiltration. The calculation was performed using TCGA data and visualised by the TIMER2.0 platform. Wilcoxon test was performed, and the *p*-value is indicated in the figure.

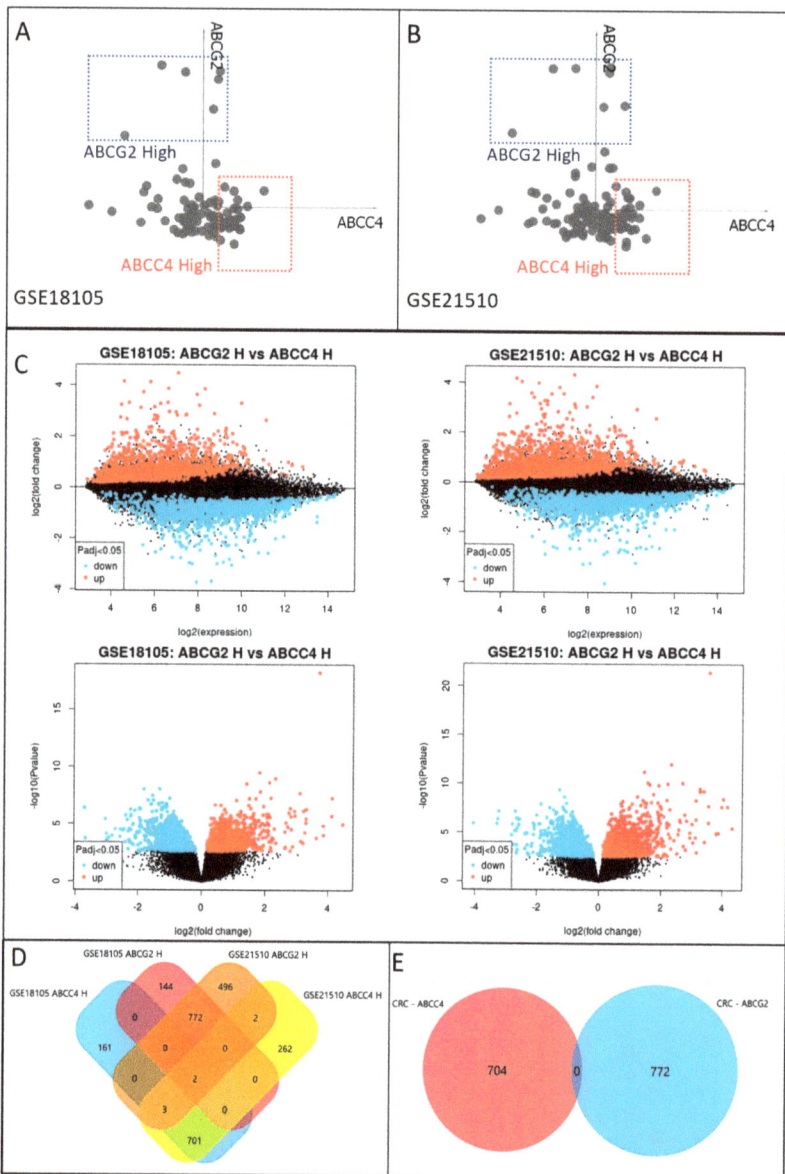

Figure 3. Identification of CRC subgroups presenting high ABCC4 (ABCC4 High) and ABCG2 (ABCG2 High) expression levels and related DEGs. Identification of CRC samples belonging to each subgroup using GSE18105 (**A**) and GSE21510 (**B**) datasets. Visualisation performed using a 2D VizRank-based algorithm and Orange data mining 3.31.1 software. Visual representation of differently expressed genes (DEGs) for ABCG2 High and ABCC4 High CRC subgroups in GSE18105 and GSE21510 analysed using the GEO2R online tool (**C**). Venn diagram of selected ABCG2 High and ABCC4 High DEGs from datasets GSE18105 and GSE21510 (**D**). Venn diagram presenting no mutual DEGs between ABCC4 High and ABCG2 High subgroups (**E**).

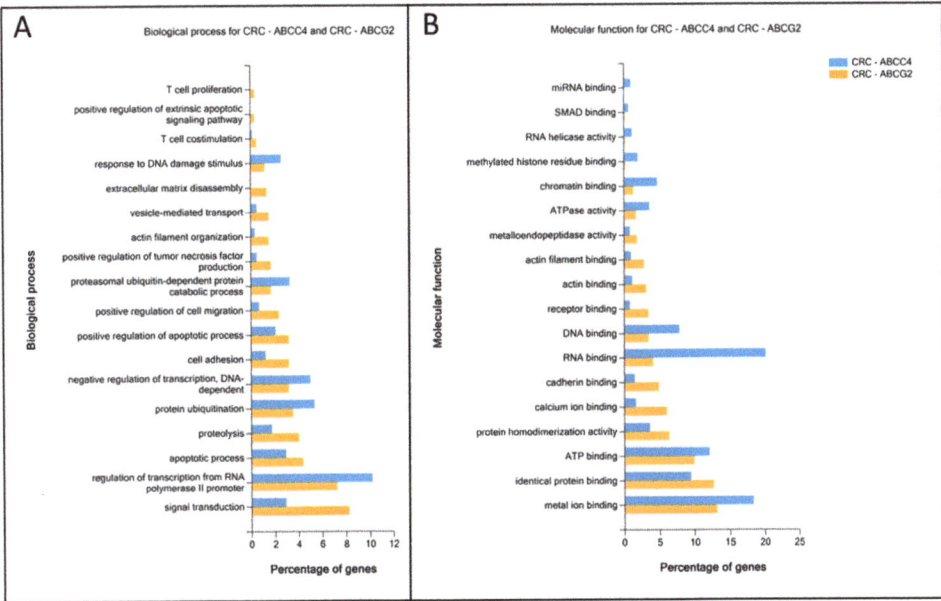

Figure 4. Enrichment analysis of ABCC4 High and ABCG2 High CRC subgroups related to DEGs. Data were analysed and visualised using the FunRich platform supported by the Gene Ontology database, depicting the total percentage of subgroup-specific DEGs enriched in Biological Process (**A**) and Molecular Functions (**B**).

Table 2. Main protein hubs observed among DEGs of ABCC4 High and ABCG2 High CRC subgroups.

	Gene	Protein	Number of Edges
ABCC4 H			
	RPS27A	ribosomal protein S27a	87
	SRSF1	Serine/arginine-rich splicing factor 1	56
	DDX3X	DEAD-box helicase family member	50
	BPTF	bromodomain PHD finger transcription factor	44
	RBBP7	RB Binding Protein 7, Chromatin Remodeling Factor	44
	POLR1B	RNA Polymerase I Subunit B	44
	HNRNPA2B1	heterogeneous nuclear ribonucleoprotein A2/B1	43
	PSMD14	proteasome 26S subunit, non-ATPase 14	42
	NOP58	ribonucleoprotein	42
	EIF2S3	eukaryotic translation initiation factor 2 subunit gamma	41
ABCG2 H			
	MAPK3	mitogen-activated protein kinase 3	53
	HIST2H2BE	histone cluster 2 H2B family member E (H2B clustered histone 21)	34
	LMNA	Lamin A/C	29
	HIST1H2BD	histone cluster 1 H2B family member D (H2B clustered histone 5)	29
	HIST1H2BK	histone cluster 1 H2B family member K (H2B clustered histone 12)	29
	HIST1H2AC	histone cluster 1 H2A family member C (H2A clustered histone 6)	29
	FYN	FYN proto-oncogene, Src family tyrosine kinase	28
	TLR4	toll-like receptor 4	28
	FLNA	filamin A	28
	HIST1H2AJ	histone cluster 1 H2B family member J (H2A clustered histone 14)	27

Additionally, using the STRING platform, we have added known proteins that interact with selected clusters, thus filling the gaps to obtain major KEGG pathways, with PPI enrichment p-value for ABCC4 High and ABCG2 High respective subgroups: 1.77×10^{-14}

and 4.28×10^{-5}, respectively. The obtained data are shown in Table 3. Interestingly, the obtained protein hub cluster network for the ABCC4 High subgroup presents high involvement in proteasome functions and RNA polymerase functions, whereas the protein hub cluster network for the ABCG2 High subgroup—in MAPK signalling pathway, focal adhesion, PD-L1 expression and PD-1 checkpoint pathway, platelet activation, natural-killer-cell-mediated cytotoxicity, apoptosis and insulin signalling pathway.

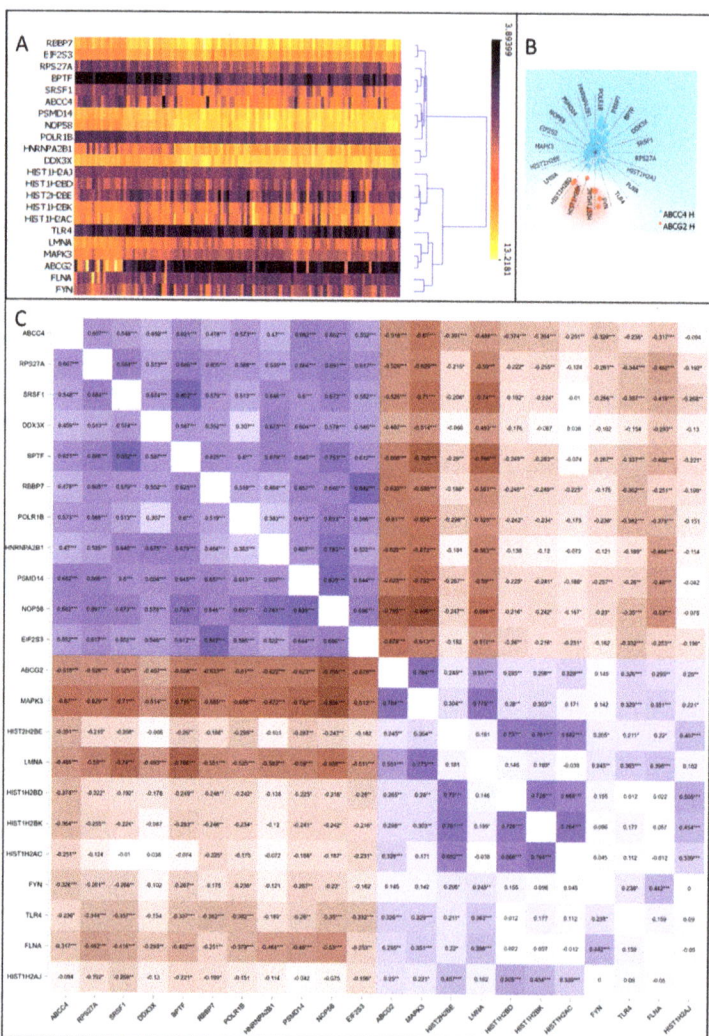

Figure 5. ABCC4 and ABCG2 correlation with top hub proteins selected from ABCC4 High and ABCG2 High CRC subgroups related to DEGs. Hierarchical clustering analysis of chosen top protein hubs, selected from DEGs using mRNA values of CRC patients from GSE18105 and GSE21510 datasets visualised using Orange data mining 3.31.1 software (**A**). Radial visualisation of clusters created by chosen top networking DEGs visualised using the FreeViz tool and Orange data mining 3.31.1 software and mRNA values of CRC patients from GSE18105 and GSE21510 datasets (**B**). Pearson correlation matrix of ABCC4, ABCG2 and chosen DEGs, using mRNA values of CRC patients from GSE18105 and GSE21510 datasets, calculated and visualised using JASP 0.16.0.0 software. * $p < 0.05$; ** $p < 0.005$; *** $p < 0.001$ (**C**).

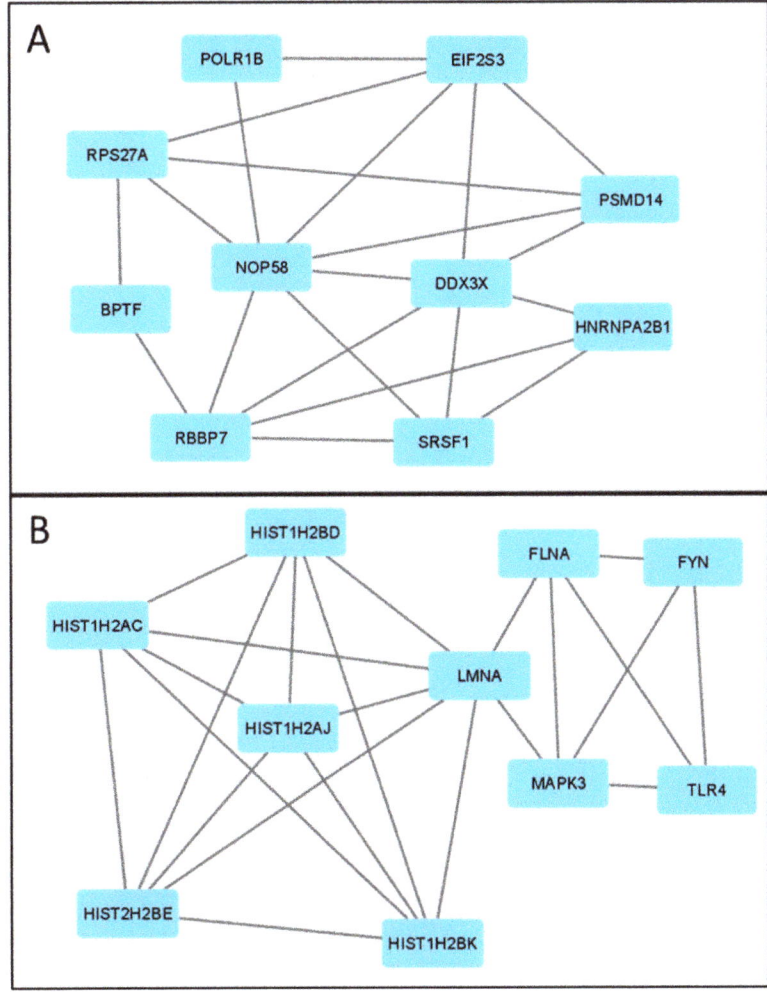

Figure 6. Protein–protein interaction network (PPI) of ABCC4 High (**A**) and ABCG2 High (**B**) CRC subgroups related to top networking DEGs. Calculated using the STRING platform and visualised by Cytoscape 3.9.1.

Table 3. Main protein hubs for ABCC4 High and ABCG2 High CRC subgroup KEGG enrichment.

	KEGG ID	Description	Strength	False Discovery Rate
ABCC4 H				
	hsa03050	Proteasome	2.14	2.26×10^{-9}
	hsa05012	Parkinson's disease	1.46	5.28×10^{-7}
	hsa05017	Spinocerebellar ataxia	1.64	5.28×10^{-7}
	hsa05014	Amyotrophic lateral sclerosis	1.29	3.48×10^{-6}
	hsa05020	Prion disease	1.35	1.47×10^{-5}
	hsa05016	Huntington's disease	1.29	2.41×10^{-5}
	hsa05010	Alzheimer's disease	1.22	5.63×10^{-5}
	hsa05169	Epstein–Barr virus infection	1.31	0.0018
	hsa03020	RNA polymerase	1.8	0.0192

Table 3. Cont.

	KEGG ID	Description	Strength	False Discovery Rate
ABCG2 H				
	hsa05034	Alcoholism	1.74	2.90×10^{-7}
	hsa05133	Pertussis	1.95	4.60×10^{-7}
	hsa05322	Systemic lupus erythematosus	1.85	9.16×10^{-7}
	hsa04620	Toll-like receptor signalling pathway	1.81	1.02×10^{-6}
	hsa05132	Salmonella infection	1.49	2.75×10^{-5}
	hsa04064	NF-kappa B signalling pathway	1.71	5.70×10^{-5}
	hsa04217	Necroptosis	1.54	0.00022
	hsa05203	Viral carcinogenesis	1.46	0.00042
	hsa05205	Proteoglycans in cancer	1.43	0.00049
	hsa05235	PD-L1 expression and PD-1 checkpoint pathway in cancer	1.65	0.0014
	hsa05142	Chagas disease	1.6	0.0018
	hsa05145	Toxoplasmosis	1.57	0.0020
	hsa05135	Yersinia infection	1.5	0.0030
	hsa05161	Hepatitis B	1.39	0.0056
	hsa05152	Tuberculosis	1.37	0.0059
	hsa05164	Influenza A	1.38	0.0059
	hsa04621	NOD-like receptor signalling pathway	1.35	0.0060
	hsa05130	Pathogenic Escherichia coli infection	1.32	0.0070
	hsa04510	Focal adhesion	1.3	0.0078
	hsa05131	Shigellosis	1.25	0.0098
	hsa05134	Legionellosis	1.68	0.0137
	hsa04010	MAPK signalling pathway	1.13	0.0185
	hsa04520	Adherens junction	1.59	0.0185
	hsa04664	Fc epsilon RI signalling pathway	1.6	0.0185
	hsa05140	Leishmaniasis	1.57	0.0185
	hsa05221	Acute myeloid leukemia	1.6	0.0185
	hsa05220	Chronic myeloid leukemia	1.54	0.0193
	hsa04012	ErbB signalling pathway	1.5	0.0226
	hsa04660	T-cell-receptor signalling pathway	1.41	0.0313
	hsa05146	Amoebiasis	1.42	0.0313
	hsa04066	HIF-1 signalling pathway	1.39	0.0327
	hsa04725	Cholinergic synapse	1.38	0.0341
	hsa04071	Sphingolipid signalling pathway	1.35	0.0366
	hsa04380	Osteoclast differentiation	1.33	0.0385
	hsa04611	Platelet activation	1.33	0.0385
	hsa04650	Natural-killer-cell-mediated cytotoxicity	1.33	0.0385
	hsa04210	Apoptosis	1.3	0.0418
	hsa04910	Insulin signalling pathway	1.29	0.0418
	hsa04145	Phagosome	1.26	0.0456
	hsa04072	Phospholipase D signalling pathway	1.25	0.0475

3.6. Analysis of Potential CRC Metastatic Organotropism Biomarkers

Finally, we decided to verify whether mRNA levels of ABCC4, ABCG2 and genes encoding major protein hubs for their respective CRC subgroups (ABCC4 High and ABCG2 High) can be used to predict metastatic organotropism. Thus, we have downloaded and analysed transcriptomic data from the GSE41568 dataset (composed of n = 133), consisting of primary CRC samples and CRC metastases to the liver, lung and omentum [34]. Samples were divided into four subgroups, Primary, Lung Met., Liver Met. and Omentum Met., and analysed using ANCOVA with Post Hoc Test and Tukey correction. The ABCC4 mRNA level presents no statistically significant changes that could distinguish metastatic sites. However, ABCG2 and six other genes encoding protein hubs (FYN, FLNA, POLR1B, RBBP7, EIF2S3 and PSMD14) were found to be potentially valuable (Figure 7A). According to our analysis, upregulation of ABCG2, FLNA and FYN with simultaneous downregulation of RBBP7 is characteristic of CRC metastasis to the liver. Thus, we may assume that the ABCG2 High CRC subgroup prefers liver metastasis. Additionally, POLR1B and EIF2S3 expression downregulation compared to primary CRC and liver metastasis was observed for CRC samples resected from the lung. Furthermore, FYN upregulation is also significant for omentum, peritoneal and abdominal wall metastasis. This metastatic site lies near the primary CRC tumour (compared to distant metastasis to the lungs or liver). It requires a different form of cancer cell migration, preferring single-cell mesenchymal migration focusing on adhesion/deadhesion and active decomposition of extracellular matrix (ECM). The protein encoded by FYN is highly involved in hsa04510 (focal adhesion) and hsa04520 (adherent junctions), as well as hsa04611 (platelet activation). Thus, to further combine the obtained data, we have developed a metastasis site discriminative model using Orange data mining 3.31.1 software and a linear projection tool based on the VizRank algorithm (Figure 7B). This model places each data point on the visualisation matrix, simultaneously analysing each attribute value (gene expression). All attributes—chosen genes—are identified on a ring surrounding the visualisation space and equally separated from one another (in this instance, 45^0 or 0.785 RAD); thus, the greater the attribute value, the closer the data point is drawn in 2D space [31]. Most primary CRC is located inside the triangle created by EIF2S3, RBBP7 and FYN and most Lung metastasis inside the triangle formed by ABCC4, PSMD14 and FLNA. The proposed method could potentially be beneficial in predicting (with some probability) metastatic progression after primary CRC biopsy. In addition, using the TIMER2.0 platform [24] and data from the TCGA database, we analysed the correlation between the expression levels of FYN, FLNA, POLR1B, RBBP7, EIF2S3 and PSMD14 and the survival of CRC patients (Figure 8). The average 5-year survival rate for CRC is 60%, a high expression of FLNA and POLR1B represents a significantly lower probability of the survival of CRC patients', but only FLNA can be considered as a prognostic biomarker with HR = 1.25 and p = 0.025.

3.7. Analysis of ABCC4 and ABCG2 Potential Chemotherapy Response Predictive Capabilities

Finally, to evaluate differences between ABCC4 and ABCG2 mRNA expression and response to the main anti-CRC chemotherapy regimens, two datasets containing mRNA expression levels of CRC patients treated with FOLFIRI (GSE62080 consisting of n = 21; 12 resistant and 9 sensitive) and FOLFOX (GSE83129 consisting of n = 23; 12 resistant, 21 sensitive) were downloaded from the GEO database. Data were analysed using previously selected and set gates for CRC subpopulations with high expression of ABCC4 and ABCG2 using Orange data mining 3.31.1 software and a VizRank-based algorithm ("linear projection") (Figure 9A,B). The ABCC4 High subgroup consists mainly of FOLFOX-sensitive samples and moderately of FOLFIRI-resistant samples, whereas the ABCG2 High subgroup is an even mix of samples with different chemotherapy responses. In addition, analysis of ABCC4 and ABCG2 mRNA expression levels revealed no statistically significant differences between FOLFIRI (Figure 9C)- and FOLFOX (Figure 9D)-resistant and -sensitive CRC patients.

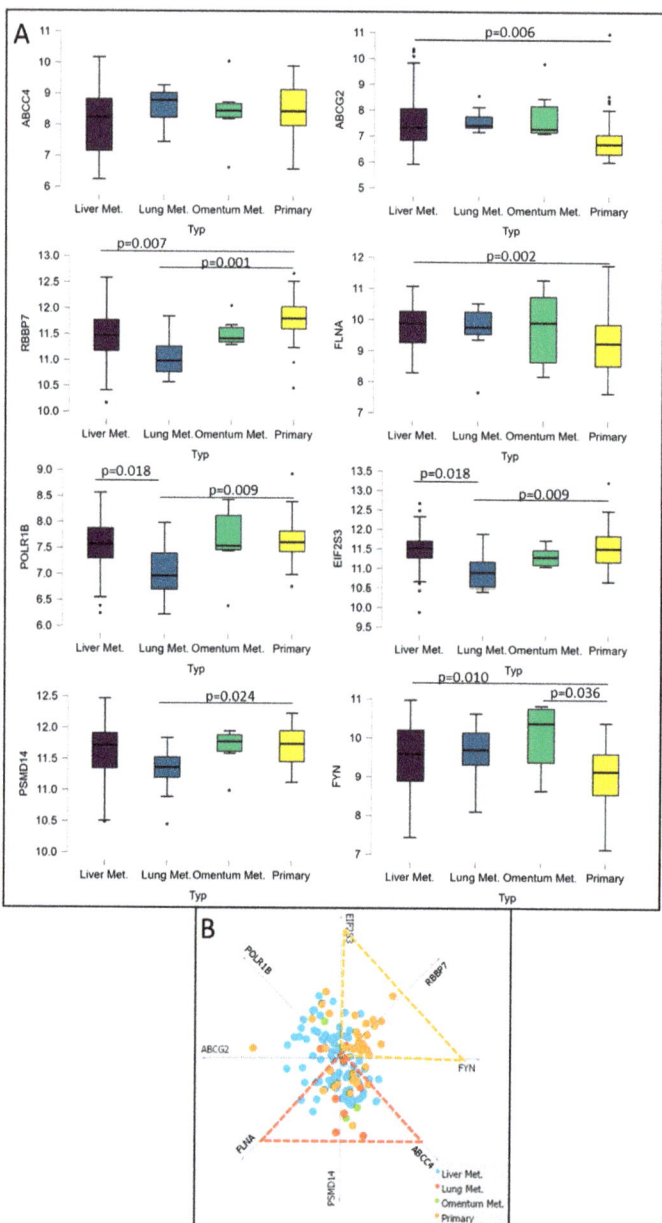

Figure 7. Selected DEGs expression level and its implication as metastatic CRC organotropism biomarkers. mRNA expression levels of selected DEGs in primary CRC, liver, lung and omentum metastases. Data downloaded from GSE41568 were calculated and visualised using JASP 0.16.0.0 software. A normality test (Shapiro–Wilk) was performed, followed by the Mann–Whitney U test (**A**)—linear projection model of primary and metastatic CRC based on the mRNA expression level of chosen DEGs. GSE41568 data were analysed and visualised using Orange data mining 3.31.1 software. Dashed lines presents region of interest formed by chosen DEGs mRNA expression consisting mostly of primary (orange) and metastatic (red) CRC (**B**).

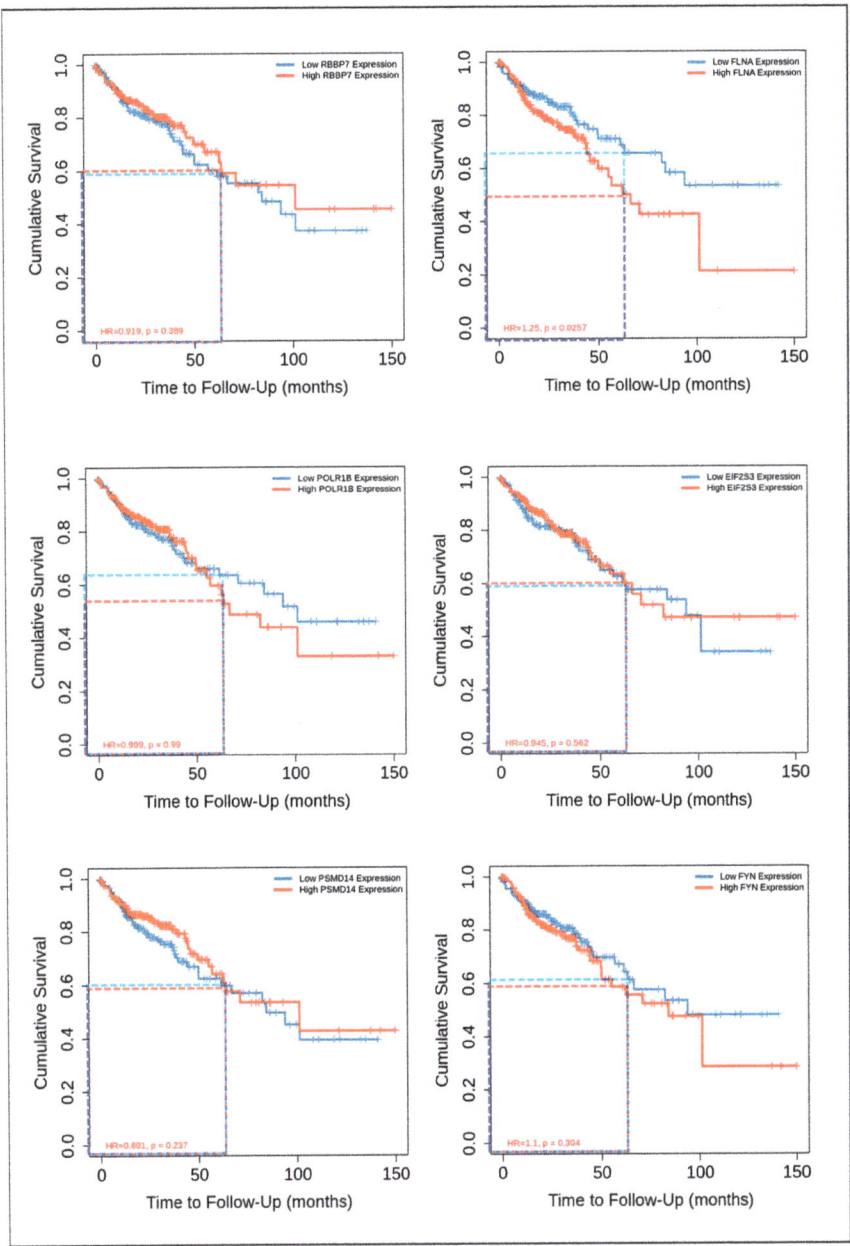

Figure 8. Selected DEGs' impact on CRC patients' survival rate. RBBP7, FLNA, POLR1B, EIF2S3, PSMD14 and FYN impact on survival rate was analysed using TCGA data and visualised by the TIMER2.0 platform. Dashed lines indicate 5-year survival rate (60 months) for CRC samples characterised by low (blue) or high (red) expression of chosen DEGs.

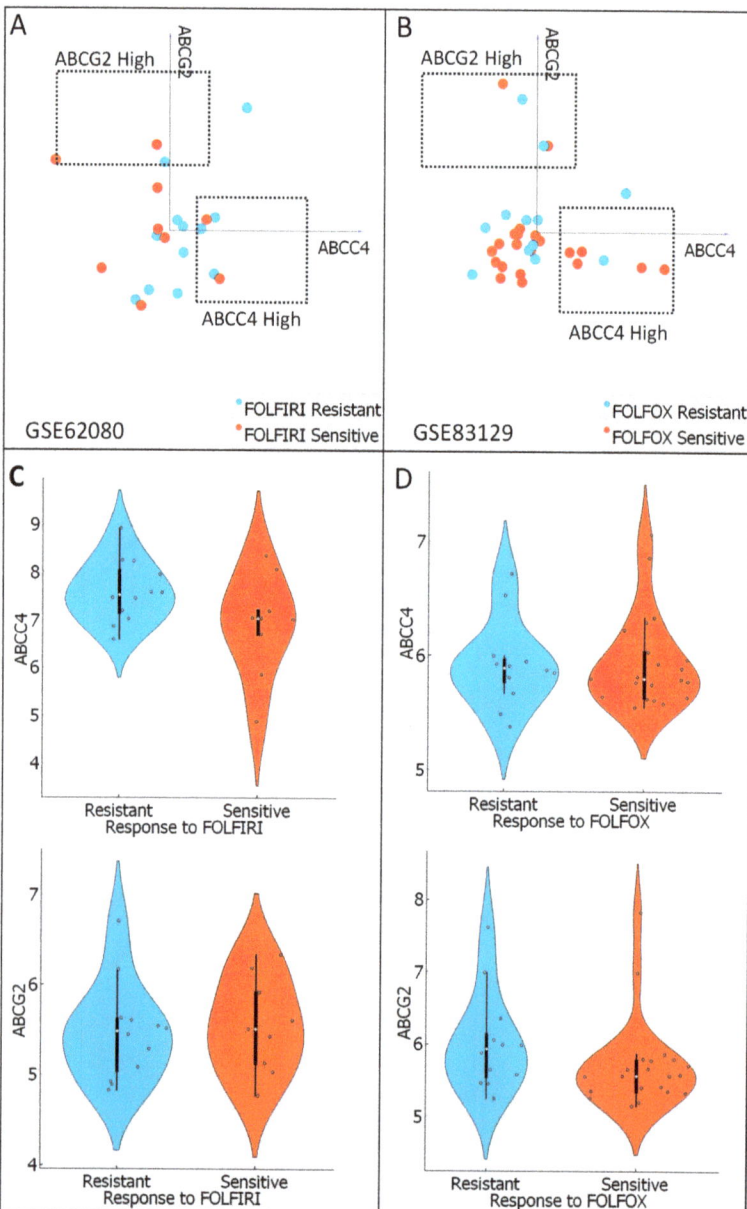

Figure 9. Chemotherapy response predictive capabilities of ABCC4 and ABCG2 mRNA expression. Data containing FOLFIRI (**A**)- and FOLFOX (**B**)-resistant and -sensitive patients' responses were downloaded from the GEO database (GSE62080 and GSE83129, respectively). Visualisation was performed using a 2D VizRank-based algorithm and Orange data mining 3.31.1 software. Dashed lines present gates set for ABCG2 High and ABCC4 High subgroups. mRNA expression of ABCC4 I ABCG2 in FOLFIRI (**C**)- and FOLFOX (**D**)-treated CRC patients' sample. Visualisation was performed using Orange data mining 3.31.1 software and the GEO database (GSE62080 and GSE83129, respectively).

4. Discussion

CRC, being one of the most common cancer types, contributes highly to cancer-related mortality. One of the most critical reasons is high molecular heterogeneity within CRC, resulting in substantial differences in treatment response to both chemo- and immunetherapy [4]. Regarding various immunotherapy schemes, CRC is considered one of the most resistant cancer types. Approximately 40–50% of CRC presents resistance to antiepidermal growth factor receptor (anti-EGFR) therapy, and only 5–10% of metastatic CRC shows a positive response to anti-PD-1/PD-L1 (anti-programmed death-1/programmed cell death ligand 1) therapy [35,36]. Thus, standard first-line treatment for CRC includes conventional, reasonably inexpensive, tissue non-specific chemotherapy based on a mix of fluorouracil and oxaliplatin or irinotecan, often leading to acquisition resistance to its components by CRC cells [5]. Different mechanisms of chemoresistance, such as systems of DNA damage repairs or overexpression of antiapoptotic factors, have been identified. However, one of the most extensively studied mechanisms is the expression of anticancer drug exporters belonging to the ABC transporter family [11,23,37]. In the case of CRC, the significance of ABCG2 protein level as the patient's potential predictive marker of resistance to irinotecan was examined. ABCG2 protein expression analysed by IHC showed that ABCG2-positive cells were mainly positioned in the cancer's invasion front, and strong membranous staining was significantly correlated with a higher Dukes' stage and distant metastases [10,38]. On the other hand, high ABCG2 expression does not contribute to higher patient mortality and negatively correlates with EMT advancement [11]. In addition, our analysis showed that ABCG2 expression did not correlate with response to FOLFOX or FOLFIRI treatment. There were no statistically significant changes in mRNA expression in the cohorts of responding and non-responding patients. In contrast, CRC patients with high ABCC4 expression and low ABCG2 expression may be considered sensitive to FOLFOX therapy and resistant to the FOLFIRI regimen. This is probably due to substrate specificity. Both proteins transport irinotecan, but neither transports oxaliplatin [39]. Recent studies prove that ABC transporters use mitochondrial-derived ATP, but not ATP from glycolysis, as the primary source of energy for drug efflux in chemo-resistant cancer cells. Importantly, often observed among various cancer types, a metabolic switch toward aerobic glycolysis (known as the Warburg effect) renders ABC proteins rather non-related to chemoresistance [37,40,41]. Thus, the correlation between the level of ABC proteins and their actual molecular function in cancers remains to be proven.

Our multi-omics analysis proves that CRC patients' sample subfractions, expressing a high level of either ABCC4 or ABCG2 followed by a low mRNA level of the second corresponding ABC transporter, are presenting different molecular and physiological functions, even though both transporters present to some extent substrate homology including active transport of irinotecan and its active metabolite SN38 [39]. The ABCG2 High CRC subgroup presents significant enrichment in positive regulation of apoptotic processes, cell adhesion extracellular matrix decomposition, actin filament assembly and cell migration. On the other hand, dysregulated genes in the ABCC4 High CRC subgroup significantly enrich processes related to DNA and RNA binding, regulation of gene expression and response to DNA damage. This observation corresponds to our previous findings, in which we have proven that during phenotypical reprogramming such as EMT, mesenchymal phenotype presenting CRC cells upregulate ABCC4 expression, simultaneously downregulating ABCG2 expression [11]. Differences in the number and composition of EMT transcription factors binding sites for both ABC transporters may explain their various expression during EMT. *ABCC4* poses 11 E-Box sequences and 3 TWIST binding sites, whereas *ABCG2*—only 6 E-Box sequences and 1 TWIST binding site [42].

Similar CAFs, Neutrophils, CD8+ and CD4+ T-cell infiltration patterns may characterise both analysed CRC subfractions. However, ABCC4 expression positively correlates with M2 macrophage infiltration, whereas ABCG2 expression level does not impact this process. Polarised M2 macrophages increase stemness and metastatic ability of CRC cells by secreting TGF-β2 and chemokine C-X-C-Motif Ligand 12 (CXCL12), which activates the

WNT/β-catenin pathway, thus promoting EMT [43]. Therefore, we suggested that due to their complex functions, ABC transporters could be considered to represent markers of specific molecular alterations or advanced reprogramming that accompany cancer progression and that more attention should be placed on the most dysregulated genes and their role in the regulation of particular processes in each analysed subpopulation.

Top networking (top hub) proteins encoded by upregulated genes in the ABCC4 High CRC subgroup are mainly involved in the regulation of nearly all stages of RNA metabolism (transcription, pre-mRNA splicing, RNA export and translation), chromatin metabolism, transcription factors binding and construction of small nucleolar ribonucleoproteins (snoRNPs) complex (composed of core RNP proteins such as NOP58, and rRNA such as SNORD27, which facilitates 2'-O-Me of A27 on 18S rRNA) [33,44,45]. Gene expression and protein levels of NOP58, BPTF and SRSF1, HNRNPA2B1 correlate with CRC progression, increased proliferation and metastasis, TNM staging, and poor prognosis of CRC patients. RNA-binding protein HNRNPA2B1 is involved in the transportation and posttranscriptional regulation of numerous cancer-progression-related micro RNA (miRNAs) and long noncoding RNA (lncRNA) through binding of the specific motifs GGAG/CCCU such as miR-934, Linc01232, miR100HG, H19 and RP11 [46,47]. Recently, it was proven that in the case of CRC, HNRNPA2B1 mediated miR-934 packaging into exosomes that macrophages take up, leading to their polarisation into TGF-β2-secreting M2 macrophages [47]. The protein encoded by the *SRSF1* gene promotes alternative splicing of BIM (also known as BCL2L11) and BIN1—isoforms that lack pro-apoptotic functions [48]. BPTF promotes CRC cell cycle progression, thus CRC proliferation and overall tumour progression by targeting Cell division cycle 25 A (Cdc25A) [49]. NOP58 is a ribonucleoprotein that is a central component for several box C/D small nucleolar RNAs (snoRNAs), such as U3, U8 and U14. Its overexpression is associated with poor cancer patients' survival, as it may regulate cell cycle mitosis, mitotic G1/S phase, mitotic G2/M phase, Rb-1 pathway, M phase, IL-10 signalling, pathways via regulation of *TP53* and P53 activity [50]. Interestingly, lncRNA ZFAS1, one of the significant EMT inducers in CRC, promotes small nucleolar RNA-mediated 2'-O-methylation via NOP58 recruitment and is also responsible for CRC tumorigenesis and further progression via DDX21-POLR1B regulatory axis [33,51,52]. Retinoblastoma-binding protein 7 (RBBP7), an important component of chromatin metabolism-regulating complex, is overexpressed in various cancer types, enhancing cancer cell proliferation, invasion and stemness, increasing cyclin-dependent kinase 4 (CDK4) expression [44,53]. The impact of DDX3X on CRC progression is somewhat enigmatic due to its involvement in all stages of RNA metabolism, which impacts different signalling pathways [45]. On the one hand, it has been reported to act as a tumour suppressor. On the other hand, DDX3X has been shown to induce EMT and subsequent CRC proliferation and migration by stabilising the mRNA of the transcription factor GATA2 [54,55]. Interestingly, the blood mRNA level of EIF2S3 was found to be a discriminating marker of CRC [56]. In addition, the expression levels of other top network proteins, such as RPS27A and PSMD14, are usually significantly higher in CRC tumours than in tumour-adjacent tissue, but unlike PSMD14, which is associated with more aggressive cancers, RPS27A correlates with smaller tumours, lower T-stage and drastically reduced apoptosis rates. [32,57].

In the ABCG2 High CRC subgroup, most top hub proteins belong to the histone cluster family. Recent studies proved that mRNA expression of HIST1H2BK, HIST1H2AG, HIST2H2AA4, HIST1H2BJ, HIST2H2BE and HIST1H2AC proteins positively correlates with each other, and their upregulation is related to the poor prognosis in glioma [58]. Additionally, HIST1H2BK correlates with metastatic CRC cytokine secretion, myeloid leukocyte migration into the tumour, and resistance to proteasome-inhibitor-based anticancer therapy [59].

Although a great deal of CRC patients present resistance to anti-EGFR therapy, it remains the primary form of immunotherapy administered to the patients [35,36]. Three (FLNA, TLR4 and FYN) of the top hub proteins for the ABCG2 High CRC subgroup are involved in the EGF–EGFR pathway. CRC tumours, characterised by high filamin A (FLNA) expression, do not respond to anti-EGFR therapy in cetuximab treatment but may respond to c-MET receptor tyrosine kinase inhibitors [60]. In squamous cell carcinoma, activation of TLR4 reversed cetuximab-induced inhibition of proliferation, migration and invasion, increasing resistance to anti-EGFR therapy [61]. As an effector of oncogenic EGFR signalling, Fyn promotes tumour growth and motility. Its silencing limits EGF-triggered cancer progression [62]. Interestingly, several multi-omics analyses prove that MAPK3 occupies one of the top networking protein positions along with EGFR in various cancers, resulting in poor prognosis [63,64].

From a clinical applicability perspective, precise discrimination of CRC patients into ABCC4/ABCG2 High subgroups may be another factor enabling the selection of correct and appropriate personalised therapy, including a mix of chemo and immunotherapy and identifying the most likely metastatic site.

5. Conclusions

Our analysis proved that ABCC4 and ABCG2 mRNA levels may be used to distinguish two molecular and physiologically different CRC subgroups that may present different susceptibilities to specific therapy. The CRC subgroup characterised by high expression of ABCC4 shows substantial dependence on EMT reprogramming (acquired via TMEM interaction) and RNA metabolism, with higher response to DNA damage stimuli and rather good response to oxaliplatin-based FOLFOX treatment that primarily focuses on the formation of DNA-platinum adducts. It may also be regulated by lncRNA ZFAS1, whereas ABCG2 high expression presenting CRC subgroup may be resistant to the anti-EGFR therapy, demonstrating higher proteolytical activity and actin-filament-related activity, thus higher ability to invade surrounding tissue. Unfortunately, the precise correlation of ABCC4 and ABCG2 mRNA expression levels with response to chemotherapy is limited by the small sample size (n) of FOLFOX- and FOLFIRI-treated patients. In addition, most of the data were obtained from Japanese (Asian) and Danish (Caucasian) patients, and accurate extrapolation to other ethnic groups is difficult and requires further investigation.

Supplementary Materials: The following supporting information can be downloaded at: https://www.mdpi.com/article/10.3390/cancers15235623/s1, Figure S1: Immune cell infiltration analysis.

Author Contributions: Conceptualisation, J.K. and J.B.; methodology, J.K.; software, J.K.; validation, J.K. and J.B.; formal analysis, J.B.; investigation, J.K.; resources, J.K. and J.B.; data curation, J.K.; writing—original draft preparation, J.K.; writing—review and editing, J.B.; visualization, J.K.; supervision, J.B.; project administration, J.B.; funding acquisition, J.B. All authors have read and agreed to the published version of the manuscript.

Funding: This research was supported by the statutory fund of the Institute of Medical Biology of the Polish Academy of Sciences.

Institutional Review Board Statement: Not applicable.

Informed Consent Statement: Not applicable.

Data Availability Statement: The data presented in this study are available in this article.

Conflicts of Interest: The authors declare that they have no competing interest.

References

1. Henry, J.T.; Johnson, B. Current and evolving biomarkers for precision oncology in the management of metastatic colorectal cancer. *Chin. Clin. Oncol.* **2019**, *8*, 49. [CrossRef]
2. Xie, Y.-H.; Chen, Y.-X.; Fang, J.-Y. Comprehensive review of targeted therapy for colorectal cancer. *Signal Transduct. Target. Ther.* **2020**, *5*, 22. [CrossRef]
3. Vatandoust, S.; Price, T.J.; Karapetis, C.S. Colorectal cancer: Metastases to a single organ. *World J. Gastroenterol.* **2015**, *21*, 11767–11776. [CrossRef]
4. Baran, B.; Mert Ozupek, N.; Yerli Tetik, N.; Acar, E.; Bekcioglu, O.; Baskin, Y. Difference Between Left-Sided and Right-Sided Colorectal Cancer: A Focused Review of Literature. *Gastroenterol. Res.* **2018**, *11*, 264–273. [CrossRef]

5. Hsu, H.-H.; Chen, M.-C.; Baskaran, R.; Lin, Y.-M.; Day, C.H.; Lin, Y.-J.; Tu, C.-C.; Vijaya Padma, V.; Kuo, W.-W.; Huang, C.-Y. Oxaliplatin resistance in colorectal cancer cells is mediated via activation of ABCG2 to alleviate ER stress induced apoptosis. *J. Cell. Physiol.* **2018**, *233*, 5458–5467. [CrossRef] [PubMed]
6. Blondy, S.; David, V.; Verdier, M.; Mathonnet, M.; Perraud, A.; Christou, N. 5-Fluorouracil resistance mechanisms in colorectal cancer: From classical pathways to promising processes. *Cancer Sci.* **2020**, *111*, 3142–3154. [CrossRef] [PubMed]
7. Bailly, C. Irinotecan: 25 years of cancer treatment. *Pharmacol. Res.* **2019**, *148*, 104398. [CrossRef] [PubMed]
8. Leslie, E.M.; Deeley, R.G.; Cole, S.P.C. Multidrug resistance proteins: Role of P-glycoprotein, MRP1, MRP2, and BCRP (ABCG2) in tissue defense. *Toxicol. Appl. Pharmacol.* **2005**, *204*, 216–237. [CrossRef] [PubMed]
9. Hlavata, I.; Mohelnikova-Duchonova, B.; Vaclavikova, R.; Liska, V.; Pitule, P.; Novak, P.; Bruha, J.; Vycital, O.; Holubec, L.; Treska, V.; et al. The role of ABC transporters in progression and clinical outcome of colorectal cancer. *Mutagenesis* **2012**, *27*, 187–196. [CrossRef] [PubMed]
10. Nielsen, D.L.; Palshof, J.A.; Brünner, N.; Stenvang, J.; Viuff, B.M. Implications of ABCG2 Expression on Irinotecan Treatment of Colorectal Cancer Patients: A Review. *Int. J. Mol. Sci.* **2017**, *18*, 1926. [CrossRef]
11. Kryczka, J.; Sochacka, E.; Papiewska-Pająk, I.; Boncela, J. Implications of ABCC4-Mediated cAMP Efflux for CRC Migration. *Cancers* **2020**, *12*, 3547. [CrossRef]
12. Przygodzka, P.; Papiewska-Pajak, I.; Bogusz, H.; Kryczka, J.; Sobierajska, K.; Kowalska, M.A.; Boncela, J. Neuromedin U is upregulated by Snail at early stages of EMT in HT29 colon cancer cells. *Biochim. Biophys. Acta* **2016**, *1860*, 2445–2453. [CrossRef]
13. Fletcher, J.I.; Haber, M.; Henderson, M.J.; Norris, M.D. ABC transporters in cancer: More than just drug efflux pumps. *Nat. Rev. Cancer* **2010**, *10*, 147–156. [CrossRef]
14. Muriithi, W.; Macharia, L.W.; Heming, C.P.; Echevarria, J.L.; Nyachieo, A.; Filho, P.N.; Neto, V.M. ABC transporters and the hallmarks of cancer: Roles in cancer aggressiveness beyond multidrug resistance. *Cancer Biol. Med.* **2020**, *17*, 253–269. [CrossRef] [PubMed]
15. Fletcher, J.I.; Williams, R.T.; Henderson, M.J.; Norris, M.D.; Haber, M. ABC transporters as mediators of drug resistance and contributors to cancer cell biology. *Drug Resist. Updat. Rev. Comment. Antimicrob. Anticancer Chemother.* **2016**, *26*, 1–9. [CrossRef] [PubMed]
16. Kryczka, J.; Boncela, J. Integrated Bioinformatics Analysis of the Hub Genes Involved in Irinotecan Resistance in Colorectal Cancer. *Biomedicines* **2022**, *10*, 1720. [CrossRef] [PubMed]
17. Makondi, P.T.; Chu, C.-M.; Wei, P.-L.; Chang, Y.-J. Prediction of novel target genes and pathways involved in irinotecan-resistant colorectal cancer. *PLoS ONE* **2017**, *12*, e0180616. [CrossRef] [PubMed]
18. Chmielewska-Kassassir, M.; Sobierajska, K.; Ciszewski, W.M.; Kryczka, J.; Zielniak, A.; Wozniak, L.A. Evening Primrose Extract Modulates TYMS Expression via SP1 Transcription Factor in Malignant Pleural Mesothelioma. *Cancers* **2023**, *15*, 5003. [CrossRef] [PubMed]
19. Uhlén, M.; Fagerberg, L.; Hallström, B.M.; Lindskog, C.; Oksvold, P.; Mardinoglu, A.; Sivertsson, Å.; Kampf, C.; Sjöstedt, E.; Asplund, A.; et al. Tissue-based map of the human proteome. *Science* **2015**, *347*, 1260419. [CrossRef]
20. Uhlen, M.; Zhang, C.; Lee, S.; Sjöstedt, E.; Fagerberg, L.; Bidkhori, G.; Benfeitas, R.; Arif, M.; Liu, Z.; Edfors, F.; et al. A pathology atlas of the human cancer transcriptome. *Science* **2017**, *357*, eaan2507. [CrossRef]
21. Li, T.; Fan, J.; Wang, B.; Traugh, N.; Chen, Q.; Liu, J.S.; Li, B.; Liu, X.S. TIMER: A Web Server for Comprehensive Analysis of Tumor-Infiltrating Immune Cells. *Cancer Res.* **2017**, *77*, e108–e110. [CrossRef] [PubMed]
22. Baran, K.; Waśko, J.; Kryczka, J.; Boncela, J.; Jabłoński, S.; Kolesińska, B.; Brzezińska-Lasota, E.; Kordiak, J. The Comparison of Serum Exosome Protein Profile in Diagnosis of NSCLC Patients. *Int. J. Mol. Sci.* **2023**, *24*, 13669. [CrossRef] [PubMed]
23. Kryczka, J.; Kryczka, J.; Czarnecka-Chrebelska, K.H.; Brzezińska-Lasota, E. Molecular Mechanisms of Chemoresistance Induced by Cisplatin in NSCLC Cancer Therapy. *Int. J. Mol. Sci.* **2021**, *22*, 8885. [CrossRef] [PubMed]
24. Li, T.; Fu, J.; Zeng, Z.; Cohen, D.; Li, J.; Chen, Q.; Li, B.; Liu, X.S. TIMER2.0 for analysis of tumor-infiltrating immune cells. *Nucleic Acids Res.* **2020**, *48*, W509–W514. [CrossRef]
25. Neophytou, C.M.; Panagi, M.; Stylianopoulos, T.; Papageorgis, P. The Role of Tumor Microenvironment in Cancer Metastasis: Molecular Mechanisms and Therapeutic Opportunities. *Cancers* **2021**, *13*, 2053. [CrossRef]
26. Shokati, E.; Safari, E. The immunomodulatory role of exosomal microRNA networks in the crosstalk between tumor-associated myeloid-derived suppressor cells and tumor cells. *Int. Immunopharmacol.* **2023**, *120*, 110267. [CrossRef]
27. Kuwahara, T.; Hazama, S.; Suzuki, N.; Yoshida, S.; Tomochika, S.; Nakagami, Y.; Matsui, H.; Shindo, Y.; Kanekiyo, S.; Tokumitsu, Y.; et al. Intratumoural-infiltrating CD4+ and FOXP3 + T cells as strong positive predictive markers for the prognosis of resectable colorectal cancer. *Br. J. Cancer* **2019**, *121*, 659–665. [CrossRef]
28. Ito, A.; Yamada, N.; Yoshida, Y.; Morino, S.; Yamamoto, O. Myofibroblastic differentiation in atypical fibroxanthomas occurring on sun-exposed skin and in a burn scar: An ultrastructural and immunohistochemical study. *J. Cutan. Pathol.* **2011**, *38*, 670–676. [CrossRef]
29. Liu, C.-Y.; Xu, J.-Y.; Shi, X.-Y.; Huang, W.; Ruan, T.-Y.; Xie, P.; Ding, J.-L. M2-polarized tumor-associated macrophages promoted epithelial-mesenchymal transition in pancreatic cancer cells, partially through TLR4/IL-10 signaling pathway. *Lab. Investig. J. Tech. Methods Pathol.* **2013**, *93*, 844–854. [CrossRef]
30. Aran, D.; Hu, Z.; Butte, A.J. xCell: Digitally portraying the tissue cellular heterogeneity landscape. *Genome Biol.* **2017**, *18*, 220. [CrossRef]

31. Leban, G.; Zupan, B.; Vidmar, G.; Bratko, I. VizRank: Data Visualization Guided by Machine Learning. *Data Min. Knowl. Discov.* **2006**, *13*, 119–136. [CrossRef]
32. Mu, Q.; Luo, G.; Wei, J.; Zheng, L.; Wang, H.; Yu, M.; Xu, N. Apolipoprotein M promotes growth and inhibits apoptosis of colorectal cancer cells through upregulation of ribosomal protein S27a. *EXCLI J.* **2021**, *20*, 145–159. [CrossRef] [PubMed]
33. Wu, H.; Qin, W.; Lu, S.; Wang, X.; Zhang, J.; Sun, T.; Hu, X.; Li, Y.; Chen, Q.; Wang, Y.; et al. Long noncoding RNA ZFAS1 promoting small nucleolar RNA-mediated 2′-O-methylation via NOP58 recruitment in colorectal cancer. *Mol. Cancer* **2020**, *19*, 95. [CrossRef]
34. Lu, M.; Zessin, A.S.; Glover, W.; Hsu, D.S. Activation of the mTOR Pathway by Oxaliplatin in the Treatment of Colorectal Cancer Liver Metastasis. *PLoS ONE* **2017**, *12*, e0169439. [CrossRef]
35. Ooi, Z.S.; Pang, S.W.; Teow, S.Y. RAS and BRAF genes as biomarkers and target for personalised colorectal cancer therapy: An update. *Malays. J. Pathol.* **2022**, *44*, 415–428. [PubMed]
36. Ooki, A.; Shinozaki, E.; Yamaguchi, K. Immunotherapy in Colorectal Cancer: Current and Future Strategies. *J. Anus Rectum Colon* **2021**, *5*, 11–24. [CrossRef]
37. Giddings, E.L.; Champagne, D.P.; Wu, M.-H.; Laffin, J.M.; Thornton, T.M.; Valenca-Pereira, F.; Culp-Hill, R.; Fortner, K.A.; Romero, N.; East, J.; et al. Mitochondrial ATP fuels ABC transporter-mediated drug efflux in cancer chemoresistance. *Nat. Commun.* **2021**, *12*, 2804. [CrossRef] [PubMed]
38. Giampieri, R.; Scartozzi, M.; Loretelli, C.; Piva, F.; Mandolesi, A.; Lezoche, G.; Prete, M.D.; Bittoni, A.; Faloppi, L.; Bianconi, M.; et al. Cancer Stem Cell Gene Profile as Predictor of Relapse in High Risk Stage II and Stage III, Radically Resected Colon Cancer Patients. *PLoS ONE* **2013**, *8*, e72843. [CrossRef]
39. Ween, M.P.; Armstrong, M.A.; Oehler, M.K.; Ricciardelli, C. The role of ABC transporters in ovarian cancer progression and chemoresistance. *Crit. Rev. Oncol. Hematol.* **2015**, *96*, 220–256. [CrossRef]
40. Warburg, O. On the Origin of Cancer Cells. *Science* **1956**, *123*, 309–314. [CrossRef]
41. DeBerardinis, R.J.; Chandel, N.S. We need to talk about the Warburg effect. *Nat. Metab.* **2020**, *2*, 127–129. [CrossRef]
42. Saxena, M.; Stephens, M.A.; Pathak, H.; Rangarajan, A. Transcription factors that mediate epithelial–mesenchymal transition lead to multidrug resistance by upregulating ABC transporters. *Cell Death Dis.* **2011**, *2*, e179. [CrossRef]
43. Shi, X.; Wei, K.; Wu, Y.; Mao, L.; Pei, W.; Zhu, H.; Shi, Y.; Zhang, S.; Tao, S.; Wang, J.; et al. Exosome-derived miR-372-5p promotes stemness and metastatic ability of CRC cells by inducing macrophage polarization. *Cell. Signal.* **2023**, *111*, 110884. [CrossRef] [PubMed]
44. Yu, N.; Zhang, P.; Wang, L.; He, X.; Yang, S.; Lu, H. RBBP7 is a prognostic biomarker in patients with esophageal squamous cell carcinoma. *Oncol. Lett.* **2018**, *16*, 7204–7211. [CrossRef] [PubMed]
45. Mo, J.; Liang, H.; Su, C.; Li, P.; Chen, J.; Zhang, B. DDX3X: Structure, physiologic functions and cancer. *Mol. Cancer* **2021**, *20*, 38. [CrossRef] [PubMed]
46. Lu, Y.; Zou, R.; Gu, Q.; Wang, X.; Zhang, J.; Ma, R.; Wang, T.; Wu, J.; Feng, J.; Zhang, Y. CRNDE mediated hnRNPA2B1 stability facilitates nuclear export and translation of KRAS in colorectal cancer. *Cell Death Dis.* **2023**, *14*, 611. [CrossRef]
47. Zhao, S.; Mi, Y.; Guan, B.; Zheng, B.; Wei, P.; Gu, Y.; Zhang, Z.; Cai, S.; Xu, Y.; Li, X.; et al. Tumor-derived exosomal miR-934 induces macrophage M2 polarization to promote liver metastasis of colorectal cancer. *J. Hematol. Oncol.J Hematol Oncol* **2020**, *13*, 156. [CrossRef] [PubMed]
48. Anczuków, O.; Rosenberg, A.Z.; Akerman, M.; Das, S.; Zhan, L.; Karni, R.; Muthuswamy, S.K.; Krainer, A.R. The splicing factor SRSF1 regulates apoptosis and proliferation to promote mammary epithelial cell transformation. *Nat. Struct. Mol. Biol.* **2012**, *19*, 220–228. [CrossRef]
49. Guo, P.; Zu, S.; Han, S.; Yu, W.; Xue, G.; Lu, X.; Lin, H.; Zhao, X.; Lu, H.; Hua, C.; et al. BPTF inhibition antagonizes colorectal cancer progression by transcriptionally inactivating Cdc25A. *Redox Biol.* **2022**, *55*, 102418. [CrossRef]
50. Wang, J.; Huang, R.; Huang, Y.; Chen, Y.; Chen, F. Overexpression of NOP58 as a Prognostic Marker in Hepatocellular Carcinoma: A TCGA Data-Based Analysis. *Adv. Ther.* **2021**, *38*, 3342–3361. [CrossRef]
51. Wang, X.; Wu, Z.; Qin, W.; Sun, T.; Lu, S.; Li, Y.; Wang, Y.; Hu, X.; Xu, D.; Wu, Y.; et al. Long non-coding RNA ZFAS1 promotes colorectal cancer tumorigenesis and development through DDX21-POLR1B regulatory axis. *Aging* **2020**, *12*, 22656–22687. [CrossRef] [PubMed]
52. O'Brien, S.J.; Fiechter, C.; Burton, J.; Hallion, J.; Paas, M.; Patel, A.; Patel, A.; Rochet, A.; Scheurlen, K.; Gardner, S.; et al. Long non-coding RNA ZFAS1 is a major regulator of epithelial-mesenchymal transition through miR-200/ZEB1/E-cadherin, vimentin signaling in colon adenocarcinoma. *Cell Death Discov.* **2021**, *7*, 61. [CrossRef]
53. Wang, R.; Huang, Z.; Lin, Z.; Chen, B.; Pang, X.; Du, C.; Fan, H. Hypoxia-induced RBBP7 promotes esophagus cancer progression by inducing CDK4 expression. *Acta Biochim. Biophys. Sin.* **2022**, *54*, 179–186. [CrossRef] [PubMed]
54. Shen, L.; Zhang, J.; Xu, M.; Zheng, Y.; Wang, M.; Yang, S.; Qin, B.; Li, S.; Dong, L.; Dai, F. DDX3 acts as a tumor suppressor in colorectal cancer as loss of DDX3 in advanced cancer promotes tumor progression by activating the MAPK pathway. *Int. J. Biol. Sci.* **2022**, *18*, 3918–3933. [CrossRef]
55. Pan, Y.; Zhu, Y.; Zhang, J.; Jin, L.; Cao, P. A feedback loop between GATA2-AS1 and GATA2 promotes colorectal cancer cell proliferation, invasion, epithelial-mesenchymal transition and stemness via recruiting DDX3X. *J. Transl. Med.* **2022**, *20*, 287. [CrossRef] [PubMed]

56. Chang, Y.-T.; Huang, C.-S.; Yao, C.-T.; Su, S.-L.; Terng, H.-J.; Chou, H.-L.; Chou, Y.-C.; Chen, K.-H.; Shih, Y.-W.; Lu, C.-Y.; et al. Gene expression profile of peripheral blood in colorectal cancer. *World J. Gastroenterol.* **2014**, *20*, 14463–14471. [CrossRef]
57. Lin, X.-H.; Li, D.-P.; Liu, Z.-Y.; Zhang, S.; Tang, W.-Q.; Chen, R.-X.; Weng, S.-Q.; Tseng, Y.-J.; Xue, R.-Y.; Dong, L. Six immune-related promising biomarkers may promote hepatocellular carcinoma prognosis: A bioinformatics analysis and experimental validation. *Cancer Cell Int.* **2023**, *23*, 52. [CrossRef]
58. Liu, W.; Xu, Z.; Zhou, J.; Xing, S.; Li, Z.; Gao, X.; Feng, S.; Xiao, Y. High Levels of HIST1H2BK in Low-Grade Glioma Predicts Poor Prognosis: A Study Using CGGA and TCGA Data. *Front. Oncol.* **2020**, *10*, 627. [CrossRef]
59. Kim, J.C.; Ha, Y.J.; Park, I.J.; Kim, C.W.; Yoon, Y.S.; Lee, J.L.; Tak, K.H.; Cho, D.-H.; Park, S.H.; Kim, S.-K.; et al. Tumor immune microenvironment of primary colorectal adenocarcinomas metastasizing to the liver or lungs. *J. Surg. Oncol.* **2021**, *124*, 1136–1145. [CrossRef]
60. Sadanandam, A.; Lyssiotis, C.A.; Homicsko, K.; Collisson, E.A.; Gibb, W.J.; Wullschleger, S.; Ostos, L.C.G.; Lannon, W.A.; Grotzinger, C.; Del Rio, M.; et al. A colorectal cancer classification system that associates cellular phenotype and responses to therapy. *Nat. Med.* **2013**, *19*, 619–625. [CrossRef]
61. Ju, H.; Hu, Z.; Lu, Y.; Wu, Y.; Zhang, L.; Wei, D.; Guo, W.; Xia, W.; Liu, S.; Ren, G.; et al. TLR4 activation leads to anti-EGFR therapy resistance in head and neck squamous cell carcinoma. *Am. J. Cancer Res.* **2020**, *10*, 454–472. [PubMed]
62. Lu, K.V.; Zhu, S.; Cvrljevic, A.; Huang, T.T.; Sarkaria, S.; Ahkavan, D.; Dang, J.; Dinca, E.B.; Plaisier, S.B.; Oderberg, I.; et al. Fyn and SRC are effectors of oncogenic epidermal growth factor receptor signaling in glioblastoma patients. *Cancer Res.* **2009**, *69*, 6889–6898. [CrossRef] [PubMed]
63. Huang, S. A novel strategy for the study on molecular mechanism of prostate injury induced by 4,4′-sulfonyldiphenol based on network toxicology analysis. *J. Appl. Toxicol. JAT* **2023**, 1–13. [CrossRef]
64. Ye, B.; Chen, P.; Lin, C.; Zhang, C.; Li, L. Study on the material basis and action mechanisms of sophora davidii (Franch.) skeels flower extract in the treatment of non-small cell lung cancer. *J. Ethnopharmacol.* **2023**, *317*, 116815. [CrossRef] [PubMed]

Disclaimer/Publisher's Note: The statements, opinions and data contained in all publications are solely those of the individual author(s) and contributor(s) and not of MDPI and/or the editor(s). MDPI and/or the editor(s) disclaim responsibility for any injury to people or property resulting from any ideas, methods, instructions or products referred to in the content.

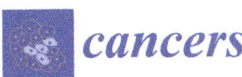

Article

Hedgehog-GLI and Notch Pathways Sustain Chemoresistance and Invasiveness in Colorectal Cancer and Their Inhibition Restores Chemotherapy Efficacy

Anna Citarella [1], Giuseppina Catanzaro [1], Zein Mersini Besharat [1], Sofia Trocchianesi [2], Federica Barbagallo [1,3], Giorgio Gosti [4,5], Marco Leonetti [4,5,6], Annamaria Di Fiore [1,2], Lucia Coppola [1], Tanja Milena Autilio [1], Zaira Spinello [1], Alessandra Vacca [1], Enrico De Smaele [1], Mary Anna Venneri [1], Elisabetta Ferretti [1], Laura Masuelli [1,†] and Agnese Po [2,*,†]

1. Department of Experimental Medicine, Sapienza University of Rome, Viale Regina Elena 324, 00161 Rome, Italy
2. Department of Molecular Medicine, Sapienza University of Rome, Viale Regina Elena 291, 00161 Rome, Italy
3. Faculty of Medicine and Surgery, Kore University of Enna, Cittadella Universitaria, 94100 Enna, Italy
4. Soft and Living Matter Laboratory, Institute of Nanotechnology, Consiglio Nazionale Delle Ricerche, Piazzale Aldo Moro 5, 00185 Rome, Italy
5. Center for Life Nano- and Neuro-Science, Istituto Italiano di Tecnologia, Viale Regina Elena 291, 00161 Rome, Italy
6. D-TAILS srl, Viale Regina Elena 291, 00161 Rome, Italy
* Correspondence: agnese.po@uniroma1.it; Tel.: +39-0649255133
† These authors contributed equally to this work.

Citation: Citarella, A.; Catanzaro, G.; Besharat, Z.M.; Trocchianesi, S.; Barbagallo, F.; Gosti, G.; Leonetti, M.; Di Fiore, A.; Coppola, L.; Autilio, T.M.; et al. Hedgehog-GLI and Notch Pathways Sustain Chemoresistance and Invasiveness in Colorectal Cancer and Their Inhibition Restores Chemotherapy Efficacy. *Cancers* **2023**, *15*, 1471. https://doi.org/10.3390/cancers15051471

Academic Editors: Rodrigo Barderas-Manchado, Cristina Díaz del Arco, María Jesús Fernández-Aceñero and Javier Martinez Useros

Received: 22 January 2023
Revised: 16 February 2023
Accepted: 22 February 2023
Published: 25 February 2023

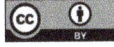

Copyright: © 2023 by the authors. Licensee MDPI, Basel, Switzerland. This article is an open access article distributed under the terms and conditions of the Creative Commons Attribution (CC BY) license (https://creativecommons.org/licenses/by/4.0/).

Simple Summary: Colorectal cancer is a leading cause of cancer-related deaths, mainly caused by resistance to therapy and metastatic spread, in turn sustained by the activation of mechanisms such as the epithelial-to-mesenchymal transition (EMT). We investigate here the role of the Hedgehog-GLI and NOTCH signaling pathways, already associated with poor prognosis in CRC, in the mechanism of chemoresistance and EMT, using monolayer and organoids from two models of common mutations in CRC: KRAS and BRAF. Our results show that treatment with the chemotherapeutic drug 5-fluorouracil activated both pathways in the investigated contexts. However, we observed a different behavior in the investigated models: in KRAS-mutated CRC, the inhibition of both the HH-GLI and NOTCH pathways is necessary to enhance chemosensitivity, while in BRAF-mutated CRC the inhibition of HH-GLI is sufficient to impair both signaling pathways and promote chemosensitivity.

Abstract: Colorectal cancer (CRC) is a leading cause of cancer-related mortality and chemoresistance is a major medical issue. The epithelial-to-mesenchymal transition (EMT) is the primary step in the emergence of the invasive phenotype and the Hedgehog-GLI (HH-GLI) and NOTCH signaling pathways are associated with poor prognosis and EMT in CRC. CRC cell lines harboring KRAS or BRAF mutations, grown as monolayers and organoids, were treated with the chemotherapeutic agent 5-Fluorouracil (5-FU) alone or combined with HH-GLI and NOTCH pathway inhibitors GANT61 and DAPT, or arsenic trioxide (ATO) to inhibit both pathways. Treatment with 5-FU led to the activation of HH-GLI and NOTCH pathways in both models. In KRAS mutant CRC, HH-GLI and NOTCH signaling activation co-operate to enhance chemoresistance and cell motility, while in BRAF mutant CRC, the HH-GLI pathway drives the chemoresistant and motile phenotype. We then showed that 5-FU promotes the mesenchymal and thus invasive phenotype in KRAS and BRAF mutant organoids and that chemosensitivity could be restored by targeting the HH-GLI pathway in BRAF mutant CRC or both HH-GLI and NOTCH pathways in KRAS mutant CRC. We suggest that in KRAS-driven CRC, the FDA-approved ATO acts as a chemotherapeutic sensitizer, whereas GANT61 is a promising chemotherapeutic sensitizer in BRAF-driven CRC.

Keywords: colorectal cancer; signaling pathways; chemoresistance; epithelial-to-mesenchymal transition; organoids

1. Introduction

Colorectal cancer (CRC) is the third most frequent cancer and the second cause of cancer-related death worldwide [1]. Mutations in KRAS and BRAF oncogenes represent the most common genetic drivers in CRC. Indeed, KRAS and BRAF mutations occur in 40% and 10% of CRC, respectively [2], and they are both associated with a poor outcome [3]. Even though they both belong to the MAPK pathway, KRAS and BRAF mutations are mutually exclusive in CRC and these two types of cancer are characterized by distinct clinical and molecular features. BRAF-mutant CRC often displays genome-wide hypermethylation, high microsatellite instability and mutation rates, while KRAS mutant CRC is associated with lower levels of microsatellite instability and gene methylation [2].

First-line and palliative treatments for metastatic CRC, bearing KRAS or BRAF mutations, include the cytotoxic chemotherapeutic agent 5-fluorouracil (5-FU) [1,4]; however, patients often present disease recurrence after 5-FU therapy [5]. Chemoresistance is conferred by a plethora of mechanisms, including the modulation of signaling pathways involved in the emergence of the cancer stem features and epithelial-to-mesenchymal transition (EMT) [6]. Other mechanisms for resistance to therapy include the inhibition of apoptosis driven by upregulation of autophagy [7], metabolic reprogramming [8], upregulation of molecules involved in drug efflux and drug metabolism and activation of alternative pathways [9].

Hedgehog-GLI (HH-GLI) and NOTCH signaling are pivotal developmental pathways involved in the regulation of multiple biological and pathological processes. The canonical HH-GLI pathway is activated upon the interaction between the extracellular ligands Shh, Ihh and Dhh and the receptor Patched (PTCH), which in turn derepresses Smoothened (Smo), thus activating the transcription factors GLI1, GLI2 and GLI3. Activated GLI translocate into the nucleus where they bind to DNA and activate the transcription of target genes [10]. In cancers, GLI1 can also be activated in a non-canonical way by the "oncogenic load" of the cancer cell [11]. NOTCH cascade is activated upon binding of ligands Jag1, Jag2, Dll1, Dll3 and Dll4 to NOTCH receptors (from 1 to 4). The binding leads to proteolytic cleavages of the NOTCH receptor, releasing the NOTCH intracellular domain (ID) into the cytoplasm. Then, NOTCH ID migrates into the nucleus where, in complex with CBF1 (also known as RPBJ), it activates its transcriptional program [12]. Downstream target genes include HES1, which is involved in EMT and transcriptionally regulates ATP-binding cassettes transporters (ABC transporters), involved in multidrug resistance [13]. Interestingly, deregulation of the NOTCH pathway was described in numerous cancerous and non-cancerous diseases, with its role being highly context-dependent [14].

Deregulated HH-GLI is involved in the development and maintenance of numerous cancers [10] and, together with NOTCH signaling, plays a crucial role in the maintenance of stem cells of the intestinal epithelia [15]. The crosstalk of HH-GLI and NOTCH signaling is fundamental for spinal cord patterning [16], and several previous reports highlighted how several molecules belonging to the NOTCH pathway regulate the key components of the HH-GLI pathway and vice versa, as reviewed Kumar et al. [17].

Both HH-GLI and NOTCH pathways were described as deregulated and associated with poor prognosis in CRC [18,19]. In this context, our previous work has described a chemoresistance mechanism operated by the HH-GLI signaling in CRC, where chemotherapy treatment resulted in aberrant activation of the HH-GLI pathway which in turn led to the transcription of ATP-binding cassette transporters (ABC transporters), involved in multidrug resistance [20].

Therefore, our current work aimed to evaluate the role of HH-GLI and NOTCH signaling pathways as regulatory molecular mechanisms responsible for chemotherapy resistance in models of KRAS- or BRAF-driven CRC.

2. Materials and Methods

2.1. Cell Cultures and Treatments

HCT116 (*KRAS G13D* mutant) and HT29 (*BRAF V600E* mutant) were obtained from American Type Culture Collection (ATCC) and grown in DMEM high glucose (supplemented with 10% (v/v) fetal bovine serum, 1% (v/v) penicillin (50 U mL^{-1})—streptomycin (50 U mL^{-1})—and 2 mM L-glutamine. Cells were routinely checked for mycoplasma contamination by testing with PCR Mycoplasma Detection Kit (Cat. G238, ABM, Richmond, BC, Canada).

Cells were treated with 10 µM GANT61 (ENZO Lifesciences, New York, NY, USA), 10 µM DAPT (Merk Life Science S.r.l., Milan, Italy), 10 µM Arsenic Trioxide (ATO) (Merck, Merk Life Science S.r.l., Milan, Italy) and 10 µM 5-Fluorouracil (5-FU).

For combined treatments, GANT61 and DAPT or Arsenic Trioxide (ATO) were administered to the cells 24 h before 5-FU.

2.2. Cell Viability by Trypan Blue Exclusion Assay

Cell proliferation was assessed by trypan blue dye exclusion test using 0.4% (w/v) Trypan Blue solution (Merk Life Science S.r.l., Milan, Italy). Blue-stained cells were scored as non-viable and unstained cells were scored as viable cells. The percentage of viable cells was obtained as the ratio between the percentage of viable cells in treated cells versus control.

2.3. Transwell Invasion Assay

Transwell invasion assay was performed using Corning® Transwell® chambers (8 µm pore size, Corning®). HCT116 and HT29 cells (2.5×10^4 in each well) were seeded in the upper chambers of the 48-well plates (Corning, Somerville, MA, USA) while lower chambers were filled with 1 mL of medium with indicated treatments. Cells in the lower chambers were fixed with 95% ethanol for 10 min, stained with crystal violet and counted.

2.4. Western Blot

Cells were lysed as previously described [20]. Lysates were separated on 8% acrylamide gel and immunoblotted using standard procedures [21]. Primary antibodies were Anti-GLI1 (L42B10, Cell Signalling Technology Inc., Boston, MA, USA), anti-PARP p85 Fragment (G7341, Promega, Madison, WI, USA) and anti-Cleaved NOTCH1 (D3B8, Cell Signalling Technology Inc., Boston, MA, USA). HRP-conjugated secondary antisera (Santa Cruz Biotechnology, Shanghai, China) were used, followed by enhanced chemiluminescence (ECL Amersham, Merk Life Science S.r.l., Milan, Italy).

2.5. RNA Isolation and Real Time qPCR

cDNA was obtained as described earlier [20]. RNA expression was analyzed on cDNAs using the ViiA™ 7 Real-Time PCR System, SensiFAST™ Probe Lo-ROX (Bioline, Memphis, TN, USA), TaqMan gene expression assay according to the manufacturer's instructions (Life Technologies, Waltham, MA, USA). mRNA quantification was expressed in arbitrary units, as the ratio of the sample quantity to the calibrator or to the mean values of control samples. All values were normalized to three endogenous controls: HPRT, GAPDH and β-ACTIN.

Primers for gene expression are listed in Supplementary Table S1. Gene expression of GLI1, HES1, c-MET, ABCG2, CD133, KRAS, BRAF, HPRT, GAPDH and β-ACTIN was assessed using Life technologies "best coverage" assays (Life Technologies, Waltham, MA, USA).

2.6. Organoids

Organoids were produced by seeding 1500 cells per well. Cells were mixed with 33% growth-factor-reduced phenol red-free Matrigel (Corning, Somerville, MA, USA). Cultures were grown using a flat-bottom 24-well microplate in advanced DMEM-F12 (Cat. 12634010, Gibco, Waltham, MA, USA) supplemented with Epidermal growth factor and Fibroblast growth factor both at final concentrations of 20 ng/µL.

For in vivo live imaging experiments, GFP-labelled organoids were obtained by transducing HCT116 with PLKO lentiviral particles carrying pTWEEN-GFP vector.

Transduced green fluorescent cells were selected by cell sorting and used for organoids production.

2.7. Whole Mount Immunofluorescence

Organoids were fixed with 4% paraformaldehyde and permeabilized with Triton X-100 in PBS (Sigma-Aldrich, St. Louis, MO, USA). Organoids were stained with anti-vimentin (ab11256, ABCAM, Cambridge, UK) antibody. Nuclei were DAPI-counterstained. Phalloidin was used for f-actin staining. Images were acquired using an LSM 900 (Zeiss, Milan, Italy) laser scanning confocal microscope with $40\times/0.75$ NA objective. Images were analyzed by using the program Zeiss ZEN 2.3 blue edition (https://www.zeiss.com/microscopy/int/products/microscope-software/zen-lite.html (accessed on 10 September 2022)).

2.8. Datasets and In Silico Analyses

Datasets available on R2 platform (https://hgserver1.amc.nl/cgi-bin/r2/main.cgi (accessed on 15 December 2021)) were interrogated to evaluate GLI1 and NOTCH1 correlation in patients carrying BRAF or KRAS mutations. In detail, Tumor Colon Mutation status (Core Exon)—Sieber—211—rma_sketch—huex10p investigated gene correlation between GENE/REPORTER1: GLI1 and GENE/REPORTER2: NOTCH1, in 29 samples of CRC-carrying braf_v600e mutation; Tumor Colon (after surgery)—Beissbarth—363—custom—4hm44k investigated gene correlation between GENE/REPORTER1: GLI1 and GENE/REPORTER2: NOTCH1, in 32 samples of CRC carrying kras_g13d mutation.

2.9. Single-Particle Tracking Analysis

Single-particle tracking (SPT) diffusibility analysis was performed in five steps. In the first step, single cells were detected from the time-lapse movies of oHCT116-treated and control group organoids using Imaris spot model. Spots were taken in each frame and were linked to the spots corresponding to the same cell in the successive frame. Frame-to-frame tracking was implemented using the linear assignment problem (LAP) method [22,23]. In the third step, MSD, the mean square distance travelled by a cell given a certain time interval (see Supplementary Figure S3), was computed from single trajectories, as described by Michalet X [24]. In the fourth step, the diffusion parameter D was calculated for each tracked cell. To this end, the MSD was plotted for different time intervals (Δt) for each cell trajectory and the slope was computed using the Least Squares Method. In the fifth step, the Kolmogorov–Smirnov test was applied on the diffusion parameters D, obtained from 5-FU-treated oHCT116 and control group organoids.

2.10. Statistical Analysis

Results are representative of at least three independent experiments and are expressed as means +/− SD. Differences were analyzed using One-way ANOVA and Two-way ANOVA tests where appropriate, using the GraphPad Prism software Version 8.0. Adjusted p-values of less than 0.05 were considered as statistically significant.

3. Results

3.1. HH-GLI and NOTCH Signaling Pathways Sustain Resistance to 5-FU in KRAS Mutant CRC Cells

5-fluorouracil (5-FU) is a chemotherapeutic agent used for adjuvant and palliative treatment of CRC; however, patients often present disease recurrence [5]. Therefore, we evaluated the role of HH-GLI and NOTCH signaling pathways as molecular mechanisms responsible for chemotherapy resistance.

KRAS mutant HCT116 CRC cells were treated with 5-FU, alone or in combination with the HH-GLI inhibitor GANT61 and/or the NOTCH inhibitor DAPT. Our results showed that GLI1 and NOTCH1 ID were significantly upregulated after 5-FU treatment (Figure 1A). HH-GLI inhibition by GANT61 resulted in the downregulation of GLI1 and, interestingly, in the upregulation of NOTCH1 ID; vice versa, NOTCH inhibition by DAPT resulted in the downregulation of NOTCH1 ID and the upregulation of GLI1 (Figure 1A).

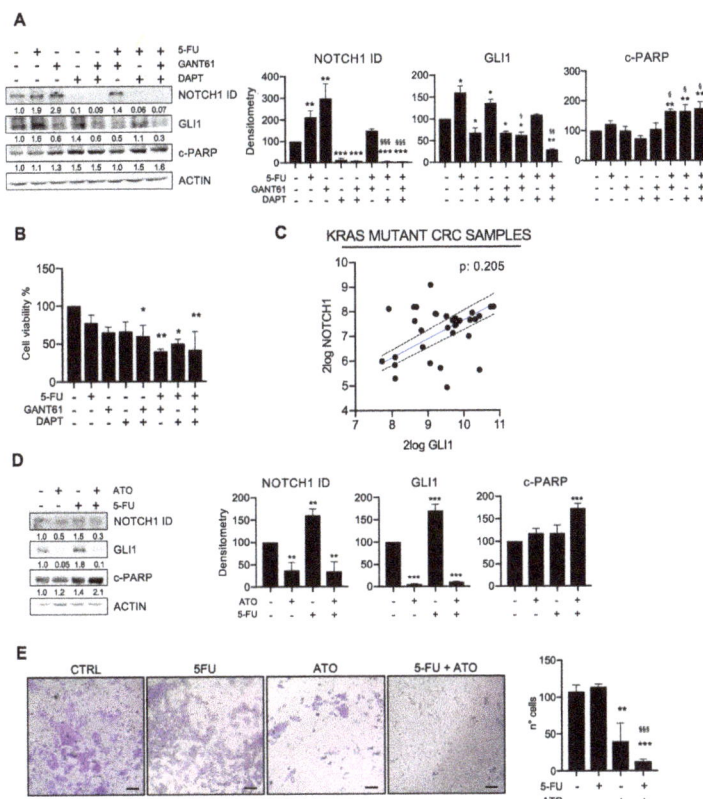

Figure 1. HH-GLI and NOTCH signaling pathways sustain resistance to 5-FU in KRAS mutant CRC cells. (A) Western blot analysis of NOTCH1 Intracellular domain (NOTCH1 ID), GLI1 and cleaved-PARP (c-PARP) in HCT116 cells after 5-FU treatment in combination with GANT61 and DAPT. Numbers indicate intensity ratio of bands. Bar graphs show densitometric quantification of the band intensity values normalized to the loading control. * $p < 0.05$; ** $p < 0.01$; *** $p < 0.001$ versus control; § $p < 0.05$ versus 5-FU; §§ $p < 0.01$; §§§ $p < 0.001$ (Two-way ANOVA test). Uncropped full scan in Supplementary Figure S4. (B) Evaluation of cell viability by Trypan Blue exclusion assay in HCT116 after 5-FU treatment with or without GANT61 and/or DAPT; * $p < 0.05$, ** $p < 0.01$ versus CTRL (One-way ANOVA test). (C) Correlation analysis between GLI1 and NOTCH1 expression from dataset interrogated on R2 platform, as indicated in main text. (D) Western blot analysis of GLI1, NOTCH1 ID and c-PARP in HCT116 cells treated with 5-FU and ATO. Numbers indicate intensity ratio of bands. Bar graphs show densitometric quantification of the band intensity values normalized to the loading control; * $p < 0.05$; ** $p < 0.01$; (Two-way ANOVA test). (E) Transwell invasion assay in HCT116 cells treated with 5-FU, ATO and the combined treatment and control group (CTRL). Scale bar 150 µm. ** $p < 0.01$; *** $p < 0.001$; versus control; §§§ $p < 0.001$ (One-way ANOVA test).

We then determined the effects of treatments with the combination of HH-GLI inhibitor, NOTCH inhibitor and 5-FU. NOTCH1 ID expression was impaired in all combined treatments that included DAPT (DAPT+GANT61, DAPT+5-FU and DAPT+GANT61+5FU), while it was unaffected by the combination of 5-FU+GANT61.

On the other hand, GLI1 was downregulated by GANT61 alone, as well as when combined with 5-FU and 5-FU+DAPT, while the combination of NOTCH inhibition and 5-FU failed to inhibit GLI1.

Overall, our results show that GLI1 and NOTCH1 ID levels were concomitantly significantly downregulated only after the combined treatment of the chemotherapeutic agent 5-FU together with the inhibition of HH-GLI and NOTCH.

In addition, we observed that the combination of HH-GLI and NOTCH pathway inhibition prevents the GLI1 upregulation and NOTCH1 activation induced by 5-FU.

To determine the effects of treatments on apoptosis, levels of cleaved PARP (c-PARP) were evaluated; our results show that c-PARP was significantly induced by the combination of 5-FU and GANT61 or DAPT, and the three drugs combined (Figure 1A).

We further analyzed the effects of treatments on cell viability, and we found it significantly impaired in cells treated with the combination of GANT61 and DAPT and with the combination of 5-FU with either GANT61 or DAPT or the combination of the three drugs (Figure 1B).

To discern potential interdependence between the HH-GLI and NOTCH signaling pathways in mutant KRAS CRC cells, we analyzed GLI1 and NOTCH1 levels in an available cohort of CRC patients carrying this mutation (Tumor Colon (after surgery)—Beissbarth—363—custom—4hm44k; https://hgserver1.amc.nl/cgi-bin/r2/main.cgi, accessed on 15 December 2021) and no correlation was found (Figure 1C).

We therefore envisioned a model where the oncogenic force of the driver gene *KRASG13D* sustains both HH-GLI and NOTCH pathways and both pathways need to be targeted to achieve a successful impairment of cells after chemotherapy.

Hence, to clarify if the KRASG13D driver mutation sustained expression of GLI1 and NOTCH, we performed silencing of KRAS in HCT116 (Supplementary Figure S1A), which resulted in the significant downregulation of GLI1 and NOTCH1 ID protein levels (Supplementary Figure S1B). KRAS silencing was also accompanied by a significant downregulation of ABCG2 and HES1, target genes of HH-GLI and NOTCH1 ID, respectively (Supplementary Figure S1C).

Arsenic Trioxide (ATO) is an organic compound approved for the therapy of adult patients with acute promyelocytic leukemia [25] and was shown to successfully inhibit both HH-GLI and NOTCH pathways [26]. ATO'sability to inhibit both GLI1 and NOTCH ID levels was confirmed in the KRASG13D-driven CRC model (Figure 1D). As previously shown, 5-FU alone was able to upregulate both GLI1 and NOTCH1 ID, while the combination with ATO impaired both signaling pathways (Figure 1D). Cleaved-PARP levels showed that apoptosis was significantly increased by the combination of ATO and 5-FU, while we observed a non-significant trend in ATO-treated cells (Figure 1D).

A pivotal feature of CRC aggressiveness relies on the epithelial-to-mesenchymal transition (EMT), a process that includes the acquisition by cancer cells of properties including motility and migration, early steps in cancer invasion and metastasis.

Therefore, we investigated whether the targeting of HH-GLI and NOTCH could impair KRAS mutant CRC's migratory ability.

We investigated the effects of the combined treatment of 5-FU and ATO on the migration ability of HCT116 cells. We observed that the migration was unaffected by 5-FU treatment, while it was impaired with ATO treatment and was completely abrogated after ATO plus 5-FU combined treatment (Figure 1E). Then, we evaluated epithelial differentiation through E-cadherin levels, which increased after the combined treatment of ATO and 5-FU (Supplementary Figure S1D).

3.2. HH-GLI Signaling Pathway Sustains Resistance to 5-FU in BRAF Mutant CRC Cells

BRAF V600E is the activating driving mutation in 10% of CRC and correlates with poor prognosis, however targeted therapy against the mutation was proven ineffective and first-line treatment includes cytotoxic chemotherapy [1]; thus, we investigated the role of the HH-GLI and NOTCH signaling pathways in 5-FU chemotherapy resistance in BRAF mutant HT29 cells.

HT29 cells were treated with 5-FU alone or in combination with the HH-GLI inhibitor GANT61 and the NOTCH1 inhibitor DAPT (Figure 2A). We observed that 5-FU induced upregulation of GLI1 and NOTCH1. GANT61 treatment resulted in the downregulation of both GLI1 and NOTCH1 ID, while DAPT treatment caused the downregulation only of NOTCH1 ID, without exerting any effect on GLI1 levels compared to control cells. The combination of GANT61 and DAPT successfully targeted both GLI1 and NOTCH1 ID. The combined treatment of GANT61 plus 5-FU was able to revert the 5-FU-induced upregulation of GLI1 and NOTCH1 ID, and the combined treatment of DAPT and 5-FU was able to revert the 5-FU-induced upregulation of NOTCH1 ID and partially of GLI1. Only when both HH-GLI and NOTCH pathways were inhibited together with 5-FU treatment were both GLI1 and NOTCH1 ID significantly downregulated (Figure 2A).

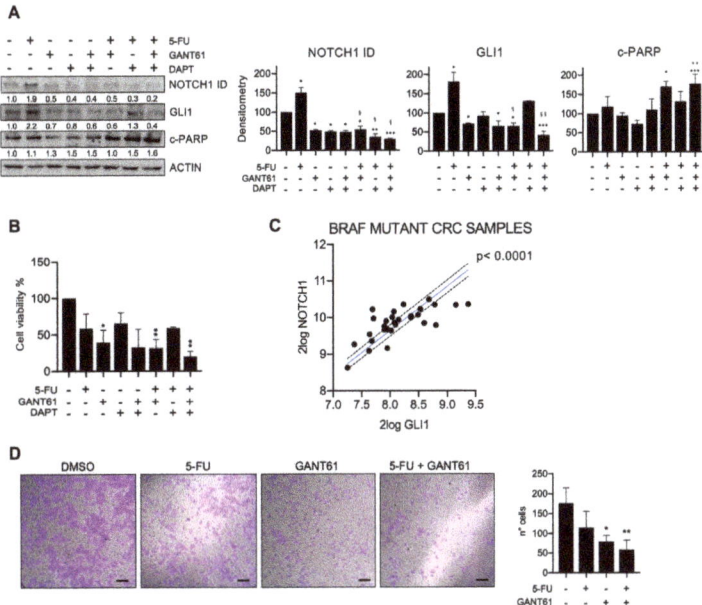

Figure 2. HH-GLI signaling pathway sustains resistance to 5-FU in BRAF mutant CRC cells. (**A**) Western blot analysis of NOTCH1 Intracellular domain (NOTCH1 ID), GLI1 and cleaved-PARP (c-PARP) in HT29 cells after 5-FU treatment in combination with GANT61 and DAPT. Numbers indicate intensity ratio of bands. Bar graphs show densitometrically quantified band intensity values normalized to the loading control; * $p < 0.05$ ** $p < 0.01$; *** $p < 0.001$; § $p < 0.05$ versus 5-FU; §§ $p < 0.01$ (Two-way ANOVA test). Uncropped full scan in Supplementary Figure S5. (**B**) Evaluation of cell viability by Tripan Blue exclusion assay in HT29 after 5-FU treatment in combination with GANT61 and DAPT; * $p < 0.05$, ** $p < 0.01$ versus CTRL (One-way ANOVA test). (**C**) Correlation analysis between GLI1 and NOTCH1 expression from dataset interrogated on R2 platform as indicated in main text. (**D**) Transwell invasion assay in HT29 cells treated with 5-FU, GANT61, the combined treatment and control group (CTRL); Scale bar 150 μm; * $p < 0.05$, ** $p < 0.01$ versus CTRL (One-way ANOVA test).

Apoptosis was evaluated through c-PARP levels; treatment with 5-FU and single inhibition of HH-GLI and NOTCH1 failed to induce apoptosis; c-PARP levels indeed increased only when cells were treated with GANT61 in combination with 5-FU, or with the combination of the three drugs (Figure 2A).

We then investigated cell viability and our results showed a significant impairment after GANT61 treatment, alone or in combination with 5-FU (Figure 2B).

Based on these results, chemotherapy resistance to apoptosis in BRAF V600E mutated cells seems to be driven by the HH-GLI signaling, which in turn sustains the activation of the NOTCH pathway. To gain more insight into the interdependence between the HH-GLI and NOTCH pathways, we interrogated GLI1 and NOTCH1 levels in a cohort of CRC patients carrying *BRAFV600E* mutation (Mutation status (Core Exon)—Sieber—211—rma_sketch—huex10p; https://hgserver1.amc.nl/cgi-bin/r2/main.cgi, accessed on 15 December 2021) and found a positive and significant correlation between GLI1 and NOTCH1 (Figure 2C). The above presented data suggest an upstream role of HH-GLI in the regulation of NOTCH signaling in the BRAF-driven CRC model.

To investigate whether BRAFV600E acted as a driver on the regulation of HH-GLI and NOTCH, we performed BRAF silencing (Supplementary Figure S2A). BRAF silencing resulted in decreased GLI1 and NOTCH1 ID protein levels (Supplementary Figure S2B).

We also evaluated mRNA levels of HH-GLI and NOTCH1 ID readout, ABCG2 and HES1, respectively, and both were significantly decreased after BRAF silencing (Supplementary Figure S2C).

The above-reported data demonstrate that chemotherapy stress induced increased levels of both HH-GLI and NOTCH1 pathways in the BRAF-driven CRC model. Interestingly, we observed that the GLI1 inhibitor GANT61 was also able to decrease NOTCH1 ID levels; conversely, the NOTCH1 inhibitor DAPT did not affect GLI1 levels.

Since we observed that the targeting of HH-GLI was able to indirectly also target the NOTCH pathway, we wondered if the combination of 5-FU and GANT61 could affect cell motility, a key feature of EMT and therefore of CRC aggressiveness.

Our experiments showed that 5-FU did not affect cell motility, while GANT61 resulted in decreased cell motility, which was further impaired by the combination of GANT61 with 5-FU (Figure 2D).

Then, we investigated the expression of two HT29 cell-specific epithelial differentiation markers, Axin and Muc2. We observed upregulation of Axin only after combined treatment, while Muc2 was affected by both 5-FU and GANT61 alone and by their combination (Supplementary Figure S2D), suggesting that treatments enhance the differentiated phenotype.

3.3. 5-FU Increases Motility of CRC Organoids

The previous set of experiments allowed us to point out the role of HH-GLI and NOTCH pathways as regulators of EMT in KRAS mutant and BRAF mutant CRC, a key feature of chemoresistance [27]. Organoid models in pre-clinical studies have become widespread due to their high reproducibility and high similarity to in vivo models [28,29]. Indeed, cell features and behavior depend on the architecture of the cell population, e.g., the cell–cell contact, the stiffness of the extracellular matrix and the interaction with the microenvironment. All these conditions concur with specific characteristics related to cell polarity, stemness and differentiation status.

Thus, to obtain CRC organoids, we seeded HCT116 and HT29 cells in Matrigel and after 7 days we observed organoid growth, as shown in Figure 3A,B. We compared basal levels of GLI1 and NOTCH1 in organoids and in 2D monolayer and our results reported higher GLI1 and HES1 expression levels in organoids, indicating that both pathways were more active in organoids compared to monolayer cellular models (Figure 3C). We then evaluated levels of the EMT marker c-MET in both organoids and monolayers and observed that c-MET was expressed at higher levels in organoids (Figure 3C). Since our results showed that 5-FU was not able to impair the migratory ability of CRC (Figures 1 and 2), and that CRC patients often present disease progression despite chemotherapy, we wondered if 5-FU itself favored aggressiveness in organoids, unleashing the migratory potential.

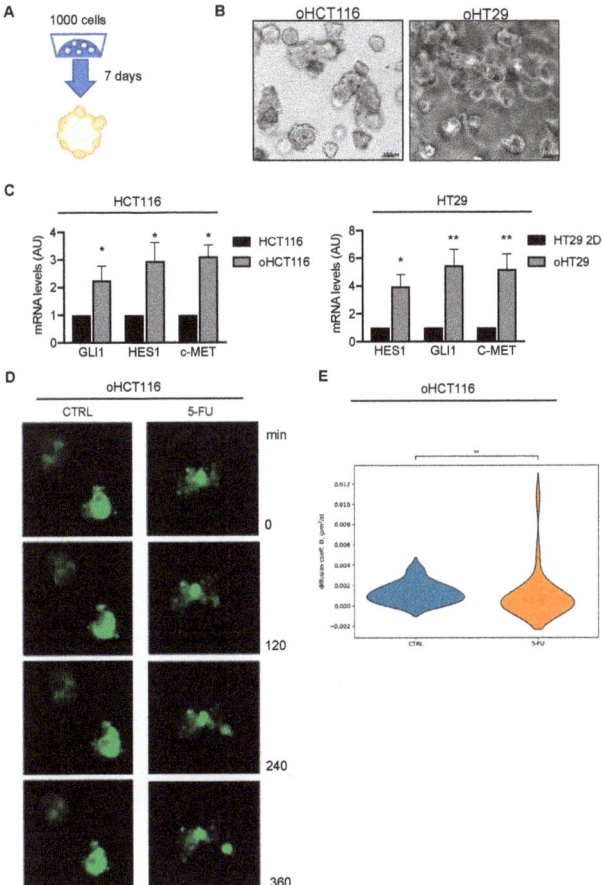

Figure 3. 5-FU increases motility in CRC organoids. (**A**) Workflow for CRC organoid growth. (**B**) Brightfield image of HCT116 and HT29 organoids (respectively oHCT116 and oHT29) after 7 days of culture. (**C**) Quantitative real-time PCR of HES1, GLI1, c-MET expressed in HCT116 and HT29 cultured in monolayer and as organoids; * $p < 0.05$ versus CTRL; ** $p < 0.01$ (Two-way ANOVA test). (**D**) Fluorescent images of GFP-labeled HCT116 on sequential hours, scale bar 200 µm. Supplementary Videos S1 and S2 of time lapse experiments are available in Supplementary Figure S3A,B. (**E**) Violin plot of the diffusion parameters obtained from the single cell trajectories for CTRL and 5-FU-treated organoids. Kolmogorov–Smirnov test p-value 0.0032.

Increased motility and migration capacity are features of EMT, thus we performed in vivo live cell imaging in the KRASG13D-driven CRC organoid model, the HCT116-derived organoids (oHCT116) at basal state and after 5-FU treatment (Supplementary Material Supplementary Video S1).

To investigate the behavior of CRC cells within organoids, we investigated the diffusion parameters that allow the motility of individual cells to be quantified. The diffusion parameters from the oHCT116 control or 5-FU-treated organoids are reported (Figure 3E) along with the single cell trajectories that were used for the calculation of the diffusion parameters (Supplementary Figure S3). Interestingly, 5-FU-treated oHCT116 cells mostly present lower diffusion parameters compared with CTRL (Figure 3D), with a long tail corresponding to a sub-group of cells presenting very high diffusion (Figure 3E). Based on these results, we believe that cells with augmented motility after chemotherapy represent a subset of aggressive cells able to initiate the metastatic process.

3.4. HH-GLI and NOTCH Inhibition Impairs 5-FU-Driven Mesenchymal Phenotype in KRASG13D-Driven CRC Organoids

We then proceeded to investigate the inhibition of HH-GLI and NOTCH by using ATO in combination with 5-FU in KRAS-driven CRC organoids, oHCT116.

Treatment with 5-FU alone did not affect organoid growth, while organoids treated with ATO were significantly smaller; the association of 5-FU and ATO further impaired organoid growth (Figure 4A). Expression levels of the EMT marker *c-MET*, cancer stemness markers *ABCG2* and *CD133a*, which is both HH-GLI target and cancer stemness marker, were significantly decreased in the combined treatment of 5-FU and ATO (Figure 4B). Interestingly, ATO was able to counteract the 5-FU-driven upregulation of ABCG2.

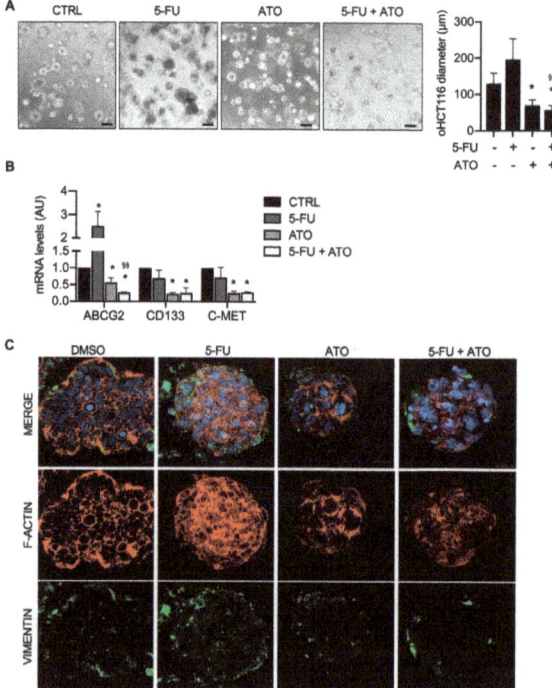

Figure 4. HH-GLI and NOTCH inhibition impairs 5-FU-driven mesenchymal phenotype in *KRASG13D*-driven CRC organoids. (**A**) Brightfield image of oHCT116 treated with 5-FU, ATO, their combination and the control group (CTRL); Scale bar 150 μm; * $p < 0.05$ versus CTRL; §§ $p < 0.01$ versus 5-FU (One-way ANOVA test). (**B**) Quantitative real-time PCR of stem markers expressed in oHCT116 treated with 5-FU, ATO, their combination and the control group (CTRL). mRNA levels of ABCG2, CD133a and c-MET expressed in oHCT116 were expressed in arbitrary units; * $p < 0.05$ versus CTRL; §§ $p < 0.01$ versus 5-FU (Two-way ANOVA test). (**C**) Whole-mount immunofluorescence staining of oHCT116 stained with phalloidin-594 (F-actin, red), vimentin (mesenchymal marker, green) and DNA (DAPI). Images were analyzed by using the program Zeiss ZEN 2.3 blue edition. Scale bar 200 μm.

Mesenchymal features were also investigated by the immunofluorescence of the EMT marker vimentin, whose levels increased after 5-FU treatment and were reduced when organoids were treated with ATO alone or in combination with 5-FU. Of note F-actin, revealed by phalloidin staining, underwent a marked rearrangement in 5-FU-treated oHCT116, where cells lost their pseudopodia, probably due to a modification in the cell polarity (Figure 4C).

3.5. HH-GLI Inhibition Impairs 5-FU-Driven Mesenchymal Phenotype in BRAFV600E-Driven CRC Organoids

We then investigated the effects of 5-FU alone or in combination with the HH-GLI blockade in the BRAFV600E-driven CRC organoids (oHT29).

Our results showed that the size of oHT29 treated with 5-FU did not differ from the control group, while organoids treated with GANT61 were smaller in size and the combination of 5-FU and GANT61 strongly impaired organoid growth (Figure 5A).

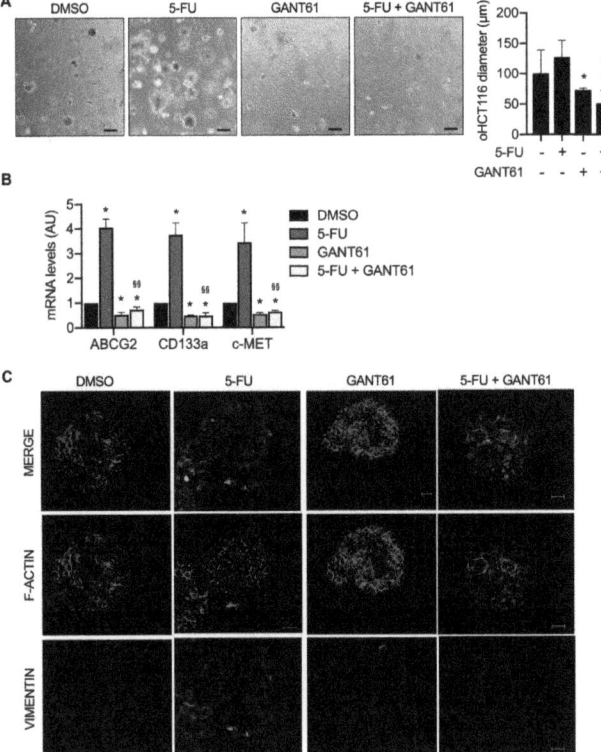

Figure 5. HH-GLI inhibition impairs 5-FU-driven mesenchymal phenotype in *BRAFV600E*-driven CRC organoids. (**A**) Brightfield image of oHT29 treated with 5-FU, GANT61, their combination and the control group (CTRL); Scale bar 150μm; * $p < 0.05$ versus Ctrl; §§ $p < 0.01$ versus 5-FU (One-way ANOVA test). (**B**) Quantitative real-time PCR of ABCG2, CD133a and c-MET expressed in oHT29 were expressed in arbitrary units. Data are representative of three independent experiments, * $p < 0.05$ versus Ctrl; §§ $p < 0.01$ versus 5-FU (Two-way ANOVA test). (**C**) Whole-mount immunofluorescence of HT29 organoids stained using phalloidin-594 (f-actin, red), vimentin (mesenchymal marker, green) and DNA (DAPI). Images were analyzed by using the program Zeiss ZEN 2.3 blue edition. Scale bar 200 μm.

Gene expression analysis showed that the levels of cancer stem cell and EMT markers *ABCG2*, *CD133* and *c-MET* significantly increased after chemotherapy treatment and were impaired by HH-GLI inhibition and the combination of 5-FU and GANT61 (Figure 5B).

To better investigate EMT, we performed whole-mount immunofluorescence staining for the mesenchymal marker vimentin and observed that vimentin levels were upregulated in 5-FU-treated organoids, they decreased with GANT61 and were strongly impaired in the combined treatment (Figure 5C).

Altogether, our experiments show that in KRAS-driven and BRAF-driven CRC, the HH-GLI and NOTCH pathways sustain the resistance to 5-FU through the activation of the EMT. Of note, ATO, the drug targeting both HH-GLI and NOTCH pathways, reverted the mesenchymal phenotype, therefore supporting the action of the chemotherapeutic drug.

4. Discussion

Despite recent advances in cancer therapy, CRC is still among the prevalent causes of cancer-related death [30]. Even though medical research has focused on identifying genetic mutations linked to CRC progression and tumor prognosis to improve patient treatment, drug resistance often occurs. One of the mechanisms conferring drug resistance is the misactivation of evolutionarily conserved pathways, such as Wingless (WNT) [31,32], phosphoinositide-3-kinase [33,34], extracellular signal-regulated kinase (ERK) [35,36], nuclear factor-κB (NF-κB) [37,38] and the Hedgehog-GLI (HH-GLI) signaling pathway [20]. The HH-GLI pathway has a crucial role in correct embryonic development and plays a role in the physiological maintenance of many tissues, including the colonic mucosa [39,40]. While canonical activation of the HH-GLI pathway transduces the signal through the Hedgehog/PTCH/SMO/GLI axis, non-canonical regulation of GLI is external to Hedgehog signaling. Of note, it was demonstrated that transforming growth factor-beta (TGF-β) [41], epidermal growth factor receptor (EGFR) [42], mitogen-activated protein kinases (MAPK) [11], β-arrestin [43] and WNT/β-catenin [44,45] were able to induce the expression of GLI, regardless of SMO activation. Since both canonical and non-canonical routes culminate with the activation of the GLI1 transcriptional program, GLI1 inhibition could be useful to prevent chemoresistance in cancer cells. Our group has previously demonstrated that HH-GLI signaling regulates the expression of ATP-binding cassette transporters (ABC transporters), which are correlated to multidrug resistance in cancer cells, providing a rationale for the consideration of the HH-GLI pathway as a therapeutic target in CRC [20]. NOTCH signaling has been reported to play a crucial role in the development of the normal mucosa [15] and its aberrant activation is related to carcinogenesis in CRC. HH-GLI and NOTCH signaling pathways together with the WNT and BMP pathways are responsible for the development of intestinal mucosa, which is the innermost layer of the colon. Stem cells, transit amplifying cells and terminally differentiated secretory cells or enterocytes, concur in the formation of the structural unit of the colon, known as the crypt of Lieberkuhn [46]. A recent paper showed that the HH-GLI blockade with GANT61 was able to inhibit NOTCH and WNT/β-catenin in cellular models of CRC [47]. Since the HH-GLI and NOTCH pathways play a fundamental role in the correct patterning of the colonic mucosa and HH-GLI is upregulated by chemotherapeutic stress, we wondered whether HH-GLI and NOTCH crosstalk could be involved in the resistance mechanism of CRC cells related to 5-FU chemotherapeutic stress.

The results of this study show how the HH-GLI and NOTCH pathways sustain CRC chemoresistance in different ways depending on the driver oncogene mutation. In detail, in KRASG13D-driven HCT116 cells we observed an upregulation of HH-GLI and NOTCH pathways after 5-FU and the inhibition of HH-GLI resulted in increased levels of NOTCH1 ID and vice versa (Figure 1A). These results, coupled with the interrogation of public datasets (Figure 1C) suggested that the HH-GLI and NOTCH signaling pathways are connected in a positive feedback loop aiming to escape apoptosis induced by 5-FU (Figure 6).

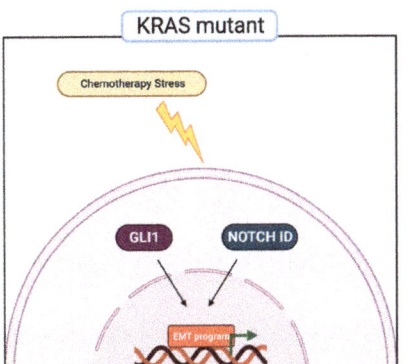 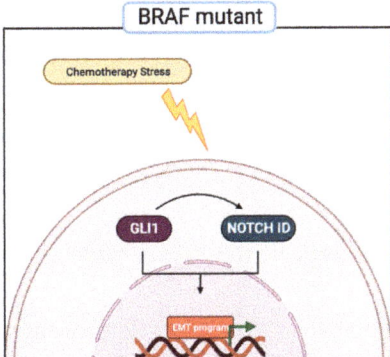

Figure 6. Hedgehog-Gli and NOTCH pathways sustain chemoresistance and the mesenchymal phenotype in CRC. Model of the activity of the Hedgehog-GLI and NOTCH pathways after chemotherapy stress in BRAFV600E and KRASG13D models. In KRAS-driven CRC, the chemotherapy stress activates both HH-GLI and NOTCH, which independently sustain the EMT program; in BRAF-driven CRC, chemotherapy stress induces the activation of the HH-GLI pathway, which in turn sustains the activation of NOTCH1 signaling, determining the acquisition of the EMT phenotype.

Importantly, the combined inhibition of HH-GLI and NOTCH was able to impair EMT, shown both as an impairment of transwell migration ability and with EMT markers in organoids (Figures 1E and 4). ATO, which was used to target both HH-GLI and NOTCH pathways, has been approved by the FDA for the therapy of adult patients with acute promyelocytic leukemia (APL). A phase I trial investigating the co-administration of ATO and 5-FU/Leucovorin in patients with advanced/relapsed CRC showed that ATO was well tolerated and that in some patients it was associated with therapeutic response and increased survival; a later study investigated GLI1 levels in biopsies from the above-mentioned clinical trial and found that it resulted to be down-modulated after ATO administration. Of note, data on the mutational status of enrolled patients are not available [48,49]. In BRAFV600E-driven CRC, both pathways were upregulated after 5-FU treatment, but importantly GANT61 downregulated not only its specific target GLI1 but also NOTCH (Figure 2A), suggesting an upstream role of HH-GLI over the NOTCH pathway (Figure 6), thus explaining the positive correlation between these two signaling pathways (Figure 2C). Importantly, HH-GLI inhibition was able to impair EMT features, both in monolayer and organoids (Figures 2D and 5).

5. Conclusions

In conclusion, our study describes for the first time two distinct models for KRAS- and BRAF-driven CRC where the HH-GLI and NOTCH signaling pathways play different roles in the chemoresistance and mesenchymal phenotype of CRC (Figure 6). Indeed, we described that in KRASG13D-driven CRC, chemotherapy resistance is directed by the concurrent activation of the HH-GLI and NOTCH pathways and the inhibition of both is crucial to revert the resistant phenotype. Conversely, in BRAFV600E-mutated CRC, the resistance to apoptosis induced by chemotherapy is mainly sustained by the HH-GLI signaling pathway. The implications of this novel information can be far-reaching if taken into consideration for the management of CRC patients, providing clinicians with further tools for the development of more effective treatment plans.

Supplementary Materials: The following supporting information can be downloaded at https://www.mdpi.com/article/10.3390/cancers15051471/s1. Supplementary Table S1. List of gene expression primers for quantitative real-time PCR. Gene expression of GLI1, HES1, c-MET, ABCG2, CD133, KRAS, BRAF, HPRT, GAPDH and β-ACTIN was assessed using Life Technologies "best coverage" assays (Life Technologies). Supplementary Figure S1. (A) Quantitative real-time PCR of KRAS in HCT116 cells after KRAS silencing (siKRAS) and control group (siCTRL). (B) Western blot analysis of KRAS, GLI1 and NOTCH1 ID in HCT116 cells after KRAS silencing (siKRAS) and control group (siCTRL). (C) Quantitative real-time PCR of ABCG2 and HES1 in HCT116 cells after KRAS silencing (siKRAS) and control group (siCTRL). (D) mRNA levels of E-cadherin (ECAD) expressed in arbitrary units in HCT116 treated with 5-FU, ATO, combined treatment and control group (CTRL). Data are representative of three independent experiments * $p < 0.05$ versus control; ** $p < 0.01$ versus 5-FU (Two-way ANOVA test). Supplementary Figure S2. (A) Quantitative real-time PCR of BRAF in HCT116 cells after BRAF silencing (siBRAF) and control group (siCTRL). (B) Western blot analysis of GLI1 and NOTCH1 ID in HT29 cells after BRAF silencing (siBRAF) and control group (siCTRL). (C) Quantitative real-time PCR of ABCG2 and HES1 in HT29 cells after BRAF silencing (siBRAF) and control group (siCTRL). (D) mRNA levels of AXIN and MUC2 expressed in arbitrary units, in HT29 treated with 5-FU, GANT61, the combined treatment and control group (CTRL). Data are representative of three independent experiments * $p < 0.05$; ** $p < 0.01$ (Two-way ANOVA test). Supplementary Figure S3. The plots show how the mean square displacement (MSD) changes for different time intervals (Δt) for each tracked single cell trajectory from either the HCT116 control group 3D organoids (CTRL) or the HCT116 5-FU-treated group (5-FU). Supplementary Figure S4. Uncropped full scan for Figure 1 (panels refer to main figure panel). Supplementary Figure S5. Uncropped full scan for Figure 2 (panels refer to main figure panel). Supplementary Video S1. time lapse of gfp transduced oHCT116 at basal state (oHCT116-gfp CTRL); Supplementary Video S2. treated with 5-FU (oHCT116-gfp 5-FU); length: 6 h.

Author Contributions: Conceptualization, A.C. and A.P.; methodology, G.G.; validation, G.C., S.T. and T.M.A.; formal analysis, Z.M.B., G.G., M.L. and L.M.; investigation, A.C., G.C., S.T., F.B., A.D.F., L.C., T.M.A., Z.S., M.A.V.; resources, M.L., E.D.S., M.A.V.; writing—original draft preparation, A.C., Z.M.B., A.P.; writing—review and editing, G.C., A.V., E.D.S., E.F. and L.M.; visualization, A.C., A.P. and L.M.; supervision, E.F., A.P.; project administration, A.P.; funding acquisition, M.L., F.B., A.V., E.F. and L.M. All authors have read and agreed to the published version of the manuscript.

Funding: This work was supported by Sapienza University of Rome (Ateneo Project 2021) (A.V.); Sapienza Ateneo 2021 RM12117A7F986146 (L.M.); Istituto Pasteur Italia—Fondazione Cenci Bolognetti (E.F.); PRIN PRIN2020 20203AMKTW (F.B.); Project LOCALSCENT, Grant PROT. A0375-2020-36549, Call POR-FESR "Gruppi di Ricerca 2020" (G.G., M.L.).

Institutional Review Board Statement: Not applicable.

Informed Consent Statement: Not applicable.

Data Availability Statement: All relevant data are included in the manuscript.

Acknowledgments: T.M.A. is fellow of Network Oncology and Precision Medicine, Dpt. Experimental Medicine, Sapienza University of Rome. Graphical abstract and Figure 6 were created with BioRender.com.

Conflicts of Interest: The authors declare no conflict of interest.

References

1. Cervantes, A.; Adam, R.; Roselló, S.; Arnold, D.; Normanno, N.; Taïeb, J.; Seligmann, J.; De Baere, T.; Osterlund, P.; Yoshino, T.; et al. Metastatic colorectal cancer: ESMO Clinical Practice Guideline for diagnosis, treatment and follow-up†. *Ann. Oncol.* **2023**, *34*, 10–32. [CrossRef]
2. Morkel, M.; Riemer, P.; Bläker, H.; Sers, C.; Morkel, M.; Riemer, P.; Bläker, H.; Sers, C. Similar but different: Distinct roles for KRAS and BRAF oncogenes in colorectal cancer development and therapy resistance. *Oncotarget* **2015**, *6*, 20785–20800. [CrossRef]
3. Li, Z.N.; Zhao, L.; Yu, L.F.; Wei, M.J. BRAF and KRAS mutations in metastatic colorectal cancer: Future perspectives for personalized therapy. *Gastroenterol. Rep.* **2020**, *8*, 192–205. [CrossRef] [PubMed]
4. Vodenkova, S.; Buchler, T.; Cervena, K.; Veskrnova, V.; Vodicka, P.; Vymetalkova, V. 5-fluorouracil and other fluoropyrimidines in colorectal cancer: Past, present and future. *Pharmacol. Ther.* **2020**, *206*, 107447. [CrossRef] [PubMed]

5. Cho, Y.H.; Ro, E.J.; Yoon, J.S.; Mizutani, T.; Kang, D.W.; Park, J.C.; Il Kim, T.; Clevers, H.; Choi, K.Y. 5-FU promotes stemness of colorectal cancer via p53-mediated WNT/β-catenin pathway activation. *Nat. Commun.* **2020**, *11*, 5321. [CrossRef] [PubMed]
6. Chen, L.; Yang, F.; Chen, S.; Tai, J. Mechanisms on chemotherapy resistance of colorectal cancer stem cells and research progress of reverse transformation: A mini-review. *Front. Med.* **2022**, *9*, 2592. [CrossRef] [PubMed]
7. Chen, J.; Na, R.; Xiao, C.; Wang, X.; Wang, Y.; Yan, D.; Song, G.; Liu, X.; Chen, J.; Lu, H.; et al. The loss of SHMT2 mediates 5-fluorouracil chemoresistance in colorectal cancer by upregulating autophagy. *Oncogene* **2021**, *40*, 3974–3988. [CrossRef]
8. Zhang, K.; Zhang, T.; Yang, Y.; Tu, W.; Huang, H.; Wang, Y.; Chen, Y.; Pan, K.; Chen, Z. N^6-methyladenosine-mediated LDHA induction potentiates chemoresistance of colorectal cancer cells through metabolic reprogramming. *Theranostics* **2022**, *12*, 4802–4817. [CrossRef]
9. Marin, J.J.G.; Macias, R.I.R.; Monte, M.J.; Herraez, E.; Peleteiro-vigil, A.; de Blas, B.S.; Sanchon-sanchez, P.; Temprano, A.G.; Espinosa-escudero, R.A.; Lozano, E.; et al. Cellular Mechanisms Accounting for the Refractoriness of Colorectal Carcinoma to Pharmacological Treatment. *Cancers* **2020**, *12*, 2605. [CrossRef]
10. Pietrobono, S.; Gagliardi, S.; Stecca, B. Non-canonical hedgehog signaling pathway in cancer: Activation of GLI transcription factors beyond smoothened. *Front. Genet.* **2019**, *10*, 556. [CrossRef]
11. Po, A.; Silvano, M.; Miele, E.; Capalbo, C.; Eramo, A.; Salvati, V.; Todaro, M.; Besharat, Z.M.; Catanzaro, G.; Cucchi, D.; et al. Noncanonical GLI1 signaling promotes stemness features and in vivo growth in lung adenocarcinoma. *Oncogene* **2017**, *36*, 4641–4652. [CrossRef]
12. Artavanis-Tsakonas, S.; Rand, M.D.; Lake, R.J. Notch Signaling: Cell Fate Control and Signal Integration in Development. *Science* **1999**, *284*, 770–776. [CrossRef]
13. Sun, L.; Ke, J.; He, Z.; Chen, Z.; Huang, Q.; Ai, W.; Wang, G.; Wei, Y.; Zou, X.; Zhang, S.; et al. HES1 Promotes Colorectal Cancer Cell Resistance To 5-Fu by Inducing Of EMT and ABC Transporter Proteins. *J. Cancer* **2017**, *8*, 2802–2808. [CrossRef] [PubMed]
14. Zhou, B.; Lin, W.; Long, Y.; Yang, Y.; Zhang, H.; Wu, K.; Chu, Q. Notch signaling pathway: Architecture, disease, and therapeutics. *Signal Transduct. Target. Ther.* **2022**, *7*, 95. [CrossRef] [PubMed]
15. Radtke, F.; Clevers, H.; Riccio, O. From Gut Homeostasis to Cancer. *Curr. Mol. Med.* **2006**, *6*, 275–289. [CrossRef]
16. Jacobs, C.T.; Huang, P. Notch signalling maintains hedgehog responsiveness via a gli-dependent mechanism during spinal cord patterning in zebrafish. *elife* **2019**, *8*, e49252. [CrossRef] [PubMed]
17. Kumar, V.; Vashishta, M.; Kong, L.; Wu, X.; Lu, J.J.; Guha, C.; Dwarakanath, B.S. The Role of Notch, Hedgehog, and Wnt Signaling Pathways in the Resistance of Tumors to Anticancer Therapies. *Front. Cell Dev. Biol.* **2021**, *9*, 857. [CrossRef] [PubMed]
18. Zhang, J.; Fan, J.; Zeng, X.; Nie, M.; Luan, J.; Wang, Y.; Ju, D.; Yin, K. Hedgehog signaling in gastrointestinal carcinogenesis and the gastrointestinal tumor microenvironment. *Acta Pharm. Sin. B* **2021**, *11*, 609–620. [CrossRef]
19. Tyagi, A.; Sharma, A.K.; Damodaran, C. A Review on Notch Signaling and Colorectal Cancer. *Cells* **2020**, *9*, 1549. [CrossRef] [PubMed]
20. Po, A.; Citarella, A.; Catanzaro, G.; Besharat, Z.M.; Trocchianesi, S.; Gianno, F.; Sabato, C.; Moretti, M.; De Smaele, E.; Vacca, A.; et al. Hedgehog-GLI signalling promotes chemoresistance through the regulation of ABC transporters in colorectal cancer cells. *Sci. Rep.* **2020**, *10*, 13988. [CrossRef]
21. Celano, M.; Schenone, S.; Cosco, D.; Navarra, M.; Puxeddu, E.; Racanicchi, L.; Brullo, C.; Varano, E.; Alcaro, S.; Ferretti, E.; et al. Cytotoxic effects of a novel pyrazolopyrimidine derivative entrapped in liposomes in anaplastic thyroid cancer cells in vitro and in xenograft tumors in vivo. *Endocr. Relat. Cancer* **2008**, *15*, 499–510. [CrossRef] [PubMed]
22. Meijering, E.; Dzyubachyk, O.; Smal, I.; van Cappellen, W.A. Tracking in cell and developmental biology. *Semin. Cell Dev. Biol.* **2009**, *20*, 894–902. [CrossRef] [PubMed]
23. Jaqaman, K.; Loerke, D.; Mettlen, M.; Kuwata, H.; Grinstein, S.; Schmid, S.L.; Danuser, G. Robust single-particle tracking in live-cell time-lapse sequences. *Nat. Methods* **2008**, *5*, 695–702. [CrossRef] [PubMed]
24. Michalet, X. Mean square displacement analysis of single-particle trajectories with localization error: Brownian motion in an isotropic medium. *Phys. Rev. E-Stat. Nonlinear Soft Matter Phys.* **2010**, *82*, 041914. [CrossRef]
25. Soignet, S.L.; Frankel, S.R.; Douer, D.; Tallman, M.S.; Kantarjian, H.; Calleja, E.; Stone, R.M.; Kalaycio, M.; Scheinberg, D.A.; Steinherz, P.; et al. United States multicenter study of arsenic trioxide in relapsed acute promyelocytic leukemia. *J. Clin. Oncol.* **2001**, *19*, 3852–3860. [CrossRef]
26. Ding, D.; Lim, K.S.; Eberhart, C.G. Arsenic trioxide inhibits Hedgehog, Notch and stem cell properties in glioblastoma neurospheres. *Acta Neuropathol. Commun.* **2014**, *2*, 31. [CrossRef]
27. Yang, L.; Shi, P.; Zhao, G.; Xu, J.; Peng, W.; Zhang, J.; Zhang, G.; Wang, X.; Dong, Z.; Chen, F.; et al. Targeting cancer stem cell pathways for cancer therapy. *Signal Transduct. Target. Ther.* **2020**, *5*, 8. [CrossRef]
28. Clevers, H. Modeling Development and Disease with Organoids. *Cell* **2016**, *165*, 1586–1597. [CrossRef]
29. Lancaster, M.A.; Knoblich, J.A. Organogenesis in a dish: Modeling development and disease using organoid technologies. *Science* **2014**, *345*, 1247125. [CrossRef]
30. Xi, Y.; Xu, P. Global colorectal cancer burden in 2020 and projections to 2040. *Transl. Oncol.* **2021**, *14*, 101174. [CrossRef]
31. Kukcinaviciute, E.; Jonusiene, V.; Sasnauskiene, A.; Dabkeviciene, D.; Eidenaite, E.; Laurinavicius, A. Significance of Notch and Wnt signaling for chemoresistance of colorectal cancer cells HCT116. *J. Cell. Biochem.* **2018**, *119*, 5913–5920. [CrossRef] [PubMed]
32. Yuan, S.; Tao, F.; Zhang, X.; Zhang, Y.; Sun, X.; Wu, D. Role of Wnt/β-Catenin Signaling in the Chemoresistance Modulation of Colorectal Cancer. *Biomed Res. Int.* **2020**, *2020*, 9390878. [CrossRef] [PubMed]

33. West, K.A.; Castillo, S.S.; Dennis, P.A. Activation of the PI3K/Akt pathway and chemotherapeutic resistance. *Drug Resist. Updat.* **2002**, *5*, 234–248. [CrossRef]
34. Deng, J.; Bai, X.; Feng, X.; Ni, J.; Beretov, J.; Graham, P.; Li, Y. Inhibition of PI3K/Akt/mTOR signaling pathway alleviates ovarian cancer chemoresistance through reversing epithelial-mesenchymal transition and decreasing cancer stem cell marker expression. *BMC Cancer* **2019**, *19*, 618. [CrossRef] [PubMed]
35. Zhao, Y.; Shen, S.; Guo, J.; Chen, H.; Yu Greenblatt, D.; Kleeff, J.; Liao, Q.; Chen, G.; Friess, H.; Sing Leung, P. Mitogen-Activated Protein Kinases and Chemoresistance in Pancreatic Cancer Cells. *J. Surg. Res.* **2006**, *136*, 325–335. [CrossRef]
36. Salaroglio, I.C.; Mungo, E.; Gazzano, E.; Kopecka, J.; Riganti, C. ERK is a Pivotal Player of Chemo-Immune-Resistance in Cancer. *Int. J. Mol. Sci.* **2019**, *20*, 2505. [CrossRef] [PubMed]
37. Godwin, P.; Baird, A.M.; Heavey, S.; Barr, M.P.; O'Byrne, K.J.; Gately, K. Targeting nuclear factor-kappa B to overcome resistance to chemotherapy. *Front. Oncol.* **2013**, *3*, 120. [CrossRef]
38. Li, Q.; Yang, G.; Feng, M.; Zheng, S.; Cao, Z.; Qiu, J.; You, L.; Zheng, L.; Hu, Y.; Zhang, T.; et al. NF-κB in pancreatic cancer: Its key role in chemoresistance. *Cancer Lett.* **2018**, *421*, 127–134. [CrossRef] [PubMed]
39. Echelard, Y.; Epstein, D.J.; St-Jacques, B.; Shen, L.; Mohler, J.; McMahon, J.A.; McMahon, A.P. Sonic hedgehog, a member of a family of putative signaling molecules, is implicated in the regulation of CNS polarity. *Cell* **1993**, *75*, 1417–1430. [CrossRef] [PubMed]
40. Bitgood, M.J.; McMahon, A.P. HedgehogandBmpGenes Are Coexpressed at Many Diverse Sites of Cell–Cell Interaction in the Mouse Embryo. *Dev. Biol.* **1995**, *172*, 126–138. [CrossRef]
41. de Reyniès, A.; Javelaud, D.; Elarouci, N.; Marsaud, V.; Gilbert, C.; Mauviel, A. Large-scale pan-cancer analysis reveals broad prognostic association between TGF-β ligands, not Hedgehog, and GLI1/2 expression in tumors. *Sci. Rep.* **2020**, *10*, 14491. [CrossRef]
42. Eberl, M.; Klingler, S.; Mangelberger, D.; Loipetzberger, A.; Damhofer, H.; Zoidl, K.; Schnidar, H.; Hache, H.; Bauer, H.C.; Solca, F.; et al. Hedgehog-EGFR cooperation response genes determine the oncogenic phenotype of basal cell carcinoma and tumour-initiating pancreatic cancer cells. *EMBO Mol. Med.* **2012**, *4*, 218–233. [CrossRef] [PubMed]
43. Miele, E.; Po, A.; Begalli, F.; Antonucci, L.; Mastronuzzi, A.; Marras, C.E.; Carai, A.; Cucchi, D.; Abballe, L.; Besharat, Z.M.; et al. β-arrestin1-mediated acetylation of Gli1 regulates Hedgehog/Gli signaling and modulates self-renewal of SHH medulloblastoma cancer stem cells. *BMC Cancer* **2017**, *17*, 488. [CrossRef] [PubMed]
44. Varnat, F.; Siegl-Cachedenier, I.; Malerba, M.; Gervaz, P.; Ruiz, I. Altaba, A. Loss of WNT-TCF addiction and enhancement of HH-GLI1 signalling define the metastatic transition of human colon carcinomas. *EMBO Mol. Med.* **2010**, *2*, 440–457. [CrossRef] [PubMed]
45. Noubissi, F.K.; Goswami, S.; Sanek, N.A.; Kawakami, K.; Minamoto, T.; Moser, A.; Grinblat, Y.; Spiegelman, V.S. Wnt signaling stimulates transcriptional outcome of the hedgehog pathway by stabilizing GLI1 mRNA. *Cancer Res.* **2009**, *69*, 8572–8578. [CrossRef]
46. Medema, J.P.; Vermeulen, L. Microenvironmental regulation of stem cells in intestinal homeostasis and cancer. *Nature* **2011**, *474*, 318–326. [CrossRef]
47. Si, Y.; Li, L.; Zhang, W.; Liu, Q.; Liu, B. GANT61 exerts anticancer cell and anticancer stem cell capacity in colorectal cancer by blocking the Wnt/β-catenin and Notch signalling pathways. *Oncol. Rep.* **2022**, *48*, 182. [CrossRef]
48. Kerl, K.; Moreno, N.; Holsten, T.; Ahlfeld, J.; Mertins, J.; Hotfilder, M.; Kool, M.; Bartelheim, K.; Schleicher, S.; Handgretinger, R.; et al. Arsenic trioxide inhibits tumor cell growth in malignant rhabdoid tumors in vitro and in vivo by targeting overexpressed Gli1. *Int. J. Cancer* **2014**, *135*, 989–995. [CrossRef] [PubMed]
49. Ardalan, B.; Subbarayan, P.R.; Ramos, Y.; Gonzalez, M.; Fernandez, A.; Mezentsev, D.; Reis, I.; Duncan, R.; Podolsky, L.; Lee, K.; et al. A phase I study of 5-fluorouracil/leucovorin and arsenic trioxide for patients with refractory/relapsed colorectal carcinoma. *Clin. Cancer Res.* **2010**, *16*, 3019–3027. [CrossRef] [PubMed]

Disclaimer/Publisher's Note: The statements, opinions and data contained in all publications are solely those of the individual author(s) and contributor(s) and not of MDPI and/or the editor(s). MDPI and/or the editor(s) disclaim responsibility for any injury to people or property resulting from any ideas, methods, instructions or products referred to in the content.

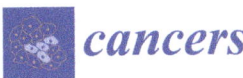

Article

Knockdown of UBQLN1 Functions as a Strategy to Inhibit CRC Progression through the ERK-c-Myc Pathway

Ruoxuan Ni [1,2,3,†], Jianwei Jiang [4,†], Mei Zhao [1,2,3], Shengkai Huang [5,*] and Changzhi Huang [1,2,3,*]

1. Department of Etiology and Carcinogenesis, National Cancer Center/National Clinical Research Center for Cancer/Cancer Hospital, Chinese Academy of Medical Sciences and Peking Union Medical College, Beijing 100021, China; 18253163755@163.com (R.N.)
2. State Key Laboratory of Molecular Oncology, National Cancer Center/National Clinical Research Center for Cancer/Cancer Hospital, Chinese Academy of Medical Sciences and Peking Union Medical College, Beijing 100021, China
3. Beijing Key Laboratory for Carcinogenesis and Cancer Prevention, National Cancer Center/National Clinical Research Center for Cancer/Cancer Hospital, Chinese Academy of Medical Sciences and Peking Union Medical College, Beijing 100021, China
4. The First Affiliated Hospital, Institute of Translational Medicine, Zhejiang University School of Medicine, Hangzhou 310058, China
5. Department of Clinical Laboratory, National Cancer Center/National Clinical Research Center for Cancer/Cancer Hospital, Chinese Academy of Medical Sciences and Peking Union Medical College, Beijing 100021, China

* Correspondence: huang1988@cicams.ac.cn (S.H.); huangcz@cicams.ac.cn (C.H.)
† These authors contributed equally to this work.

Simple Summary: The mortality rate of CRC is higher than that of other malignant tumors because of its high late-diagnosis rate. Searching for new diagnostic biomarkers for CRC is very important clinically. Accumulating evidence has demonstrated that UBQLN1 plays an important role in many biological processes. However, the role of UBQLN1 in CRC progression is still elusive. In this study, we found that UBQLN1 was significantly highly expressed in CRC tissues compared with normal tissues. In addition, reduced UBQLN1 inhibited CRC cell proliferation, colony formation, and EMT in vitro and CRC cells' tumorigenesis and metastasis of nude mice in vivo. Moreover, the knockdown of UBQLN1 reduced the expression of c-Myc by downregulating the ERK-MAPK pathway. Collectively, the knockdown of UBQLN1 inhibits the progression of CRC through the ERK-c-Myc pathway, which provides new insights into the mechanism of CRC progression. UBQLN1 may be a potential prognostic biomarker and therapeutic target of CRC.

Abstract: Purpose: Colorectal cancer (CRC) is characterized by the absence of obvious symptoms in the early stage. Due to the high rate of late diagnosis of CRC patients, the mortality rate of CRC is higher than that of other malignant tumors. Accumulating evidence has demonstrated that UBQLN1 plays an important role in many biological processes. However, the role of UBQLN1 in CRC progression is still elusive. Methods and results: we found that UBQLN1 was significantly highly expressed in CRC tissues compared with normal tissues. Enhanced/reduced UBQLN1 promoted/inhibited CRC cell proliferation, colony formation, epithelial–mesenchymal transition (EMT) in vitro, and knockdown of UBQLN1 inhibited CRC cells' tumorigenesis and metastasis in nude mice in vivo. Moreover, the knockdown of UBQLN1 reduced the expression of c-Myc by downregulating the ERK-MAPK pathway. Furthermore, the elevation of c-Myc in UBQLN1-deficient cells rescued proliferation caused by UBQLN1 silencing. Conclusions: Knockdown of UBQLN1 inhibits the progression of CRC through the ERK-c-Myc pathway, which provides new insights into the mechanism of CRC progression. UBQLN1 may be a potential prognostic biomarker and therapeutic target of CRC.

Keywords: UBQLN1; ERK-c-Myc pathway; colorectal cancer; cancer progression

Citation: Ni, R.; Jiang, J.; Zhao, M.; Huang, S.; Huang, C. Knockdown of UBQLN1 Functions as a Strategy to Inhibit CRC Progression through the ERK-c-Myc Pathway. *Cancers* **2023**, *15*, 3088. https://doi.org/10.3390/cancers15123088

Academic Editors: María Jesús Fernández-Aceñero, Rodrigo Barderas-Manchado, Javier Martinez Useros and Cristina Díaz del Arco

Received: 15 May 2023
Revised: 31 May 2023
Accepted: 2 June 2023
Published: 7 June 2023

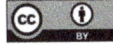

Copyright: © 2023 by the authors. Licensee MDPI, Basel, Switzerland. This article is an open access article distributed under the terms and conditions of the Creative Commons Attribution (CC BY) license (https://creativecommons.org/licenses/by/4.0/).

1. Introduction

Colorectal cancer (CRC) is a globally important disease that ranks as the third most diagnosed malignancy worldwide [1–3]; it has the second highest incidence among malignant tumors in China and ranks first among digestive tract tumors, according to the latest report from the National Cancer Center [4]. For a long time, due to the frequent diagnosis of CRC at an advanced stage, mortality ranks second among cancers globally [5,6]. Therefore, it is critical to find novel biomarkers for early diagnosis, as well as new directions for the treatment of CRC.

UBQLN1 belongs to the family of ubiquitin-like proteins and plays an important role in regulating protein degradation [7,8]. In eukaryotes, UBQLN1 connects proteasomes and ubiquitinated proteins to stimulate the degradation of ubiquitinated and misfolded proteins via autophagy regulation [9,10]. The inactivation of UBQLN1 function can induce the pathological process of a variety of human neurodegenerative diseases, such as Alzheimer's disease and Huntington's disease [11,12]. In addition, UBQLN1 is related to the occurrence and progression of a variety of human tumors. UBQLN1 is abnormally upregulated in breast cancer, and the knockdown of UBQLN1 inhibited the invasion and stemness of breast cancer cells through the AKT pathway [13]. In non-small cell lung carcinoma, loss of UBQLN1 repressed EMT [14]. Upregulated UBQLN1 predicts a poor prognosis in hepatocellular carcinoma patients and induced PGC1β degradation in a ubiquitination-independent manner to reduce mitochondrial biogenesis [15]. However, the expression of UBQLN1 in colorectal cancer and the corresponding mechanism of action have not yet been reported.

KRAS mutation is found in approximately 35–45% of colorectal cancers [16]. Mutant KRAS was reported to cause activation of the ERK signaling pathway [17]. Previous research has shown that activation of the ERK pathway could promote c-Myc protein stability by post-translational phosphorylation [18].

In this study, we noted enhanced expression of UBQLN1 in CRC samples compared with normal samples. Moreover, we found that overexpression/knockdown of UBQLN1 promoted/inhibited the proliferation, migration, invasion, and epithelial–mesenchymal transition (EMT) of CRC cells in vitro and knockdown of UBQLN1 inhibited CRC cell's tumorigenesis as well as metastasis in vivo. Furthermore, we demonstrated that the knockdown of UBQLN1 inhibited cell progression by downregulating the ERK-c-Myc signaling pathway.

2. Materials and Methods

2.1. Cell Lines and Cell Culture

HCT-116, SW480, and HEK-293T cells were preserved by Huang Changzhi's laboratory and cultured in DMEM with 10% fetal bovine serum (FBS). DLD1, HCT-8, LoVo cell was preserved by Huang Changzhi's laboratory and cultured in RPMI-1640 with 10% FBS. All cells were grown at 37 °C with 5% CO_2 in cell incubator.

2.2. Plasmid Constructions

Human cDNA of Ubqln1 was cloned using Q5 high-fidelity DNA polymerase Kit (New England Biolabs, MA, USA). The full-length cDNA of Ubqln1 was constructed into pLVX-Puro vector. The Ubqln1 full-length primers were as follows: forward, 5′-AAGTCTAGAGAATTCGGATCCATGGCCGAGAGTGGTGAAAGC-3′; reverse, 5′-AACAAGCTTCCATGGCTCGAGCTATGATGGCTGGGAGCCCAG-3′. Short hair-pin RNA (shRNA) targeting Ubqln1 was initially inserted into the BamH I and EcoR I sites of pSIH1 plasmid, forming the pSIH1-shUBQLN1 plasmids. Three pairs of shUBQLN1 sequences were as follows: shUBQLN1.1: sense: 5′-GTTTTTCAATGTCTAAGTCGTCCCA AAAGAGAACTTTTTGGGACGACTTAGACATTGCCTAG-3′; antisense: 5′-GCAATGTCT AAGTCGTCCCAAAAAGTTCTCTTTTGGGACGACTTAGACATTGAAAAACTTAA-3′; shUBQLN1.2: sense: 5′-GTTTTTGAGGGTTGAAAGGAGGTTGTTAGAGAACTTAACAA CCTCCTTTCAACCCTCCCTAG-3′; antisense: 5′-GGAGGGTTGAAAGGAGGTTGTTAA

GTTCTCTAACAACCTCCTTTCAACCCTCAAAAACTTAA-3′; and shUBQLN1.3: sense: 5′-GTTTTTGGAGTCGATGTCTTAGGTCTTAGAGAACTTAAGACCTAAGACATCGACT CCCCTAG-3′; antisense: 5′-GGGAGTCGATGTCTTAGGTCTTAAGTTCTCTAAGACCT AAGACATCGACTCCAAAAACTTAA-3′.

Human cDNA of c-Myc was cloned using Q5 high-fidelity DNA polymerase Kit (New England Biolabs, MA, USA). The full-length cDNA of c-Myc was constructed into pLVX-Puro vector. The c-Myc full-length primers were as follows: forward, 5′-CCGGAATTCCTGGATTTTTTTCGGGTAGTG-3′; reverse, 5′-CCGCTCGAGTTACGCACA AGAGTTCCGTAG-3′.

2.3. Establishment of Stable Expression Cell Lines

Lentivirus was produced using packaging system psPAX2, pMG2G, and pLVX-Ubqln1-Puro (pSIH1-shUBQLN1) plasmid at the ratio of 4:2:4, transfected by Lipofectamine 2000 (Invitrogen) in HEK-293T cells.

Cells were plated in 6-well plates and infected with lentivirus assisted by 8 µg/mL poly-brene (Sigma-Aldrich, St. Louis, Missouri, USA) for 36 h, and were then selected by puromycin for two weeks. Expression of Ubqln1 in stable cell lines was verified by Western blot.

2.4. Cell Counting Kit-8 (CCK-8) Assay

CCK-8 assay was carried out to assess cell proliferation. CCK-8 reagent (Meilunbio, Dalian, China) was added to 96-well plates with cells seeded in at a ratio of 1:10, and then spectrometric absorbance at 450 nm was measured after incubation at 37 °C for 1 h.

2.5. Colony Formation Assay

For colony formation assay, every 400 cells were seeded into 6-well plate and then incubated at 37 °C until colonies were macroscopic. Next, colonies were stained with 0.5% crystal violet, and the number of colonies was counted.

2.6. Cell Invasion and Motility Assay

To investigate cell motility and invasion capabilities, a total of 2×10^5 colorectal cancer cells were added to the upper chamber of cell culture insert (pore size, 8 µm; Corning, NJ, USA) coated with diluted Matrigel basement membrane matrix (BD, Franklin Lakes, NJ, USA) and grown in serum-free medium. In the lower chamber, 600 µL of cell culture medium supplemented with 10% FBS was added. As a result of PBS wash, non-attached cells were removed after being incubated for 24 h in 5% CO_2 at 37 °C. We fixed attached cells in 4% paraformaldehyde for 30 min and stained them with 0.5% crystal violet. Five visual fields at ×100 magnification were randomly selected, and the number of cells in fields was recorded. The mean value was calculated from three independent experiments performed in triplicate.

2.7. Western Blot

Cells were washed with ice-cold PBS and lysed in lysis buffer. BCA protein concentration determination was used to quantify total protein contents. A total of 20 µg of protein were loaded on SDS-PAGE and transferred to PVDF membrane. After blocking in 5% BSA, PVDF membrane was incubated with specific primary antibodies (anti-β-actin, 1:1000, Abclonal Technology, Wuhan, China; anti-UBQLN1, 1:1000, Proteintech, Wuhan, China; anti-GAPDH, anti-E-cadherin, anti-MMP-9, anti-VIMENTIN, anti-t-ERK1/2, anti-p-ERK1/2, anti-MEK1, anti-p-MEK1, and anti-c-MYC, 1:1000, Cell Signaling Technology, MA, USA) overnight. After washing, membrane was incubated with secondary antibody for 1 h. Finally, blots were visualized with enhanced chemiluminescent (NCM Biotech, Suzhou, China) by GE ImageQuant LAS 4000.

2.8. Nude Mice Xenograft and Metastasis Experiments

Nude mice (5 weeks old) were purchased from Beijing Huafukang Bioscience and raised in SPF laboratory animal room. All animal experiments were approved by the Animal Care and Use Committee of the Chinese Academy of Medical Sciences Cancer Hospital, and conducted in accordance with guidelines of the National Animal Welfare Law of China.

In nude mice xenograft experiment, LoVo-shCTRL and LoVo-shUBQLN1.2 cells at their exponential growth phase were harvested and washed twice in 0.9% saline water, and then resuspended in 0.9% saline water at a density of 3×10^7 cells/mL. Cell suspension (0.1 mL, 3×10^6 cells) was subcutaneously injected into the right flank of 5- to 6-week-old male BALB/c nude mice (4 mice in each group). Mice were humanely euthanized when the subcutaneous tumors reached 10 mm in diameter.

In nude mice metastasis experiment, LoVo-shCTRL and LoVo-shUBQLN1.2 cells at their exponential growth phase were harvested and washed twice in 0.9% saline water, and then resuspended in 0.9% saline water at a density of 1.5×10^7 cells/mL. Cell suspension (0.1 mL, 1.5×10^6 cells) was injected into tail veins of nude mice (5 mice in each group). Mice were humanely euthanized when the mice were raised to 40–50 days.

2.9. Statistical Analysis

Data were described as mean ± SD from at least 3 independent experiments. Student's *t*-test was used to assess statistical differences between groups. Differences with *p* value less than 0.05 were considered to be statistically significant. Statistical analysis of data was performed using GraphPad Prism 8.0 and SPSS 17.0 software.

3. Results

3.1. UBQLN1 Enhanced Expression in Colorectal Cancer Tissues and Is Correlated with Poor Prognosis

To assess the overall profile of UBQLN1 expression in colorectal cancer, we analyzed the UBQLN1 gene expression level in a Gene Expression Omnibus (GEO) dataset (GSE106582), and these data were analyzed via a scatter plot. UBQLN1 showed significantly increased expression in 77 colorectal cancer tissues compared with 117 healthy control tissues (Figure 1A).

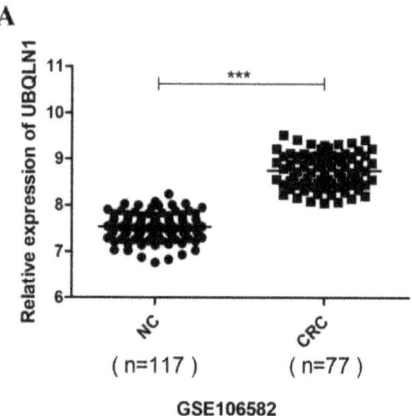

Figure 1. *Cont.*

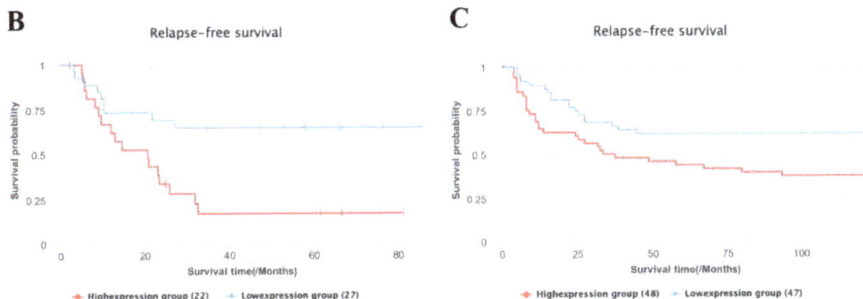

Figure 1. UBQLN1 enhanced expression in colorectal cancer tissues and is correlated with poor prognosis. (**A**) UBQLN1 mRNA expression levels of colorectal cancer samples and normal control were analyzed by quantitative RT-PCR; (**B,C**) relapse-free survival (RFS) of colon cancer patients (**B**) and colorectal cancer patients (**C**) based on UBQLN1 mRNA expression was analyzed by lnCAR database. Data are shown as mean ± SD; *** $p < 0.001$ based on Student's t-test.

We used the lnCAR database (https://lncar.renlab.org/, accessed on 7 August 2020) to access prognosis data for those colorectal patients with high levels of UBQLN1 expression. Prognostic values, including two relapse-free survival (RFS) values of UBQLN1 mRNA expression, respectively, in colon cancer samples and colorectal cancer tissues, were estimated. We found that the mRNA expression level of UBQLN1 was negatively correlated with RFS in colon cancer (Figure 1B; analysis ID: CR_O19, $p = 0.0056$) and colorectal cancer (Figure 1C; analysis ID: CR_O16, $p = 0.0172$).

3.2. UBQLN1 Promoted CRC Cell Proliferation In Vitro

UBQLN1 protein expression level was measured in five CRC cell lines (DLD1, HCT-8, HCT-116, LoVo, and SW480) by Western blot, respectively (Figure 2A). The results showed that among five CRC cell lines, the expression level of three cell lines (HCT-8, LoVo, and SW480) was higher compared to another two (DLD1 and HCT-116).

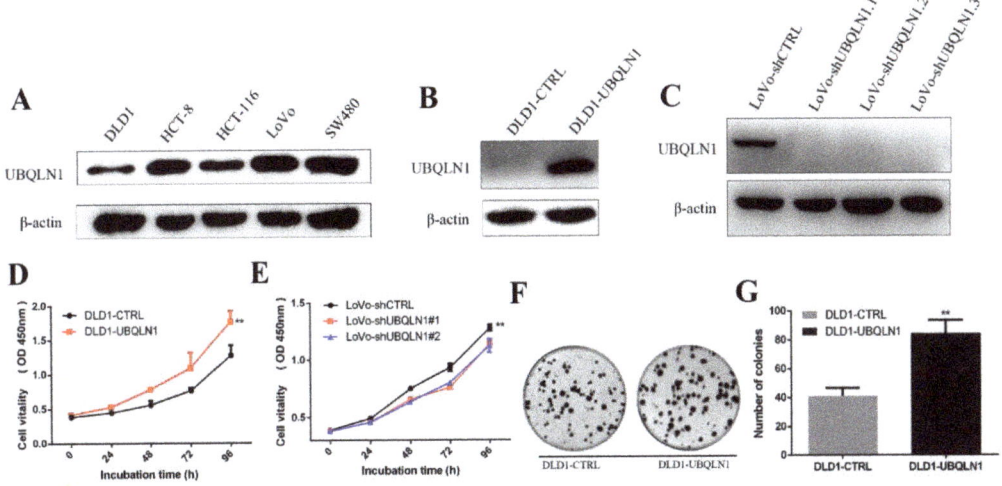

Figure 2. *Cont.*

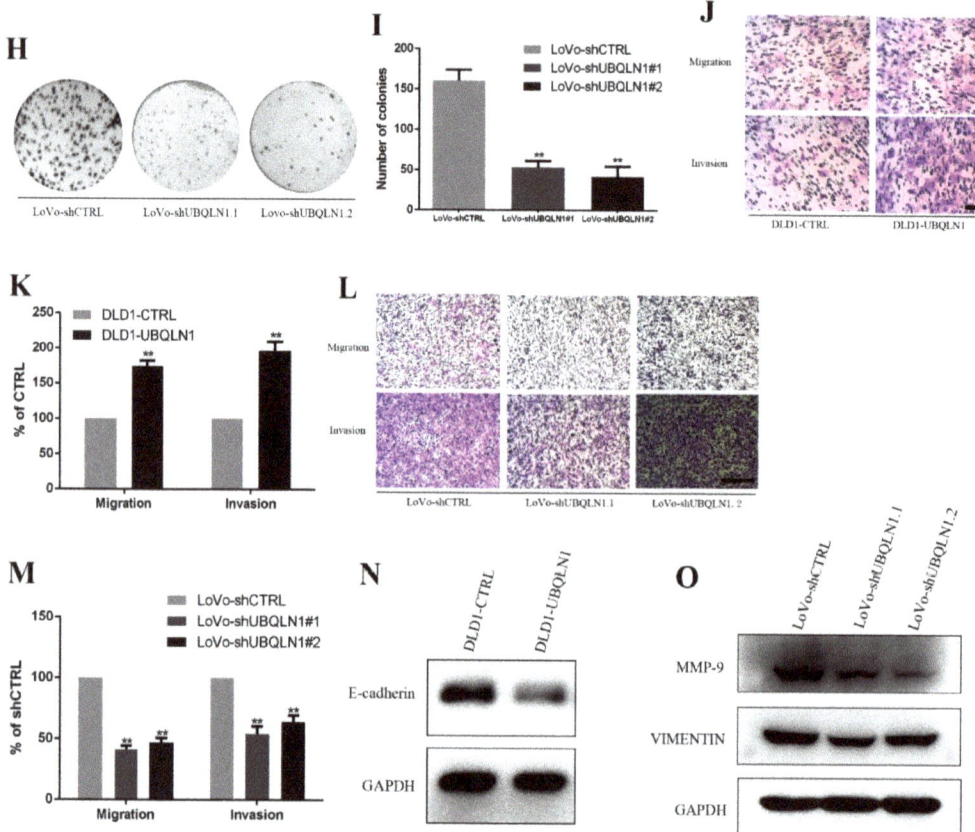

Figure 2. UBQLN1 promoted colorectal cancer cell progression in vitro. (**A**) UBQLN1 protein expression levels were detected in different cell lines by Western blot; (**B**) colorectal cancer cell line DLD1 was used to establish UBQLN1 over-expression cell line; (**C**) colorectal cancer cell line LoVo was used to establish UBQLN1 silencing cell line; (**D,E**) CCK-8 assay was performed to detect cell proliferation in DLD1-UBQLN1 (**D**) and LoVo-shUBQLN1 (**E**); (**F,G**) colony formation assay was performed in DLD1-UBQLN1 to detect cell colony formation ability and results were displayed as represent figures (**F**) and statistical graph (**G**); (**H,I**) colony formation assay was performed in LoVo-shUBQLN1 to detect cell colony formation ability and results were displayed as represent figures (**H**) and statistical graph (**I**); (**J,K**) Transwell and Matrigel assays were performed in DLD1-UBQLN1 to detect cell vitality and mobility and results were displayed as represent figures (**J**) and statistical graph (**K**), and the scale bars represent 50 μm; (**L,M**) Transwell and Matrigel assays were performed in LoVo-shUBQLN1 to detect cell vitality and mobility, results were displayed as figures (**L**) and statistical graph (**M**), and the scale bars represent 50 μm; (**N,O**) Western blot was performed to detect EMT marker proteins in UBQLN1 over-expression cell line DLD1 (**N**) and UBQLN1 silencing cell line LoVo (**O**). Data are shown as mean ± SD; n = 3 independent experiments; and ** $p < 0.01$ based on Student's t-test.

To identify the functional role of UBQLN1 in CRC cells, we established two CRC cell lines that stably enhanced/reduced UBQLN1, whose expression level was assayed by Western blot (Figure 2B,C). CCK-8 assay and colony-formation assay were performed to examine the effect on the cell's abilities of proliferation and colony formation brought by UBQLN1. As shown, DLD1-UBQLN1 and LoVo-shUBQLN1 cells, which increased/decreased UBQLN1, exhibited higher/lower ability of proliferation than that of control cells, i.e., DLD1-CTRL and LoVo-CTRL (Figure 2D,E), as well as the ability of colony formation (Figure 2F–I).

3.3. UBQLN1 Promoted CRC Cells' EMT In Vitro

To ascertain whether over-expression/knockdown of UBQLN1 would influence cell epithelial–mesenchymal transition (EMT) capacities, a transwell migration and invasion assay were performed. Over-expression of UBQLN1 increased the numbers of migrated and invaded cells through the bottom of the transwell with or without matrigel (Figure 2J,K). In contrast, the knockdown of UBQLN1 decreased migrated and invaded cells' numbers (Figure 2L,M). Meanwhile, Western blot assay was used to detect EMT marker E-cadherin, VIMENTIN, and MMP-9. The protein level of E-cadherin was reduced in DLD1-UBQLN1 cells compared with the control level (Figure 2N), and the protein level of VIMENTIN and MMP-9 was reduced in LoVo-shUBQLN1 cells compared with the control level (Figure 2O), suggesting that UBQLN1 may also enhance CRC cells' EMT.

3.4. Reduced UBQLN1 Inhibited CRC Cells' Tumorigenesis and Metastasis In Vivo

To investigate the role of UBQLN1 in CRC carcinogenesis in vivo, a CRC xenograft model was established by implanting LoVo-shCTRL and LoVo-shUBQLN1 cells subcutaneously into the right flanks of nude mice. The results showed the tumors of the mice injected with LoVo-shCTRL cells after injection for four weeks (Figure 3A,B). The average weight of the tumors taken from the mice injected with LoVo-shCTRL cells was 245 milligrams, while that of the tumors from the ones injected with LoVo-shUBQLN1 cells was 158 milligrams (Figure 3C). Additionally, Tumor growth curves indicated that reduced UBQLN1 inhibited tumor growth in terms of volumes (Figure 3D).

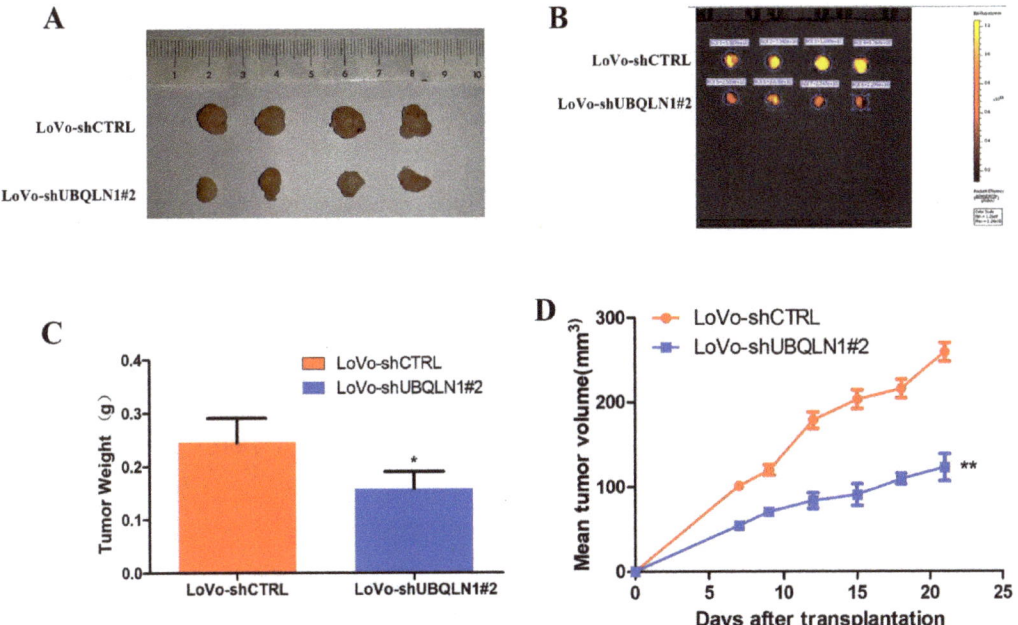

Figure 3. *Cont.*

Figure 3. Reduced UBQLN1 inhibited CRC cells' tumorigenesis and metastasis in vivo. (**A,B**) Nude mice were subcutaneously injected with UBQLN1 silencing cell line LoVo and its control cells. The transplanted tumors were dissected out. (**C**) tumors' weights were measured after dissection. (**D**) tumors' volumes were measured during growth process. (**E,F**) nude mice were injected with UBQLN1 silencing cell line LoVo and its control cells through tail vein to establish distant metastasis model. The nude mice were sacrificed by anesthesia, and their liver metastasis was observed. Results were displayed as figures (**E**) and statistical graph (**F**). Data are shown as mean ± SD; n = 3 independent experiments; and * $p < 0.0.5$, ** $p < 0.01$ based on Student's *t*-test.

Moreover, to detect the role of UBQLN1 in CRC metastasis in vivo, LoVo-shCTRL and LoVo-shUBQLN1 cells were injected into nude mice through the tail vein, respectively. The visible metastatic foci point in the liver of the mice injected with LoVo-shUBQLN1 cells was significantly less than those in the control group (Figure 3E,F). The results indicated that reduced UBQLN1 inhibited CRC cells' tumorigenesis and metastasis in vivo.

3.5. Knockdown of UBQLN1 Suppressed ERK-c-Myc Signaling Pathway in CRC

Approximately 50% of patients with metastatic colorectal cancer has mutations in the RAS gene, including HRAS, KRAS, and NRAS mutations, most of which are KRAS mutations [19–21]. KRAS mutations can abnormally activate the MAPK signaling pathway, causing the continuous activation of downstream ERK1/2 and promoting colorectal cancer malignant progression [22,23]. As we determined that the knockdown of UBQLN1 inhibited CRC cells' progression both in vitro and in vivo, Western blot was used to detect the activity of ERK1/2, a downstream effector of RAS in the MAPK pathway. As shown, the phosphorylation level at site Thr202/Tyr204 of ERK1/2 protein was decreased, while the total protein level of ERK1/2 was changeless after knocking down UBQLN1 in CRC cells (Figure 4A). Meanwhile, Western blot was used to detect the activity of MEK1, an intermediator in signal transmission between RAS and ERK1/2. As shown, the phosphorylation level at site Thr286 of the MEK1 protein was decreased, while the total protein level of MEK1 was changeless after knocking down UBQLN1 in CRC cells (Figure 4B). Previous research has shown that c-Myc is a potential target of the ERK1/2-MAPK pathway [24]; thus, we detect the effect of UBQLN1 on c-Myc. We found that the protein level of c-Myc was decreased after knocking down UBQLN1 in LoVo cells (Figure 4C). Nextly, we sought to validate whether the knockdown of UBQLN1 reduces the expression of c-Myc through ERK-MAPK suppression. ERK1/2 activator tert-Butylhydroquinone (tBHQ, 50 μM) was used to treat LoVo-shUBQLN1 cells for 48 h. Western blot analysis showed activating the ERK signaling pathway reversed the decreased c-Myc protein expression brought by the knockdown of UBQLN1 (Figure 4D). Those results suggested the knockdown of UBQLN1 attenuated expression of c-Myc through the ERK1/2 signaling pathway.

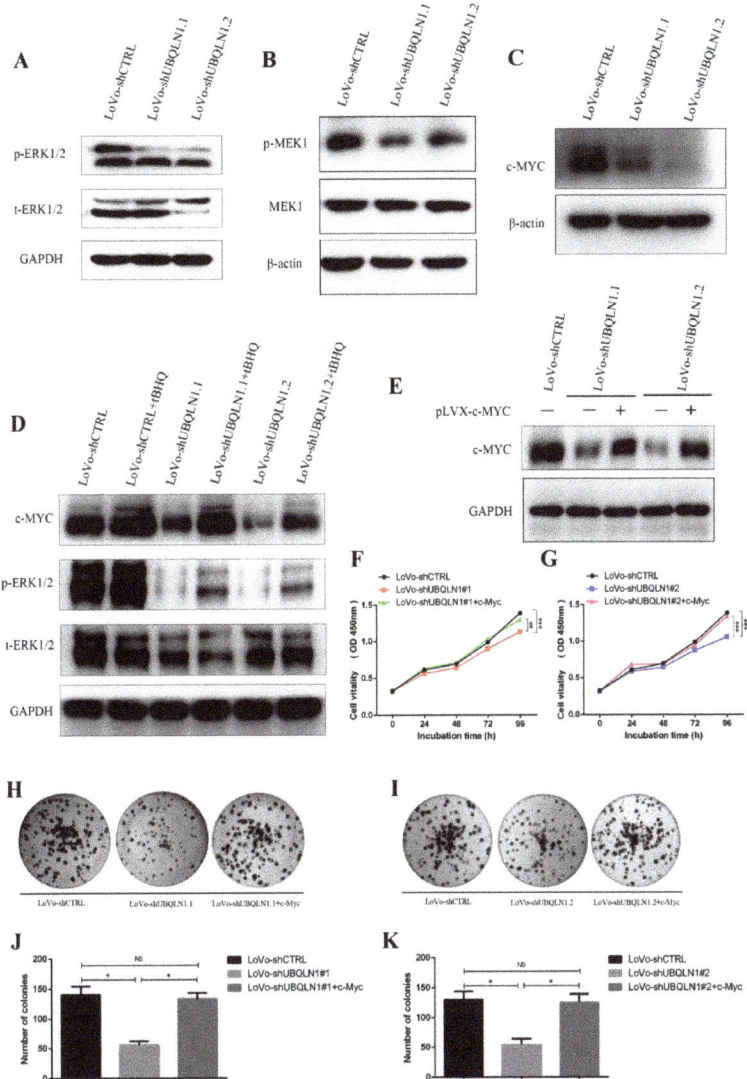

Figure 4. Knockdown of UBQLN1 inhibited colorectal cells' malignant progression through ERK-c-Myc signaling pathway. (**A**,**B**) Western blot was performed to detect influence of UBQLN1 silencing on ERK-MAPK pathway; (**C**) Western blot was performed to detect influence of UBQLN1 silencing on expression of c-MYC; (**D**) Western blot was performed to detect relativity between ERK-MAPK pathway and c-MYC in UBQLN1 silencing cell line LoVo; (**E**) UBQLN1 silencing cell line LoVo was used to establish c-MYC over-expression cell line; (**F**,**G**) CCK-8 assay was performed to detect cell proliferation in LoVo-shUBQLN1 followed by c-MYC over-expression; (**H**–**K**) Colony formation assay was performed to detect cell colony formation ability in LoVo-shUBQLN1 followed by c-MYC over-expression; and results were displayed as figures (**H**,**I**) and statistical graph (**J**,**K**). Data are shown as mean ± SD; n = 3 independent experiments; and NS $p \geq 0.05$, * $p < 0.05$, ** $p < 0.01$, and *** $p < 0.001$ based on Student's t-test.

3.6. Knockdown of UBQLN1 Inhibited CRC Cells' Malignant Progression through ERK-c-Myc Signaling Pathway

To specify whether UBQLN1 loss inhibited CRC cells' progression through the ERK-c-Myc signaling pathway, we overexpressed c-Myc in UBQLN1-deficient CRC cells (Figure 4E). The CCK-8 and colony formation assay showed LoVo cells' abilities of proliferation and colony forming were restored to normal levels upon elevation of c-Myc in UBQLN1-deficient cells, establishing a strong connection between UBQLN1 and c-Myc (Figure 4F–K). We also confirmed the correlation between knockdown of UBQLN1 and ERK-c-Myc pathway in SW480 (Figure S1). These results confirmed that c-Myc is the downstream target of UBQLN1 that mediates proliferation by UBQLN1 loss. Above all, the knockdown of UBQLN1 inhibited CRC cells' malignant progression through the ERK-c-Myc signaling pathway.

4. Discussion

UBQLN1 is a member of the UBQLN family, which plays important roles in protein degradation [7,25]. In our study, we found that over-expression of UBQLN1 promoted colorectal cancer cell progression, including proliferation, migration, and invasion, and vice versa. We also found knockdown of UBQLN1 downregulated the ERK-c-Myc pathway. Moreover, enhanced c-MYC rescued colorectal cancer cell progression caused by UBQLN1 silencing. To our knowledge, this is the first report to show that UBQLN1 played a role in colorectal cancer and was correlated with the ERK-c-Myc pathway.

As a member of the mitogen-activated protein kinases (MAPK) family, extracellular-signal-regulated kinases (ERK) are a type of serine/threonine protein kinase, including ERK1 and ERK2 [26]. The Ras/Raf/MEK/ERK signal transduction pathway follows the three-stage enzymatic cascade of MAPKs [27–29]. Ras acts as an upstream activating protein, which is activated after external stimulation and transmits the signal to Raf, namely MAPKKK. MEK acts as MAPKK to receive the signal [30]. Additionally, then the phosphorylated ERK is translocated to the nucleus, which mediates the transcriptional activation of Elk-1, c-fos, and c-Jun [29,31,32]. Finally, extracellular signals are transmitted to the nucleus, mediating cells to participate in a variety of life activities. Our study revealed that the knockdown of UBQLN1 inhibited the phosphorylation levels of ERK1/2 and MEK1, suggesting UBQLN1 could regulate the ERK pathway.

Previous studies have shown that activation of the ERK pathway could upregulate the expression level of c-Myc [24]. The *Myc* gene is the first proto-oncogene discovered in Burkitt lymphoma [33]. The *Myc* gene family members include *b-Myc, l-Myc, n-Myc, s-Myc,* and *c-Myc,* among which *c-Myc* is the most widely studied [34]. Previous studies observed the amplification or over-expression of the *c-Myc* gene in gastric cancer [35], breast cancer [36], cervical cancer [37], and other cancers, suggesting that the abnormal activation of the *c-Myc* gene is closely related to the occurrence and development of malignant tumors [38,39]. Similarly, our study revealed that the knockdown of UBQLN1 reduced protein expression of c-MYC and activated the ERK pathway, mediated by the tBHQ-rescued expression of c-Myc caused by UBQLN1 silencing.

Our study identified the knockdown of UBQLN1 down-regulated c-Myc by reducing the phosphorylation level of the ERK pathway. Furthermore, we found enhanced c-MYC rescued colorectal cancer cell progression caused by UBQLN1 silencing. These findings suggested that the knockdown of UBQLN1 inhibited colorectal cancer cell progression through ERK-c-Myc pathway.

5. Conclusions

The knockdown of UBQLN1 inhibits the progression of CRC through the ERK-c-Myc pathway, which provides new insights into the mechanism of CRC progression. UBQLN1 may be a potential prognostic biomarker and therapeutic target of CRC.

Supplementary Materials: The following supporting information can be downloaded at https://www.mdpi.com/article/10.3390/cancers15123088/s1. Figure S1: Knockdown of UBQLN1 inhibited colorectal cells' malignant progression through ERK-c-Myc signaling pathway; Figure S2: Densitometric analysis.

Author Contributions: Conceptualization, R.N. and J.J.; investigation, R.N. and J.J.; data curation, R.N. and M.Z.; writing—original draft preparation, R.N. and J.J.; writing—review and editing, R.N., J.J., S.H. and C.H.; supervision, S.H. and C.H.; funding acquisition, S.H. and C.H. All authors have read and agreed to the published version of the manuscript.

Funding: This research was funded by the National Natural Science Foundation of China (Grant no. 81872038) (Grant no. 81902503), CAMS Innovation Fund for Medical Sciences (CIFMS) (Grant no. 2021-I2M-1-014), and the Fundamental Research Funds for the Central Universities (Grant no. 3332019056).

Institutional Review Board Statement: All animal protocols were approved by the Animal Care and Welfare Committee of the National Cancer Center, Chinese Academy of Medical Sciences Cancer Hospital (protocol code 20/286-2482, 26 August 2020).

Data Availability Statement: Not applicable.

Acknowledgments: We greatly thank Hong Lin and Longmei He for their experimental skills.

Conflicts of Interest: The authors declare no conflict of interest.

References

1. Biller, L.H.; Schrag, D. Diagnosis and Treatment of Metastatic Colorectal Cancer: A Review. *JAMA* **2021**, *325*, 669–685. [CrossRef] [PubMed]
2. Keum, N.; Giovannucci, E. Global burden of colorectal cancer: Emerging trends, risk factors and prevention strategies. *Nat. Rev. Gastroenterol. Hepatol.* **2019**, *16*, 713–732. [CrossRef] [PubMed]
3. Sung, H.; Ferlay, J.; Siegel, R.L.; Laversanne, M.; Soerjomataram, I.; Jemal, A.; Bray, F. Global Cancer Statistics 2020: GLOBOCAN Estimates of Incidence and Mortality Worldwide for 36 Cancers in 185 Countries. *CA Cancer J. Clin.* **2021**, *71*, 209–249. [CrossRef]
4. Wei, W.; Zeng, H.; Zheng, R.; Zhang, S.; An, L.; Chen, R.; Wang, S.; Sun, K.; Matsuda, T.; Bray, F.; et al. Cancer registration in China and its role in cancer prevention and control. *Lancet Oncol.* **2020**, *21*, e342–e349. [CrossRef] [PubMed]
5. Arnold, M.; Sierra, M.S.; Laversanne, M.; Soerjomataram, I.; Jemal, A.; Bray, F. Global patterns and trends in colorectal cancer incidence and mortality. *Gut* **2017**, *66*, 683–691. [CrossRef] [PubMed]
6. Ladabaum, U.; Dominitz, J.A.; Kahi, C.; Schoen, R.E. Strategies for Colorectal Cancer Screening. *Gastroenterology* **2020**, *158*, 418–432. [CrossRef]
7. Marín, I. The ubiquilin gene family: Evolutionary patterns and functional insights. *BMC Evol. Biol.* **2014**, *14*, 63. [CrossRef]
8. Kurlawala, Z.; Shah, P.P.; Shah, C.; Beverly, L.J. The STI and UBA Domains of UBQLN1 Are Critical Determinants of Substrate Interaction and Proteostasis. *J. Cell. Biochem.* **2017**, *118*, 2261–2270. [CrossRef]
9. Chen, X.; Ebelle, D.L.; Wright, B.J.; Sridharan, V.; Hooper, E.; Walters, K.J. Structure of hRpn10 Bound to UBQLN2 UBL Illustrates Basis for Complementarity between Shuttle Factors and Substrates at the Proteasome. *J. Mol. Biol.* **2019**, *431*, 939–955. [CrossRef]
10. Lipinszki, Z.; Kovács, L.; Deák, P.; Udvardy, A. Ubiquitylation of Drosophila p54/Rpn10/S5a regulates its interaction with the UBA-UBL polyubiquitin receptors. *Biochemistry* **2012**, *51*, 2461–2470. [CrossRef]
11. Bertram, L.; Hiltunen, M.; Parkinson, M.; Ingelsson, M.; Lange, C.; Ramasamy, K.; Tanzi, R.E. Family-based association between Alzheimer's disease and variants in UBQLN1. *N. Engl. J. Med.* **2005**, *352*, 884–894. [CrossRef] [PubMed]
12. Rutherford, N.J.; Lewis, J.; Clippinger, A.; Thomas, M.A.; Adamson, J.; Cruz, P.E.; Cannon, A.; Xu, G.; Golde, T.E.; Shaw, G.; et al. Unbiased screen reveals ubiquilin-1 and -2 highly associated with huntingtin inclusions. *Brain Res.* **2013**, *1524*, 62–73. [CrossRef]
13. Feng, X.; Cao, A.; Qin, T.; Zhang, Q.; Fan, S.; Wang, B.; Song, B.; Yu, X.; Li, L. Abnormally elevated ubiquilin-1 expression in breast cancer regulates metastasis and stemness via AKT signaling. *Oncol. Rep.* **2021**, *46*, 236. [CrossRef]
14. Shah, P.P.; Lockwood, W.W.; Saurabh, K.; Kurlawala, Z.; Shannon, S.P.; Waigel, S.; Zacharias, W.; Beverly, L.J. Ubiquilin1 represses migration and epithelial-to-mesenchymal transition of human non-small cell lung cancer cells. *Oncogene* **2015**, *34*, 1709–1717. [CrossRef]
15. Xu, J.; Ji, L.; Ruan, Y.; Wan, Z.; Lin, Z.; Xia, S.; Tao, L.; Zheng, J.; Cai, L.; Wang, Y.; et al. UBQLN1 mediates sorafenib resistance through regulating mitochondrial biogenesis and ROS homeostasis by targeting PGC1β in hepatocellular carcinoma. *Signal Transduct. Target. Ther.* **2021**, *6*, 190. [CrossRef] [PubMed]
16. Van Cutsem, E.; Köhne, C.-H.; István Láng; Folprecht, G.; Nowacki, M.P.; Cascinu, S.; Shchepotin, I.; Maurel, J.; Cunningham, D.; Tejpar, S.; et al. Faculty Opinions recommendation of Cetuximab plus irinotecan, fluorouracil, and leucovorin as first-line treatment for metastatic colorectal cancer: Updated analysis of overall survival according to tumor KRAS and BRAF mutation status. *J. Clin. Oncol.* **2011**, *29*, 2011–2019. [CrossRef] [PubMed]

17. Waters, A.M.; Der, C.J. KRAS: The Critical Driver and Therapeutic Target for Pancreatic Cancer. *Cold Spring Harb. Perspect. Med.* **2018**, *8*, a031435. [CrossRef]
18. Qin, Y.; Hu, Q.; Ji, S.; Xu, J.; Dai, W.; Liu, W.; Xu, W.; Sun, Q.; Zhang, Z.; Ni, Q.; et al. Homeodomain-interacting protein kinase 2 suppresses proliferation and aerobic glycolysis via ERK/cMyc axis in pancreatic cancer. *Cell Prolif.* **2019**, *52*, e12603. [CrossRef]
19. Zhu, G.; Pei, L.; Xia, H.; Tang, Q.; Bi, F. Role of oncogenic KRAS in the prognosis, diagnosis and treatment of colorectal cancer. *Mol. Cancer* **2021**, *20*, 143. [CrossRef]
20. Hofmann, M.H.; Gerlach, D.; Misale, S.; Petronczki, M.; Kraut, N. Expanding the Reach of Precision Oncology by Drugging All KRAS Mutants. *Cancer Discov.* **2022**, *12*, 924–937. [CrossRef]
21. Moore, A.R.; Rosenberg, S.C.; McCormick, F.; Malek, S. RAS-targeted therapies: Is the undruggable drugged? *Nat. Rev. Drug Discov.* **2020**, *19*, 533–552. [CrossRef] [PubMed]
22. Drosten, M.; Barbacid, M. Targeting the MAPK Pathway in KRAS-Driven Tumors. *Cancer Cell* **2020**, *37*, 543–550. [CrossRef] [PubMed]
23. Roberts, P.J.; Stinchcombe, T.E. KRAS mutation: Should we test for it, and does it matter? *J. Clin. Oncol.* **2013**, *31*, 1112–1121. [CrossRef] [PubMed]
24. Chen, J.; Ding, C.; Chen, Y.; Hu, W.; Lu, Y.; Wu, W.; Zhang, Y.; Yang, B.; Wu, H.; Peng, C.; et al. ACSL4 promotes hepatocellular carcinoma progression via c-Myc stability mediated by ERK/FBW7/c-Myc axis. *Oncogenesis* **2020**, *9*, 42. [CrossRef]
25. Satoh, J.; Tabunoki, H.; Ishida, T.; Saito, Y.; Arima, K. Ubiquilin-1 immunoreactivity is concentrated on Hirano bodies and dystrophic neurites in Alzheimer's disease brains. *Neuropathol. Appl. Neurobiol.* **2013**, *39*, 817–830. [CrossRef]
26. Fang, J.Y.; Richardson, B.C. The MAPK signalling pathways and colorectal cancer. *Lancet Oncol.* **2005**, *6*, 322–327. [CrossRef]
27. Molina, J.R.; Adjei, A.A. The Ras/Raf/MAPK pathway. *J. Thorac. Oncol.* **2006**, *1*, 7–9. [CrossRef]
28. Roberts, P.J.; Der, C.J. Targeting the Raf-MEK-ERK mitogen-activated protein kinase cascade for the treatment of cancer. *Oncogene* **2007**, *26*, 3291–3310. [CrossRef]
29. Yuan, J.; Dong, X.; Yap, J.; Hu, J. The MAPK and AMPK signalings: Interplay and implication in targeted cancer therapy. *J. Hematol. Oncol.* **2020**, *13*, 113. [CrossRef]
30. Yaeger, R.; Corcoran, R.B. Targeting Alterations in the RAF–MEK Pathway. *Cancer Discov.* **2019**, *9*, 329–341. [CrossRef]
31. Han, J.; Liu, Y.; Yang, S.; Wu, X.; Li, H.; Wang, Q. MEK inhibitors for the treatment of non-small cell lung cancer. *J. Hematol. Oncol.* **2021**, *14*, 1. [CrossRef] [PubMed]
32. Yue, J.; López, J.M. Understanding MAPK Signaling Pathways in Apoptosis. *Int. J. Mol. Sci.* **2020**, *21*, 2346. [CrossRef] [PubMed]
33. Thorley-Lawson, D.A.; Allday, M.J. The curious case of the tumour virus: 50 years of Burkitt's lymphoma. *Nat. Rev. Microbiol.* **2008**, *6*, 913–924. [CrossRef] [PubMed]
34. Dang, C.V. MYC on the path to cancer. *Cell* **2012**, *149*, 22–35. [CrossRef]
35. Liu, M.; Yao, B.; Gui, T.; Guo, C.; Wu, X.; Li, J.; Ma, L.; Deng, Y.; Xu, P.; Wang, Y.; et al. PRMT5-dependent transcriptional repression of c-Myc target genes promotes gastric cancer progression. *Theranostics* **2020**, *10*, 4437–4452. [CrossRef]
36. Figueiredo, J.C.; Knight, J.A.; Cho, S.; Savas, S.; Onay, U.V.; Briollais, L.; Goodwin, P.J.; McLaughlin, J.R.; Andrulis, I.L. Polymorphisms cMyc-N11S and p27-V109G and breast cancer risk and prognosis. *BMC Cancer* **2007**, *7*, 99. [CrossRef]
37. Chen, M.; Liang, X.; Liang, Z.; Zhao, L. Study on the effect and mechanism of NFKBIA on cervical cancer progress in vitro and in vivo. *J. Obstet. Gynaecol. Res.* **2021**, *47*, 3931–3942. [CrossRef]
38. Martelli, A.M.; Evangelisti, C.; Paganelli, F.; Chiarini, F.; McCubrey, J.A. GSK-3: A multifaceted player in acute leukemias. *Leukemia* **2021**, *35*, 1829–1842. [CrossRef]
39. Tsai, C.-C.; Su, Y.-C.; Bamodu, O.A.; Chen, B.-J.; Tsai, W.-C.; Cheng, W.-H.; Lee, C.-H.; Hsieh, S.-M.; Liu, M.-L.; Fang, C.-L.; et al. High-Grade B-Cell Lymphoma (HGBL) with *MYC* and *BCL2* and/or *BCL6* Rearrangements Is Predominantly BCL6-Rearranged and BCL6-Expressing in Taiwan. *Cancers* **2021**, *13*, 1620. [CrossRef]

Disclaimer/Publisher's Note: The statements, opinions and data contained in all publications are solely those of the individual author(s) and contributor(s) and not of MDPI and/or the editor(s). MDPI and/or the editor(s) disclaim responsibility for any injury to people or property resulting from any ideas, methods, instructions or products referred to in the content.

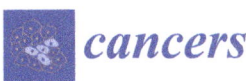

Review

Prognostic Biomarkers of Cell Proliferation in Colorectal Cancer (CRC): From Immunohistochemistry to Molecular Biology Techniques

Aldona Kasprzak

Department of Histology and Embryology, University of Medical Sciences, Swiecicki Street 6, 60-781 Poznan, Poland; akasprza@ump.edu.pl; Tel.: +48-61-8546441; Fax: +48-61-8546440

Simple Summary: This review aims to shed light on the proliferative markers important in the everyday clinical management of colorectal cancer (CRC), ranging from simple methods of assessing cellular proliferation (e.g., DNA ploidy, BrdUrd/IdUrd/tritiated thymidine binding index) to the use of immunohistochemistry (IHC) and modern molecular biology techniques (e.g., qRT-PCR, in situ hybridization, RNA/DNA sequencing) for the detection of genetic and epigenetic markers. Among the examined markers, the prognostic utility was demonstrated for aneuploidy and the overexpression of IHC markers (e.g., TS, cyclin B1, and D1, PCNA, and Ki-67). Classical genetic markers of prognostic significance mostly comprise mutations in commonly examined genes such as *APC*, *KRAS/BRAF*, *TGF-β*, and *TP53*. Chromosomal markers include CIN and MSI, while CIMP is indicated as a potential epigenetic marker with many other candidates such as *SERP*, *p14*, *p16*, *LINE-1*, and *RASSF1A*. Modern technology-based approaches to study non-coding fragments of the human genome have also yielded some candidates for CRC prognostic markers among the lncRNAs (e.g., SNHG1, SNHG6, MALAT-1, CRNDE) and miRNAs (e.g., miR-20a, miR-21, miR-143, miR-145, miR-181a/b). With growing knowledge of the human genome structure and the rapid development of molecular biology techniques, it is hoped that a panel of reliable prognostic markers could improve the assessment of survival as well as allow for the better estimation of the treatment outcomes for CRC patients.

Abstract: Colorectal cancer (CRC) is one of the most common and severe malignancies worldwide. Recent advances in diagnostic methods allow for more accurate identification and detection of several molecular biomarkers associated with this cancer. Nonetheless, non-invasive and effective prognostic and predictive testing in CRC patients remains challenging. Classical prognostic genetic markers comprise mutations in several genes (e.g., *APC*, *KRAS/BRAF*, *TGF-β*, and *TP53*). Furthermore, CIN and MSI serve as chromosomal markers, while epigenetic markers include CIMP and many other candidates such as *SERP*, *p14*, *p16*, *LINE-1*, and *RASSF1A*. The number of proliferation-related long non-coding RNAs (e.g., SNHG1, SNHG6, MALAT-1, CRNDE) and microRNAs (e.g., miR-20a, miR-21, miR-143, miR-145, miR-181a/b) that could serve as potential CRC markers has also steadily increased in recent years. Among the immunohistochemical (IHC) proliferative markers, the prognostic value regarding the patients' overall survival (OS) or disease-free survival (DFS) has been confirmed for thymidylate synthase (TS), cyclin B1, cyclin D1, proliferating cell nuclear antigen (PCNA), and Ki-67. In most cases, the overexpression of these markers in tissues was related to worse OS and DFS. However, slowly proliferating cells should also be considered in CRC therapy (especially radiotherapy) as they could represent a reservoir from which cells are recruited to replenish the rapidly proliferating population in response to cell-damaging factors. Considering the above, the aim of this article is to review the most common proliferative markers assessed using various methods including IHC and selected molecular biology techniques (e.g., qRT-PCR, in situ hybridization, RNA/DNA sequencing, next-generation sequencing) as prognostic and predictive markers in CRC.

Citation: Kasprzak, A. Prognostic Biomarkers of Cell Proliferation in Colorectal Cancer (CRC): From Immunohistochemistry to Molecular Biology Techniques. *Cancers* **2023**, *15*, 4570. https://doi.org/10.3390/cancers15184570

Academic Editors: Javier Martinez Useros, Cristina Díaz del Arco, Rodrigo Barderas-Manchado and María Jesús Fernández-Aceñero

Received: 21 July 2023
Revised: 4 September 2023
Accepted: 13 September 2023
Published: 15 September 2023

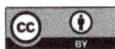

Copyright: © 2023 by the author. Licensee MDPI, Basel, Switzerland. This article is an open access article distributed under the terms and conditions of the Creative Commons Attribution (CC BY) license (https://creativecommons.org/licenses/by/4.0/).

Keywords: colorectal cancer; cell proliferation; genetic and epigenetic markers; cell cycle-related antigens; prognostic markers; cyclins; PCNA; Ki-67 antigen; ncRNAs; immunohistochemistry; qRT-PCR; RNA/DNA sequencing

1. Introduction

Colorectal cancer (CRC) remains a major medical challenge worldwide, ranking third in prevalence and second among cancer-related death causes [1–4]. The high mortality rate persists in European countries, but also affects several other regions around the world such as the Caribbean, East Asia (China), and South America (Uruguay), indicating a continuously high incidence as well as lackluster detection and treatment methods [3]. An increase can also be observed in CRC incidence in younger people (under 50 years of age), with those predisposed to CRC generally classified as 'medium' and 'high' risk groups [1,3,5,6]. Moreover, the incidence of CRC is positively correlated with the levels of the human development index (HDI) [6].

The development of CRC is a multistage process. The numerous genetic alterations in CRC are reflected in morphological features that can be visualized by various molecular techniques [7–9]. A significant role in tumor initiation, growth, and metastasis is now attributed to cancer/tumor-initiating cells (CICs/TICs) or cancer stem cells (CSCs), which are capable of self-renewal and differentiation. Numerous studies support the 'CSC hypothesis', in which the essence of carcinogenesis is progressive colonic SC overpopulation. Research is ongoing into the biology of these cells, the identification of their molecular markers, and the mechanisms of CSC proliferation, differentiation, and resistance to treatment in CRC [10–15].

There are several theories regarding the sequence of events in the formation of CRC [16]. The first pathway of the 'adenoma–carcinoma sequence' describes a sequence of morphological alterations, from hyperplasia through dysplasia to the formation of malignant, invasive foci [7,17]. Pre-cancerous lesions, in this case, comprise adenomatous polyps [7], with the 'adenoma–carcinoma sequence' concept supplemented by early dysplastic lesions, known as aberrant crypt foci (ACF) [18,19]. The second theory of CRC formation, known as the mutator pathway, took its origin from the 1992 discovery of genetic alterations in patients with Lynch syndrome (LS), also known as hereditary non-polyposis CRC (HNPCC) [20].

Approximately 15% of CRC arises from genetic alterations. Several syndromes can be distinguished in the etiology of CRC, associated with a high lifetime risk of CRC due to the inheritance of mutations in a single gene. Specific 'Mendelian' CRC syndromes include familial adenomatous polyposis (FAP), with gene mutation of the adenomatous polyposis coli (*APC*) gene, LS genes (*MSH2, MLH1, MSH6, PMS2*), Peutz–Jeghers syndrome (*LKB1/STK11*), juvenile polyposis (*SMAD4, BMPR1A*), *MUTYH*-associated polyposis, and hereditary mixed polyposis (*GREM1*). All of these conditions, except for *MUTYH*-associated polyposis, are inherited in a dominant manner. However, there is a recessive version of HNPCC in which both copies of one of the DNA mismatch repair (*MMRs*) genes are mutated (reviewed in [21]).

A third theory of CRC development, the serrated pathway or hyperplastic polyp-carcinoma sequence, considers hyperplastic polyps (HPs) together with a subgroup of serrated polyps (SPs) as precursors of CRC [22]. It is now recognized that up to 10–30% of CRC cases arise through this alternative pathway, characterized by its genetic and epigenetic profile [23–27].

From a clinical perspective, people with LS or colorectal polyposis syndromes are at the most significant risk of developing CRC. LS accounts for 1–3% of all cases, with people affected with this syndrome characterized by an absolute CRC risk ranging from 30 to 70% [28]. Increased risk also applies to people with colorectal adenomatous polyps, inflammatory bowel disease, a history of CRC, or cases of this cancer in close family members under the age of 50. Low to moderate risk of developing CRC applies to virtually the entire population, associated with age over 50 years and the consequences of an unhealthy lifestyle leading to obesity and other metabolic disorders, resulting in the production of a number of tumor-promoting proteins [12,29]. Obesity prevention, especially among the young human population, is an important preventive factor for CRC. A recent meta-analysis showed that overweight and obesity may be more potent risk factors for CRC and, possibly, other cancers than the previous epidemiological studies suggested [30].

Together with changes in chromatin structure and DNA methylation, gene mutations in CRC lead to the dysregulation of signaling pathways responsible for cell proliferation, apoptosis, metabolism, differentiation, and survival [16,21,31,32].

The 'adenoma–carcinoma sequence' is mainly characterized by a loss of proliferation control. In turn, in the serrated neoplasia pathway, a failure of apoptosis mechanisms is the most characteristic factor. However, asymmetric proliferation (shift of the zone of proliferation from the base to the lateral side) is typical of the architecturally distorted serrated crypt, a characteristic of sessile serrated lesions (SSLs) [22].

CRC is a typically malignant tumor characterized by genetic/epigenetic mutations in mutator genes (i.e., genes whose alterations accelerate mutations in other genes). However, the molecular and cellular alterations associated with the immortality (abnormal maintenance of proliferation) and autonomy of colorectal cells, as with other malignancies, remain unknown (reviewed in [33]). Studies also suggest that the mechanism linking abnormalities at the genetic (e.g., *APC* mutations) and cellular level (e.g., hyperplasia, dysplasia) between tumor initiation to metastasis is the excessive number of colonic CSCs. It also considers the symmetrical division of CSCs as an essential mechanism driving tumor growth, which may have therapeutic implications for patients with advanced CRC [34].

Due to the above, searching for optimal methods to evaluate tumor proliferation and for more sensitive markers with potential prognostic significance seems crucial. A prognostic factor is a variable that indicates the predicted natural course of the disease and can be used to estimate the chance of recovery or the likelihood of recurrence. Prognostic significance is particularly relevant to progression-free survival (PFS) and overall survival (OS). Prognostic factors are classified into tumor-related, host-related, and environmental [35,36].

The aim of this article was to review the most common proliferative markers assessed by various methods including immunohistochemistry (IHC) and selected molecular biology techniques (e.g., qRT-PCR, in situ hybridization, RNA/DNA sequencing, next-generation sequencing) as prognostic and predictive CRC markers.

2. Molecular Mechanisms of Colorectal Cancerogenesis

At the core of the classical pathway of CRC development ('adenoma–carcinoma sequence') are genetic alterations of several suppressor genes such as *APC*, responsible for the development of FAP, and a gene known as colorectal mutant cancer protein (*MCC*) [37,38]. *APC* mutations usually result in activation of the canonical Wnt pathway [39]. Further genes include deleted in colorectal cancer *(DCC)*, encoding members of the CAM immunoglobulin family of adhesion proteins [40], similar to neural cell adhesion molecules (NCAMs) [41]. Its product acts as a netrin 1 receptor [42] and is often silenced in CRC through the loss of heterozygosity or epigenetic mechanisms [43]. *TP53* and the *K-ras* (*K-RAS*, *KRAS*) and *BRAF* protooncogenes are also implicated in the development of CRC, playing a role in the MAPK signaling pathway [5,9,44]. However, further studies have indicated that alterations in the three 'classical' carcinogenesis genes (*APC*, *K-RAS*, *TP53*) affect only about 10% of CRC, as this cancer is characterized by considerable genetic heterogeneity [23].

Thus, according to the conventional pathway theory of colorectal carcinogenesis, the first step involves *APC* changes, resulting in increased cell proliferation and polyp formation. In the next step, genetic alterations of *K-RAS* result in further clonal tissue proliferation and increased polyp size. This is followed by polyp proliferation due to *DCC* mutations. *TP53* mutations with telomerase activation are reported in approximately 70%

of CRC cases. Mutation in the *TP53* leads to malignancy, resulting in metastasis to the surrounding tissues and distant organs [5,16,44].

Nowadays, it is known that at the molecular level, chromosomal instability (CIN) (~70–85%), extensive DNA methylation known as CpG island methylator phenotype (CIMP) (~17% CRC), and microsatellite instability (MSI) (~15% CRC) are the most common factors in the classical pathway of colorectal carcinogenesis [9,17,23,32]. The presence of CIN in tumors results in the accumulation of mutations in oncogenes and tumor suppressor genes (*APC*, *TP53*, *KRAS*, and *BRAF*). However, more than 24 mutated genes have currently been associated with CRC [45], with the number possibly higher due to the development of modern testing techniques including single-cell next-generation sequencing (NGS) [46].

In contrast to CIN, in MSI, morphological changes are associated with minor aneuploidy, with LS serving as a typical example (3% CRC) [20]. The main characteristic of these lesions is the mutation of *MMR* genes, namely *MLH1*, *MSH2*, *MSH6*, and *PMS2*, with no congenital polyps in the CRC development sequence. The process of neoplastic transformation, however, is similar to that in the CIN pathway (i.e., with a prior development of adenoma (AD)). On the LS (mutator pathway), the development of CRC can occur through (1) sporadic adenomas that acquire secondary *MMR* deficiency (dMMR); (2) flat intramucosal lesions that arise directly from dMMR crypts; (3) LS-specific adenomas that arise from flat lesions as a result of secondary *APC* mutations [47]. A subgroup of hypermutating carcinomas that do not show MSI features has also been demonstrated. In addition, families with oligopolyposis and MS stable (MSS) at a young age but without *APC* or *MYTYH* (*MYH*) mutations have been identified. Investigations of further mechanisms responsible for the hypermutation revealed germline exonuclease domain (EDM) mutations of *POLE* and *POLD1* genes, associated with a high risk of multiple ADs and CRC, resulting in a condition known as polymerase proofreading-associated polyposis (PPAP). Somatic *POLE* EDMs have also been found in sporadic CRC, although very few *POLD1* somatic EDMs have been described [48].

In the third concept, the so-called serrated pathway ('hyperplastic polyp–carcinoma sequence'), HPs, together with a subgroup of serrated polyps (SPs), have been recognized as precursors of CRC [22]. It is now known that as many as 10-30% of CRCs arise through this alternative pathway, characterized by their own genetic and epigenetic profile [23–27]. The most recent classification of serrated colorectal lesions (formerly known as sessile serrated polyp/adenoma) describes them as precursors of various molecular CRC subtypes [22,49]. In these lesions, hypermethylation of cytosine residues within CpG islands can sometimes be observed. Point mutations of B-Raf protooncogene serine/threonine kinase (*BRAF*), promoter methylation of multiple genes, and MSI have also been described in the serrated pathway [24]. In turn, the molecular mechanisms of the CIMP pathway are not well understood. These cancers are characterized by a poorer prognosis but can be detected earlier, as aberrant DNA methylation is already present [50]. Morphologically, the CIMP pathway is associated with lesions with a characteristic microscopic 'serrated' mucosal edge structure, previously identified as hypertrophic benign polyps. These polyps are currently known as sessile serrated adenomas/polyps (SSA/Ps) and have been recognized as major precursor lesions for CRC. They can arise from HPs or de novo from normal mucosa [24,25]. Serrated polyposis syndrome (SPS) is also a risk factor for CRC, characterized by large and multiple serrated polyps throughout the colon. The most common genetic variants associated with CRC susceptibility in SPS patients are rs4779584-GREM1, rs16892766-EIF3H, and rs3217810-CCND2 [51].

Interestingly, the MSS/CIMP-negative subset has been shown to evolve through the classical 'adenoma–carcinoma sequence'. In contrast, the MSI/CIMP-positive and MSS/CIMP-positive subsets often develop through the 'serrated pathway' [23]. As indicated by a recent cohort study (~30,000 participants) evaluating 40 established CRC susceptibility subtypes, common genetic variants play a potential role in conventional and serrated CRC pathways. The occurrence of different sets of variants for these two pathways demonstrates the etiological heterogeneity of CRC [52]. It should be noted that a third concept of CRC development (in addition to the conventional tubular/villous adenoma–carcinoma and the serrated adenoma–carcinoma pathways) has been proposed (although much less common), namely, cancer formation in the mucosal domain of gut-associated lymphoid tissue (GALT) [53].

There are currently four molecular subtypes of CRC, the so-called consensus molecular subtypes (CMS) (i.e., CMS1—immunological, CMS2—canonical, CMS3—metabolic, and CMS4—mesenchymal). Considering the clinical features, biology, and gene signatures of colon cancer subtypes (CCS), the CCS3 subtypes, whose precursors are SSAs, have the worst prognosis (defined by the shortest disease-free survival, DFS). Using the CR-Cassigner signature to classify the TCGA dataset, they are known as the stem-like and transit-amplifying (TA) (including cetuximab-resistant TA) subtypes [54].

Among the numerous molecular markers of CRC (more than 100 differentially expressed), most are overexpressed during tumorigenesis. Functionally, they are involved in various biological signaling pathways including those related to cell proliferation [55].

3. Cellular Proliferation Models versus Colorectal Carcinogenesis Theories

Complex cell cycle (mitotic cycle) mechanisms regulate proliferation, survival, and death. The processes and factors involved in cell cycle regulation in mammalian cells in physiology and tumorigenesis have been well-characterized in numerous reviews [56–59]. The cell cycle is primarily driven by the activation of serine/threonine cyclin-dependent kinases (Cdks) by cyclins and the phosphorylation and dephosphorylation of Cdks [56,57,60]. In human cells, there are 20 different Cdks and about 30 cyclin genes [57,61], which, in addition to participating in the cell cycle process, are also involved in transcription and pre-mRNA splicing [62]. In addition to Cdks, which drive cell passage through the phases of the cell cycle, there are also kinase inhibitors that regulate it and prevent it from progressing. The concentration of Cdks in the cell is constant, while the concentration of cyclins varies according to the cycle phase. The most significant role in cell cycle progression and its timely and precise regulation is attributed to the ubiquitin–proteasome system [59].

Cell cycle genes encoding proteins that stimulate the cell cycle are known as protooncogenes, and those that inhibit the cell cycle are the suppressor genes. In a cancer cell, genetic changes result in the conversion of protooncogenes to oncogenes, and the loss of function of some suppressor genes. This leads to a steady production of proteins that induce cell division (products of oncogenes) and a deficiency of proteins that inhibit this process (suppressor genes products). According to the clonal theory of oncogenesis, tumor formation starts from a single cell. Furthermore, there is a close relationship between tumor development and the inhibition of apoptosis, which ensures cell immortality [63]. Dysregulation proliferation, apoptosis, and autophagy factors also include altered Ca^{2+} transmission [64].

According to the somatic mutation theory (SMT) of carcinogenesis, external cancer-causing agents (e.g., environmental, chemical, radiation, carcinogens) damage the DNA of a single cell, leading to the generation of mutations. These, in turn, through successive rounds of cell proliferation and clonal selection, drive the process of carcinogenesis. In contrast, tissue organization field theory (TOFT) recognizes that proliferation and motility are the default states of all cells [65]. Among the current 10 hallmarks of cancer, in addition to 'genomic instability and mutations', 'non-mutational epigenetic reprogramming', and 'polymorphic microbiomes' are 'sustaining proliferative signaling', 'enabling replicative immortality', and 'resisting cell death' [66].

Unlike normally differentiating cells, cancer cells can enter the proliferation or tumorigenesis pathway from the G0 to G1 phase (the G0 repose model) [67]. This hypothesis assumes that in a tumor, there are non-proliferating cells in the G0 phase, forming a resting compartment (quiescent, Q). The fate of these cells was dual, either re-entering the cycle through the G1 phase with growth factors, cytokines, oxygenation, and nutrients or cell death (after exiting the G0 phase and Q compartment) [67,68]. In tumor tissues, the proliferative process predominates, resulting in a greater withdrawal (especially in the absence of nutrients, hypoxia) of cells from the G1 to G0 phase. This greater number of cells in the G0 phase is characteristic of solid tumors including CRC. Another proliferation model (the growth retardation model) assumed that, under unfavorable conditions, the withdrawal of cells to the G0 phase could occur in any stage of the cycle, not only in the G1 phase [69]. A few years later, a multilevel model of cancer cell proliferation, known as the proliferation plane model, was proposed [70]. It assumes the existence of different subpopulations of cells that differ in growth rate, rates of cycling, and recruitment to the cycle within a single population. A modification of this model is the so-called Wilson's integrated tumor growth model, which also assumes different subpopulations of cells in the tumor but also various factors affecting tumor growth (e.g., differentiation, apoptosis, tumor microenvironment (TME) factors) [68]. The advantage of both models is the potential prognostic and predictive significance of a subpopulation of slowly proliferating cells in the tumor and the depiction of the molecular mechanisms controlling the division cycle of tumor cells. These cells may include CSCs that reside in the G0 phase (like SCs of normal tissues) or proliferate very slowly.

The assessment of proliferation in CRC, especially in a prognostic and diagnostic context, has been the focus of scientists and clinicians for a number of years. The difficulty in interpreting many findings in this area is related to the enormous heterogeneity of the tumor in terms of genotype, phenotype, morphology, and cell metabolism [46]. Interestingly, while epithelial cells in the large intestine have a longer lifespan and proliferate slower than in the small intestine (5–21 days versus 3–4 days) [71,72], colon cancer is far more common than small intestinal cancers (10% versus <1% of all cancers) [4]. This discrepancy between proliferation characteristics and the risk of uncontrolled, malignant tissue transformation is called 'the proliferation paradox' [73]. For example, patients with FAP are ~30 times more likely to develop CRC than duodenal cancer. Studies by Tomasetti and Vogelstein suggest that this occurs as there are ~150 times more SC divisions in the colon than in the duodenum. The risk of CRC would be very low (even with the *APC* mutation) if the SCs of the colonic epithelium were not constantly dividing [74]. Thus, both SCs and non-SCs, which may differentiate into an SC-like cell phenotype, are suggested to be involved in colon carcinogenesis [75]. In the 'top–down' model of CRC heterogeneity involving intestinal SCs (ISCs), tumor initiation would start at the top of the crypt, where *APC*-mutated cells are observed and spread laterally and downward toward the normal crypt [76]. The second model of carcinogenesis is the spread of cancer 'from the bottom up.' In patients with a familial predisposition to *APC* mutations, dysplastic lesions have been observed on the tissue surface and then within individual crypts. Hence, this direction of lesion spread involving ISCs is not excluded [77].

The tissue heterogeneity of CRC is explained in two ways, namely (1) in the CSC model and (2) in the clonal evolution model. In the former, tumor cells are organized hierarchically. Some of them are CSCs, which retain the ability to proliferate, while their progeny 'differentiate' into non-proliferating lineages [10,13]. It was in colon cancer that the different subpopulations of CSCs/CICs/TICs, which are responsible for the different stages of CRC development in primary CRC (pCRC), were first distinguished [14]. Previous studies indicated that in the progression from normal to the mutated epithelium of AD, aldehyde dehydrogenase 1 (ALDH1)-positive cells restricted to the normal crypt bottom increased in number and became distributed further up the crypt. This marker was therefore found to be a favorable marker of CSCs responsible for tumor progression [12]. The role of CSCs with a leucine-rich repeat-containing G-protein-coupled receptor 5 (Lgr5)(+) phenotype, essential for tumor growth and metastasis formation (e.g., in the liver), has also been demonstrated in growing CRC tumor tissues [78–80]. Genetic experiments have confirmed that these dynamic CSCs are at the top of the hierarchy of human CRC cells, and this organization resembles that of the normal colonic epithelium [78].

Interestingly, ablation of Lgr5(+) CSCs did not inhibit the growth of the primary tumor, as Lgr5(+) CSCs were continuously replenished by proliferative Lgr5(−) cancer cells, but resulted in reduced liver metastasis (CRLM) [79]. There has long been research evaluating other colon markers of CSCs and the mechanisms controlling the rate of division and self-renewal, which may confer tumor growth and be the cause of chemoresistance [81,82]. In a rat model, it has been shown that only 1 in 25 cells, or 1 in 262 cells, have the characteristics of CSCs in the whole CRC cell population [11,12]. Moreover, the CSC480 CRC stem cell line exhibited an elevated expression of CSC markers such as CD44, ALDH1, and Sox2 compared to the grade 3–4 colon adenocarcinoma cell line (SW480). In addition, the quiescent cells were detected in a heterogeneous tumor cell population using the proliferation marker 5-ethynyl-2′-deoxyuridine (EdU) and a label-retaining cell protocol. Most of the normal fetal human colon epithelial cell line (FHC) resided in this quiescent state. These cells are characterized by extremely slow cell division, as evidenced by the increased expression of ALDH1 compared to other cell lines. In addition, elevated ATP-binding cassette superfamily G member 2 (ABCG2) expression was also present in the FHC cells compared to the SW480 and CSC480 cells. This may support reports that quiescent cells are resistant to chemotherapy (CTx) [82].

The clonal evolution model assumes that genetic and epigenetic changes occur over time in individual cancer cells and that if such changes confer a selective advantage, they will allow particular cancer cell clones to compete with other clones. Clonal evolution can lead to genetic heterogeneity, resulting in phenotypic and functional differences between cancer cells within a single patient [13]. While initial studies suggested that colorectal tumors were monoclonal, later research has shown that the majority (up to 76%) of human early microadenomas are polyclonal [10,83,84].

Clinical observations have prompted more intensive research into the cellular and environmental mechanisms affecting the tumor cell proliferation rate. Proliferative abnormalities of the normal colonic mucosa have been proposed as a possible marker of increased susceptibility to CRC development (particularly an upward shift of the proliferative compartment in the normal mucosa of CRC patients) [85]. Significant differences in the effects of the same therapy (CTx and RT) in patients with the same type of CRC have also been noted [86–88]. Attention has been drawn to the predictive (efficacy of different treatment options, individualization of treatment) and prognostic values (treatment outcome) of proliferation rates as a biological CRC feature. The prevailing view was that the pool of rapidly proliferating and mature tumor cells within the tumor was responsible for treatment failure [86]. Increased proliferation rates were considered as one of the determining factors in the accelerated repopulation of malignant tumors including CRC [89,90]. Therefore it was necessary to assess the tumor growth rate as early as possible (i.e., before treatment) to prevent recurrence. Although the prognostic significance of rapid tumor cell proliferation has not been demonstrated, there is a consensus that rapidly proliferating tumors should be treated with accelerated RT regimens. When it comes to CRC, there are huge discrepancies regarding how RT should be administered in rectal cancer (RC). There is no international consensus regarding the preoperative RT irradiation schedule for RC [91].

The main culprits of treatment resistance, metastasis, and relapse in CRC appear to be CSCs [92,93]. These cells are mostly 'quiescent' and poorly differentiated and thus can easily survive CTx. The high heterogeneity of TICs was first shown in colon cancer, with only specific subpopulations (self-renewing long-term TICs, LT-TICs) leading to the development of metastatic disease. Other examples of this subgroup include tumor transient amplifying cells (T-TACs) and rare delayed contributing TICs (DC-TICs) [14]. Moreover, abnormal activation of multiple cellular pathways (e.g., Wnt, Notch, Hedgehog, PI3K/AKT) in CRC can result in the emergence of CSCs characterized by excessive self-renewal, increased invasiveness, and resistance to treatment [92].

It appears that varied therapy effects did not occur due to differences in the proliferation rates between CSCs and more differentiated tumor cells as the therapy-induced deaths did not depend on the proliferative status of the cells. These results confirm that CSCs are selectively resistant to conventional CTx due to reduced mitochondrial priming [94]. Studies indicate that these cells arise from normal proliferating colonic crypt SCs. The marker of these cells, encoded by the *LGR5* gene, is overexpressed during CRC development. At the same time, *LGR5* is associated with Wnt pathway activation and the *c-MYC* protooncogene, and may be a prognostic factor in CRC [95].

4. Methods to Assess Cell Proliferation in Colorectal Cancer

In clinical practice and basic research, several methods exist for assessing the growth rate of normal and tumor cells. The most common is the assessment of (1) the "density" of ongoing mitoses in the tissue material, known as the mitotic index (the percentage of mitoses in the assessed pool of tumor cells per 1 mm^2), the so-called mitotic rate, the rate at which cells enter the mitotic phase (M phase) (% of the cells/h) [96–98]; (2) the percentage of cells in the S phase by calculating the so-called bromo-, iododeoxyuridine labeling index (LIBrdIUdR) [99–102] with in vitro tritiated thymidine [103,104], or with a new thymidine analog, 5-ethynyl-2-deoxyuridine (EdU) labeling [82]; (3) IHC expression of classical proliferative markers (e.g., cyclins, proliferating cell nuclear antigen (PCNA), and Ki-67 [105–109]); (4) computed tomography (CT) with dual-layer spectral detector CT [110] or positron emission tomography (PET) [111–113].

The cancerogenic process of the colonic mucosa is associated with the development of cell proliferation abnormalities, which precede the onset of morphological alterations such as epithelial dysplasia. Individuals with gastrointestinal (GI) tract cancer risk factors and animals exposed to carcinogens mainly show an increase in the cell proliferation rate and abnormalities in the distribution of proliferating cells. The so-called extension of the proliferative compartment was observed even when the mucosa was not yet affected by morphological abnormalities. This proliferative feature seems to be related to the presence of defects in cell differentiation [114]. There is also a report in which a significantly lower expression of multi-gene proliferation signature (GPS) was observed in CRLMs, confirming lower levels of their proliferation using qRT-PCR and Ki-67 immunostaining. According to the authors, slow proliferation is a biological feature of both CRLMs and primary tumors with metastasis capacity [115]. In the context of the stem cell hypothesis of CRC development, in vitro studies based on the exposure of CSC480 cells to a 2 h pulse of 10 µg EdU have recently allowed for the identification of as many as five different cell populations, of which the EdU-negative and CD44-positive population may represent the 'true' CSC lineage [82].

In formalin-fixed, paraffin-embedded tissues, changes in DNA content or the expression of proteins involved in the cell cycle in dysplastic, precancerous, and neoplastic tissues of the human colon were most often comparatively assessed. However, changes in the expression of IHC markers (e.g., PCNA, p53, Ki-67) at different developmental stages of CRC were not always clear enough to serve as reliable prognostic markers [31,116,117].

4.1. Assessment of Mitosis in Cancer Tissues

The mitosis count/mitotic index in pathological samples allows for the assessment of tumor proliferative activity, facilitates tumor classification and diagnosis, assesses grade malignancy, determines aggressive behavior, allows for intratumoral lymphocyte counts, and may present prognostic significance [98,118]. The preferred sites for mitosis counting include invasive fronts (rich in viable tumor cells) or the periphery of the tumors. The tissue area for counting mitotic activity for different tumors was standardized as the number of mitoses in a fixed number of high-power fields (HPFs) (typically 10 fields of view at × 400 magnification) [118]. HPFs for digital pathology, different from glass-slide HPFs in conventional light microscopy, require re-evaluation [119]. The current recommendation for CRC is not to report the number of mitoses in HPFs, but to report them per square millimeter [98], or per 2 mm^2 (this is approximately equivalent to 10 HPFs on modern microscopes) [97,118].

4.2. DNA Ploidy and Percentage of Cells in S Phase

Aneuploidy refers to an abnormal number of chromosomes in a cell, different from a multiplication of the haploid set, resulting from several genetic alterations. It reflects both gain/loss of whole chromosomes and unbalanced chromosome rearrangements (e.g., deletions, amplifications, translocations of large genome regions) [120]. For more than 100 years, aneuploidy has been postulated as a tumor-promoting factor, and its clinical relevance is still highlighted as a prognostic marker [121,122]. Interestingly, it has been suggested that tissue SCs have also developed their distinct response to aneuploidy, being able to survive and proliferate as aneuploid [121].

DNA content and ploidy were evaluated as prognostic factors in CRC [123–126], with DNA aneuploidy demonstrated to be a feature of tumors with a higher proliferation rate [124,126,127]. On the other hand, ploidy alone, determined by flow cytometry (FCM), had no prognostic significance in CRC (DFS). In a group of more than 400 CRC patients, it was shown that nearly 73% of patients showed aneuploid tumors. Still, the DNA pattern was not correlated with either age, gender, location, differentiation, or stage of the tumors [128].

Review studies [129,130] and a meta-analysis [127] indicate a significant association of aneuploidy with tumor progression and a worse prognosis. An older meta-analysis (2007) showed that patients undergoing surgical resection of aneuploid CRC have a higher risk of death after five years [129]. Later meta-analysis (2015) including more than 7000 CRC patients showed a higher prevalence of aneuploidy in late versus early stage sporadic CRC (OD 1.51, 95% CI 1.37–1.67), indicating that genomic instability increases with CRC progression. In 54.1% of studies, a significant effect of aneuploidy on prognosis was described for OS, disease-specific survival (DSS), and recurrence (relapse)-free survival (RFS). Hence, aneuploidy may be considered as a tumor stage-specific prognostic marker [127].

Other methods to assess the proliferation of different cell populations in CRC include evaluating the number of cells in which DNA synthesis occurs using LIBrdIUdR, with tritiated thymidine [103,104] and EdU labeling [82]. Such procedures allow in vivo calculation of the S-phase fraction labeling index (LI), the duration of the S phase (Ts), and the potential tumor doubling time (Tpot) [131].

Evaluation of the binding index of BrdUrd/IdUrd/tritiated thymidine, etc., is possible (1) following the use of monoclonal antibodies (mAbs) against thymidine analogs in FCM or (2) by using the IHC method. Although these method variations are inexpensive and easy to perform, they are characterized by high subjectivity in the evaluation of specimens, poor reproducibility of results, and the lack of standardization between centers [104,124,128,132].

Studies from the 1990s showed that examining only the total and aneuploid LI in CRC is not sufficient as an indicator of proliferation, as Ts also can vary between tumors and even within a single tumor (from 4.0 to 28.6 h). The mean Tpot ranged from 1.7 to 21.4 days. None of the cellular kinetic parameters correlated with Dukes' classification or histologic examination [133]. Wilson et al. showed that while IUdR assessed by FCM (IUdRfmc) and assessed by IHC (IUdRimm) correlated with each other, and their LIs were significantly higher in aneuploid than diploid tumors, no prognostic property of these markers was demonstrated [124]. Similar results were reported by other authors [126]. On the other hand, Palmqvist et al., using both IUdR detection techniques (FCM + IHC), demonstrated that patients with Dukes' B tumors with higher IUdR LI (in invasive margin) and/or low Tpot (at both the invasive margin and the luminal border) had longer survival [100]. FCM studies on the prognostic value of the DNA index or S-phase fraction also did not demonstrate prognostic significance for disease recurrence in CRC stages II and III [125], survival in the overall group, or within stages [132]. In contrast, the kinetic parameters assessed by Michel et al. using in vivo injection of Brd and FCM, were independent prognostic factors in diploid tumors. These included lymph node (LN) involvement, ploidy, and Tpot in all tumors, and Tpot only in diploid tumors [131].

In summary, most studies failed to demonstrate the prognostic value of the CRC proliferation markers assessed. Moreover, using these methods, more accurate results for evaluating normal and tumor cell proliferation are obtained after analyzing material at different stages of CRC development. On the other hand, performing such tests before and during treatment allows one to predict the outcome of CRC radiotherapy. For example, BrdUrd LI before RT treatment of RC was not a predictor of early clinical and pathological tumor response. In contrast, the BrdUrd LI ratio before/after RT was correlated with the inhibition of proliferation in responsive tumors. Thus, the rapid growth rate of preoperatively irradiated rectal cancer was a favorable prognostic factor [134].

4.3. Immunohistochemical Methods for the Detection of Proliferative Markers

The immunohistochemical (IHC) technique is based on antibodies against specific antigens in tissues and cells. In histopathology, IHC testing is most commonly performed on formalin-fixed, paraffin-embedded tissues that can be stored for long periods of time [135,136]. Increasingly, tissue microarrays (TMAs), which contain selected tissue material from tumors, normal tissues (control), and tumor metastases on a single slide, are being used for IHC. Although the cost of producing TMAs remains high, their selection saves labor time and the number of reagents used (including sometimes expensive antibodies), allowing for better result reproducibility [137]. The markers most commonly used to assess tumor proliferation rate (including CRC) are discussed below.

4.3.1. Thymidylate Synthase (TS) in CRC

Thymidylate synthase (TS, EC 2.1.1.45) is an enzyme protein required to synthesize and repair DNA. It catalyzes the conversion of $2'$-deoxyuridine-5-monophosphate (dUMP) to deoxythymidine-$5'$-monophosphate (dTMP), which is phosphorylated to the triphosphate state (dTTP), a direct precursor for DNA synthesis. It is also an important cellular target for cytotoxic drugs of the fluoropyrimidine group, which are widely used to treat solid tumors [138]. The first clinically used TS inhibitor was the 5-fluorouracil (5-FU) antimetabolite drug, a metabolite of 5-fluorouracil, fluoro-deoxyuridine monophosphate, which forms a ternary complex with TS and 5,10-methylenetetrahydrofolate [139].

IHC studies of TS are used to determine proliferative indices and drug resistance [138]. The role of ectopic production of human TS in the neoplastic transformation of mouse cells in vitro and in vivo has also been demonstrated, suggesting a role for TS as an oncogene [140]. Overexpression of TS is responsible for the resistance of tumor cells to TS-targeted chemotherapeutics and correlates with response to targeted CTx [141–144]. With the generation of mAbs against TS, particularly TS 106 and TS 109, it was possible to use IHC methods to detect TS in normal and tumor tissues. The color reaction is granular and occurs in the cytoplasm of cells. TS has been shown to be overexpressed in tumors including CRC. The prognostic significance of this IHC marker has also been studied [141–143,145–147].

Observations on the prognostic role of TS indicate that increased tissue expression of TS may serve as an independent factor of poor prognosis for DFS and OS [141,143,145,146,148–150] or RFS and OS [147]. However, there are also results in which the prognostic role of TS in the survival of CRC patients could not be proven. Moreover, it was shown that high levels of Ki-67 were associated with increased (decreased) survival in patients with a low (high) expression of TS [142]. The meta-analysis by Popat et al. showed that tumors with high TS levels appeared to have worse OS compared to tumors with low TS levels (HR 1.74, 95% CI 1.34 to 2.26) [151].

The predictive role of TS in CRC adjuvant therapy has also been investigated in various combinations (e.g., 5-FU-based CTx, oxaliplatin followed by 5-FU). One study showed a significantly higher degree of TS immunoreactivity in primary tumors compared to corresponding metastases. Still, the response rates after CTx for metastatic disease were similar for patients with low and high levels of TS shown in their primary tumors. In contrast, response rates were found to be higher in patients with low versus high TS in metastatic disease (71% and 23%, respectively) [152]. Thus, TS levels in primary tumors cannot be reliably used to predict the response to adjuvant therapy [147,152]. An opinion questioning the benefit of TS labeling for predicting the effect of 5-FU in CRC can also be found in a review paper [139].

Moreover, while an extensive prospective analysis showed that high TS levels in the tumor were associated with improved DFS and OS after adjuvant treatment of CRC, TS expression in the tumor did not predict the benefit of 5-FU-based CTx [153]. However, a recent study by Badary et al. showed that high TS expression is a predictor of early failure in CRC therapy. Hence, high TS expression may help identify patients who will benefit less from oxaliplatin and 5-FU CTx (FOLFOX) [143].

4.3.2. Cyclins in CRC

The human cyclin family includes about 30 genes encoding protein products containing the so-called cyclin box. Only a few subfamilies of these proteins (A-, B-, C-, D-, and E-cyclins) play a role in cell cycle regulation [57,58,61,154]. Others distinguish between 'primary' cyclins (A, B1, D1, D3, and E), crucial for cell cycle progression, and 'secondary' cyclins (C and H), with indirect cell cycle-related effects. Few papers have addressed the secondary prognostic role of cyclins in cancer including CRC [155].

Cyclin A can activate two different Cdks, playing a role in both the S phase and mitosis (M) [156], controlling various phenomena related to DNA replication and progression through the G2 phase [58]. Cyclin B is a regulator of the mitotic phase, responsible for M phase entry and chromosome segregation. In turn, cyclin C, encoded by the *CCNC* gene, is involved in G1/S progression. It forms complexes with cdk8 and cdk19, modulating DNA initiation and duplication by binding Mdm2 binding protein (MTBP), an interaction required for proper entry into the M phase with complete DNA replication [157]. D-type cyclins are a major determinant of cell cycle initiation and progression in many cell types. Cyclins D1, D2, and D3 (encoded by *CCND1*, *CCND2*, and *CCND3*) are identified as cell type-specific G1 mitogen sensors. The E-type cyclins control DNA replication. Cyclin E1, encoded by the human *CCNE1* gene, interacts mainly with Cdk1 and Cdk2 and plays an essential role in transition of human cells from G1 to the S phase [58,158].

In some studies, cyclin A (A2) overexpression was observed in 77–80% of CRC cases [159,160]. In rectal cancer, a linear correlation was observed between cyclin A and Ki-67-positive cell expression, whereas no such relationship was found between TS and cyclin A [161]. Several publications have recognized cyclin A overexpression as an independent unfavorable prognostic factor in CRC patients [159,160,162]. There are also reports showing that high cyclin A expression was independently associated with improved survival [155], and its level above the median predicted a better prognosis in CRC patients (HR 0.71, 95% CI 0.53–0.95) [163].

Cyclin B (B1) is classified as a mitotic cyclin [164,165]. Its elevated expression may promote the development of CRC, but its prognostic significance is controversial. Decreased expression of this cyclin has been shown in pCRC cases characterized by large size, mucinous type, deep invasion, or short postoperative survival. High cyclin B1 expression has been associated with increased p53 levels in ADs, and high Ki-67 in ADs and primary carcinomas [164]. Cyclin B1 is overexpressed and promotes cell proliferation in early-stage CRC [165,166]. No correlation was found between cyclin B1 expression and DFS or OS [165]. Other authors have reported that after CRC cells invade surrounding tissues and metastasize to distant tissues, cyclin B1 expression is reduced. Furthermore, it was observed that patients with a low level of cyclin B1 had lower survival rates than those with a high level of cyclin B1 expression. Suppression of cyclin B1 may promote tumor cell migration and invasion and reduce E-cadherin expression. Cyclin B1 may thus promote tumor growth but inhibit metastasis in CRC [166]. As shown in a recent meta-analysis regarding the prognostic role of cyclin B1 in solid tumors, in CRC, elevated cyclin B1 expression was associated with better prognosis, reflected by favorable 5-year OS of CRC (OR 0.49, 95% CI 0.30–0.82) [167].

Cyclin C overexpression was observed in 88% of CRCs, and *CCNC* (qRT-PCR) amplification was independently associated with poor prognosis. The association between *CCNC* amplification and impaired survival appears independent of its gene product [155]. However, further studies on the role of cyclin C itself as a prognostic factor in CRC are lacking. In contrast, a study by Firestein et al. found the expression of Cdk8, a kinase functionally related to cyclin C, in 70% of CRCs. This expression was independently associated with β-catenin activation, female gender, and fatty acid synthase (FASN) overexpression. Cdk8 expression also significantly increased the colon cancer-related mortality. However, no such association was observed among RC patients. These data support a potential association between Cdk8 and β-catenin and suggest that CDK8 may identify a subgroup of CRC patients with poor prognoses [168].

D-type cyclins play a central role in cell cycle entry. Changes in the activity of the D-Cdk4/6 cyclin complex are an almost universal feature of cancer cells [60]. Their expression increases in response to oncogenic alterations in key oncogenic pathways (e.g., K-RAS, PI3K/AKT, WNT) [58]. Overexpression of cyclin D1 is observed in CRC, particularly in advanced disease [160,169–171]. However, opinions are divided on the prognostic significance of this cyclin. Overall, more than 20 publications have been published on the prognostic value of cyclin D1 expression in case–control studies, as reviewed by other authors [171]. Maeda et al. showed a shortening of both OS and DFS, and an increase in the CRC recurrence rate in patients with strong cyclin D1 expression [172]. In the study by Bahnassy et al., as mentioned, cyclin D1 overexpression in CRC, similarly to cyclin A, was also correlated with shorter OS. This study indicated that cyclin D1 amplification was also associated with reduced OS. Both cyclin D1 and cyclin A were independent prognostic factors in CRC patients [160]. Another study showed an association between increased cyclin D2 and D3 expression and vascular invasion, CRLM, and decreased DSS [173]. In turn, a study by Mao et al. showed that positive cyclin D1 expression was associated with shorter survival in patients with colon adenocarcinoma [174]. Another publication demonstrated worse 5-year survival in patients with positive cyclin D1 expression in advanced-stage CRC (III, IV) [169]. Moreover, a recent study showed that cyclin D1 and epidermal growth factor receptor (EGFR) overexpression and late pathological stage after surgery were characterized by shorter relapse-free time (RFT) [175]. It has also been shown that the early recurrence of CRC in high-risk Duke B and Duke C stages is associated with high cyclin D1 expression [176]. However, some studies reported no prognostic role for cyclin D1 in RC or CC [155,177–180]. Finally, some studies have considered cyclin D1 overexpression to be a good predictor of survival [181,182], both in terms of cytoplasmic and nuclear expression [183].

There are also two meta-analyses on the prognostic significance of cyclin D1. One of them (2014) showed that cyclin D1 overexpression is a factor for poor prognosis in CRC, both in terms of OS (HR 0.73, 95% CI 0.63–0.85) and DFS (HR 0.60, 95% CI 0.44–0.82) [170]. Another meta-analysis (2022) confirmed these results, reporting both shorter OS (HR 0.36, 95% CI 0.94–0.22) and DFS (HR 0.46, 95% CI 0.77–0.20) [184].

In contrast, in a study by Jun et al. based on a large cohort of pCRC patients (n = 495), in which high cyclin D1 expression was observed in nearly 80% of patients, high cyclin D1 expression was a marker for better OS and RFS. Multivariate analysis showed that cyclin D1 overexpression and the young age of patients remained independent predictors of higher OS rate. In turn, high cyclin D1, female gender, CTx, absence of nodal metastasis, and lower T category remained independent predictors of better RFS. The authors believe that cyclin D1 expression can be a favorable prognostic indicator in CRC patients [171].

Studies on the prognostic role of cyclin E in CRC have also been conducted, most often together with other markers of cellular proliferation (e.g., cyclin D1 and Ki-67) [176,179,185,186]. Ioachim et al. demonstrated cyclin E overexpression in 30% of CRC patients, but the prognostic significance in determining the risk of recurrence and OS was not confirmed [179]. Elevated cyclin E expression correlated with increasing TNM staging and decreasing tumor differentiation. In turn, PFS and median survival were reduced in patients with positive cyclin E expression [185]. Another group found cyclin E expression in a similar proportion of CRC patients (~35%) but did not report prognostic significance in CRC as a single marker [186].

The data in Table 1, arranged chronologically, show variable results regarding the tissue expression of various cyclins in CRC. In general, the overexpression of these cell cycle markers is detected in most patients (up to almost 90%). When it comes to the evaluation of the prognostic value of cyclins, most data concern cyclins A (A2), B (B1), and D (D1). However, as with other tissue markers, the data are not consistent. Cyclins of the D family show the strongest association with signaling pathways involved in CRC development (e.g., KRAS, PI3K/AKT, WNT). Moreover, while some studies have also associated cyclin D1 overexpression with poor prognosis, some present results describe no prognostic significance or indicate cyclin D1 as a good prognostic factor. In conclusion, examining the expression of these proteins alone seems insufficient to determine the prognosis for survival of CRC patients. Hence, further research is needed to determine the role of cyclin C and E as prognostic markers in CRC.

Table 1. Cyclins and their potential prognostic value in colorectal cancer (CRC).

Type of Cyclin	Material (No. of Cases) and Method	Findings	Year of Publication	Ref. No.
A (A2)	CRC (73); IHC, SI	Mean: 12.26 ± 5.8; SI was correlated with tumor differentiation; ↑expression correlated with ↓OS; ↑expression is an independent negative prognostic factor (HR 7.82, 95% CI, 0.02–60.12) (UA) and (HR 13.89; 95% CI 1.01–190.58) (MA)	1999	[159]
	CRC (60); IHC, SI	↑Expression associated with ↓OS; independent prognostic factor	2004	[160]
	CRC (167); IHC	(+) Expression (61.1%); (+) expression correlated with ↓survival; (+) expression, LN meta, and Dukes' stage were independently associated with unfavorable prognosis	2004	[162]
	CRC (219); IHC; qRT-PCR	(+) Expression (83%), extra gene copies (6.2%); correlation with stage and differentiation; ↑expression independently associated with improved survival (UA), (HR 0.57, 95% CI 0.33–0.98) (MA)	2005	[155]
	CRC (790); IHC	Expression above the median predicted an improved patient prognosis (HR 0.71, 95% CI 0.53–0.95); cell proliferation and (+) expression were prognostic indicators of patient outcome	2011	[163]
B (B1)	C (22), ADs (62); CAs in ADs (17), pCRC (194), LN meta (21); IHC	↑B1 expression from C through ADs to pCRC; ↑expression with increasing degree of dysplasia in ADs, from peripheral ADs to central CAs, and from primary to metastatic foci; ↓in pCRC with large size, mucinous type, deep invasion, or short PPS time	2003	[164]
	CRC (342); IHC	↑Expression (78.7%); no association with histopathologic features; no impact on OS and DFS (UA)	2004	[165]
	CRC (219); IHC, qRT-PCR	(+) Expression (83%), extra gene copies (9%); no prognostic value	2005	[155]
	CRC (150); WB; qRT-PCR; IHC	↑mRNA expression (92.7%); ↑expression negatively related to LN and distant meta, and TNM; ↓expression associated with poor OS	2015	[166]
C	CRC (219); IHC; qRT-PCR	↑Expression (88%), extra gene copies (26.9%); ↑expression correlated with *CCNC* amplification; protein expression tends to associate with DSS; *CCNC* amplification related to an unfavorable prognosis, (HR 1.72, 95% CI 1.00–2.94) (MA)	2005	[155]

Table 1. Cont.

Type of Cyclin	Material (No. of Cases) and Method	Findings	Year of Publication	Ref. No.
D (D1, D3)	CRC (123); IHC	↑D1 expression correlated with poor OS and DFS; an independent predictor of disease recurrence	1998	[172]
	CRC (90); IHC	Nuclear/cytoplasmic expression of cyclin D1; no prognostic value	1998	[177]
	CRC (73); IHC, SI	Mean: 6.9 ± 6.3; SI correlated with tumor differentiation; ↑in LN meta vs. those without; ↑in advanced than in early CAs; ↑expression tends to associate with poor prognosis	1999	[159]
	CRC (126); IHC	(+) Expression (58.7%); cytoplasmic (HR 0.56, 95% CI 0.31–1.0) or nuclear level (HR 0.24, 95% CI 0.07–0.81) related to ↑survival	2001	[183]
	RC (160); IHC, (+) at the 10% level	(+) D1 expression (48%); no prognostic role of this marker	2002	[178]
	CRC (60); IHC, SI	↑SI within deeply invasive tumors and LN meta; ↑expression and D1 amplification associated with ↓OS; independent prognostic factor	2004	[160]
	CRC (219); IHC; qRT-PCR	(+) D1 expression (11%) and extra gene copies (55%), cyclin D3 (36%) and extra gene copies (20.5%); no prognostic role of these markers	2005	[155]
	CC and RC (363), Dukes' A–D, TMA; IHC	(+) Nuclear staining of cyclin D1 reflected better survival	2005	[182]
	CRC (97); IHC, (+) at >5% cells	↑Expression (5.9%); ↑levels in mucous differentiation; ↑expression correlated with stage, LN meta; no prognostic value	2008	[179]
	CC (602), stage I–IV; IHC	↑Expression (55%) was related to low cancer-specific mortality (HR 0.57, 95% CI 0.39–0.84) (MA), and for low overall mortality (HR 0.74, 95% CI 0.57–0.98); ↑expression related to ↑survival	2009	[181]
	CRC (84), TMA; cyclin D1, D2, D3; IHC	D2 expression at the margin associated with vascular invasion, LN meta, and CRLM; ↑D2 and D3 associated with vascular invasion, CRLM, and ↓DSS (cyclin D2)	2010	[173]
	CRC (169); IHC	(+) D1 expression related to shorter survival	2011	[174]
	CRC (117), TMA; IHC	↓Nuclear expression associated with negative lymphovascular invasion; no prognostic value of cyclin D1	2015	[180]
	CRC with meta (1205); IHC	↑Expression (46.7%); ↑D1, EGFR expression, late stage after S indicated ↓RFT (UA); no independent factor of prognosis (MA)	2019	[175]
	CC (102); IHC	(+) Expression of cyclin D1 correlated with a worse 5-yrs survival rate in pts with advanced stage (III, IV)	2019	[169]
	CRC (101), Dukes' B and C stages; IHC	↑Expression more often in DFS ≤24 group vs. ≥48 group and had 5.2 higher odds of having DFS <24 mo; ↑expression correlated with early recurrence in high-risk Duke's B and C stage	2021	[176]
E	CRC (219); IHC, qRT-PCR	(+) Expression (25%) and extra gene copies (19.1%); no prognostic value	2005	[155]
	CRC (97); IHC, (+) at >5% cells	↑Expression (30%); (+) correlation with p21waf1/cip1, PCNA-LI and Ki-67; no prognostic value	2008	[179]
	CRC (200), benign alterations (200); IHC; RT-PCR	↑Expression with TNM and decreasing tumor differentiation; (+) expression correlated with shorter PFS and median survival	2016	[185]
	CRC (31), TMA; IHC	(+) Expression (34.78%); no prognostic role of this marker	2016	[186]
	CC (102); IHC	(+) Correlation with cyclin D1; no prognostic role	2019	[169]

Legend: ↑/↓—increase (overexpression)/decrease; </>—lower/higher; (+)/(−)—positive/negative; ADs—adenomas; C—control, normal mucosa; Cas—carcinomas; CC—colon cancer; CCNC—cyclin-C encoded gene; CI—confidence interval; CRLM—CRC liver metastasis; DFS—disease-free survival; DSS—disease-specific survival; (p)CRC—(primary) colorectal cancer; EGFR—epidermal growth factor receptor; HR—hazard ratio; IHC—immunohistochemistry; LI—labeling index; LN(s)—lymph node(s); MA—multivariate analysis; meta—metastasis; mo—months; no.—number; OS—overall survival; PCNA—proliferating cell nuclear antigen; PFS—progression-free survival; PPS—postoperative patient survival; pts—patients; RFT—relapse-free time; qRT-PCR—quantitative real-time polymerase chain reaction; RT-PCR—reverse transcriptase-polymerase chain reaction; S—surgery; SI—staining index; UA—univariate analysis; WB—Western blot analysis; yrs—years.

4.3.3. Proliferating Cell Nuclear Antigen (PCNA) in CRC

In eukaryotic cell physiology, PCNA plays a vital role in DNA replication and many replication-associated processes. It is a 36 kDa non-histone nuclear protein, accompanying delta and epsilon DNA polymerase. It is referred to as a cyclin, playing a prominent role in cell proliferation. It is mainly produced in proliferating and transformed cells as a specific marker of cell division [187]. PCNA expression is detected in all phases of the cell cycle, confirming the function of this polypeptide in DNA repair, synthesis, and regulation [108].

There is a significant variability of results regarding PCNA expression in 'adenoma–carcinoma sequence' changes in CRC. Either no increase in PCNA-positive cells was detected in adenocarcinoma [116], or a gradual increase in PCNA expression was shown in HP-AC lesion sequences [117]. Some authors observed high PCNA expression in more aggressive forms of ADs, which can progress to malignant lesions [188]. As for the value of PCNA expression in predicting CRC, results also vary. One publication recognized PCNA as an independent predictor of relapse and shorter survival in CRC patients [189]. Choi et al. demonstrated a significantly higher relapse rate in CRC patients, with higher-than-average PCNA-LI. Also, the four-year survival rates in cases with higher-than-average PCNA-LI were considerably worse than those with lower-than-average PCNA-LI [190]. Other studies either failed to demonstrate the prognostic value of PCNA in this cancer [123,124,191] or showed an inverse relationship between the percentage of PCNA-positive cells and the survival time of CRC patients [192]. Increased PCNA-LI of tumors was often associated with tumor progression (venous invasion, lymph node metastasis, or liver metastasis), while higher PCNA-LI was also associated with less differentiated tumors. Thus, PCNA testing could have prognostic significance for assessing higher malignant potential [193]. However, Neoptolemos et al., in RC studies, showed that PCNA-LI was not prognostic in this cancer subtype and that patients with the smallest LI exhibited the worst survival times [191]. In contrast, Nakamura et al. showed longer survival for CRC patients with lower PCNA expression, which was true for both CEA-positive and serum CEA-negative patients [194]. Some authors have indicated that while higher proliferation is associated with a higher incidence of rectal ADs, PCNA-LI is not useful for predicting future colorectal neoplasia [195]. Others have found lower PCNA-LI expression to be a good predictor of survival, especially in combination with HLA-DR expression [196]. Studies of the entire cell cycle panel (e.g., cyclins D1, E, cyclin-dependent kinase (CDK) inhibitors: p21 and p27) and other cell cycle regulators including PCNA have not proven the prognostic value of any of them in terms of predicting the risk of relapse or OS. These molecules have mainly been considered as cell growth regulators during colorectal carcinogenesis [179]. Moreover, studies by Guzinska et al. confirmed correlations between PCNA expression and lymph node metastasis and tumor location (lower in RC). However, the prognostic value of PCNA was not evaluated [197].

The only available meta-analysis on the level of immunohistochemical PCNA expression as a prognostic factor in CRC considered OS, cancer-specific survival (CSS), and DFS in 1372 CRC patients [198]. It showed that patients with high PCNA expression were characterized by shorter OS (HR 1.81, 95% CI 1.51–2.17) and CSS (HR 1.99, 95% CI 1.04–3.79). However, there was no significant association between PCNA and DFS. Thus, it was shown that high PCNA expression can predict a poor prognosis in CRC patients. However, this analysis needs to be confirmed in a larger number of studies based on bigger groups of patients.

Table 2 shows, in chronological order, the results that illustrate the difficulty in forming a clear opinion on the prognostic significance of PCNA. The tissue expression of PCNA was studied simultaneously with various histopathological classifications and/or with other tumor biomarkers (e.g., CEA, HLA-DR, Bcl-2) to analyze the interactions of these proteins and/or to expand the panel of prognostic factors in CRC.

Table 2. Prognostic value of proliferating cell nuclear antigen (PCNA) in colorectal cancer (CRC).

S No.	Material (No. of Cases) and Methods	Findings	Prognostic Role	Year of Publication	Ref. No.
1.	CRC (40); IHC, PI	↑PI in both cancer and epithelial cells of adjacent C crypts in those who died vs. survivors	PI is an independent predictor of recurrence and poor survival in both groups	1993	[189]
2.	CRC (82) and LN meta (18); IHC, q estimation	Similar to the median and range of the % of (+) cells in primary tumors and LN meta	An inverse relationship between the % of (+) cells and survival times	1993	[192]
3.	CRC (60) and ADs (35); IHC; FCM for DNA content	Mean: 38% (ADs); mean: 50.4% (CRC); aneuploid ACs had a tendency to poorer prognosis, especially in Dukes' C female pts	Can be an indirect indicator of cells in the S phase; is not an independent prognostic factor	1994	[123]
4.	CRC (125); IHC, LI, image analysis	LI without significant correlation with clinical characteristics (stage, grade, age, sex, fixity)	No prognostic role for survival	1994	[124]
5.	CRC (49); IHC, LI	↑LI of tumors with venous invasion (mean: 51.7%); with LN meta (mean: 50.5%); with meta to the liver (mean: 55.2%); ↑LI associated with less differentiated tumors	Evaluation of LI at the invasive tumor margin may help identify CRC with ↑malignant potential	1994	[193]
6.	CRC biopsies (50); FCM, LI	LI from 38.7% to 53.0%; in diploid tumors (27), the median LI in G0/G1: 71.5%, in S: 10.5%, in G2/M: 17.4%	Is expressed throughout the cell cycle; prognostic role—probable	1995	[108]
7.	CC (50) and 40 RC; IHC (79), LI	LI improved the prediction of survival when used with histopathological classification (Dukes' or Jass') (MA)	Little prognostic power of LI (UA); not predictive for RC; ↓LI related to the worst prognosis	1995	[191]
8.	CRC (57); IHC, LI	↑Deep invasion, CRLM, and ↑stages with ↑LI (>49.4%) vs. ↓LI; ↑survival curves for pts with (−) CEA and ↓LI vs. pts with (+) CEA and ↑LI; ↑survival curves for pts with (+) CEA and ↓LI vs. pts with (+) CEA and ↑LI	Serum CEA and PCNA LI for cancer pts are useful in the evaluation of tumor progression and prognosis	1996	[194]
9.	CRC (86); IHC, LI	↑LI with stage, histologic differentiation, lymphatic and vascular invasion, LN meta, and CRLM; ↑LI in tumors with DNA aneuploidy	↑Recurrence rate with LI > than the mean LI; ↓4-yr survival rates for overall and curative pts with LI > than the mean LI	1996	[190]
10.	CRC (59); IHC, LI	Lesions combining HLA-DR expression and a relatively ↓LI had the best prognosis	HLA-DR expression with ↓LI is an important outcome predictor	1998	[196]
11.	CRC (47); IHC, >60% nuclei (+)	(+) Correlation with Bcl-2, LN meta, and tumor location	May be an indicator of the development of LN meta	2009	[197]

Legend: ↑/↓—increase/(overexpression)/decrease; (−)/(+)—negative/positive; </>—lower/higher; AC(s)—adenocarcinoma(s); AD(s)—adenoma(s); AS1—antisense to PCNA; C—control, normal mucosa; CRLM—CRC liver metastasis; FCM—flow cytometry; HLA-DR—human leukocyte antigen–DR isotype, major histocompatibility complex, class II, DR alpha; HP(s)—hyperplastic polyp(s); LN(s)—lymph node(s); meta—metastases; No.—number; PI—proliferating index; pTNM—pathological tumor/node/metastasis; pts—patients; q—quantitative; ROC—receiver operating characteristic curve; RR—risk ratio; S No.—study number.

4.3.4. Ki-67 Antigen in CRC

The prototype of the Ki-67 antigen was the IgG1 class, murine mAb, directed against the nuclear fraction of the Hodgkin's lymphoma-derived cells (L428) [106,199]. Recognition of the structure of the Ki-67 protein (pKi-67) has enabled this protein to be placed in a new category of cell cycle-related, nuclear non-histone proteins. pKi-67 is encoded by the *MKI67* gene on chromosome 11 (10q26) and has two major splice variants of 320 and 352 kDa [200]. The pioneering generation of anti-Ki-67 mAbs [199], characterization of the Ki-67 antigen using molecular biology techniques [201] and experimental studies demonstrated the presence of pKi-67 in the S, G2, and M phases of the cell cycle, and its absence in the G0 phase [105]. Thus, Ki-67 exhibits the so-called growth fraction in non-cancerous cells and tumors, indicating it as a marker of cellular proliferation [105,202]. It is worth mentioning that Ki-67 positivity does not always indicate that the cell entered the division phase. It can also signify a transition into a quiescent state and the possibility of entering the cell cycle after removing the inhibiting factor. Subcellular localization during interphase shows the presence of Ki-67 mainly in the cell nucleus, while in mitosis, it is translocated to the surface of chromosomes [106]. Recent studies have also indicated the extranuclear translocation of pKi-67 in non-cancerous cells to eliminate the protein, with initial accumulation in the endoplasmic reticulum (ER) and later in the Golgi apparatus. This mechanism is less effective in cancer cells [203].

Numerous publications over the years have discussed the role of Ki-67 as a marker of proliferation [106,202,204–206] and thus as a prognostic factor in many diseases, primarily cancer (including CRC) [207]. At the same time, studies have been conducted on the structure and biological role of pKi-67 in normal cells [207–210]. The multifactorial regulation of Ki-67 in non-cancerous and cancerous human cells has been described [203,206,210]. The role of Ki-67 in cell cycle progression is debated, most notably its almost opposite role in the initial phase of mitosis (prometaphase) (chromosome individualization) and exit from mitosis (chromosome clustering) [211]. Ki-67 has been shown to form repulsive molecular brushes during the early stages of mitosis [212]. In turn, the brushes collapse during mitotic exit, and Ki-67 promotes chromosome clustering [213]. Other significant advancements regarding the structure and functional role of pKi-67 in recent years include the demonstration of (1) the putative role of this protein in the higher-order organization of perinucleolar chromatin [208]; (2) the involvement of pKi-67 in the early stages of rRNA synthesis in vivo [209]; (3) the involvement of Ki-67 as a PP1 interacting protein (PIP) in the phosphorylation of nucleophosmin/B23 by casein kinase II (CKII) and the organization of the perichromosomal layer [214]; (4) the role in the generation of a spherical and electrostatic charge barrier, enabling independent chromosome mobility and efficient interaction with the mitotic spindle [212]; (5) the role in the spatial organization of heterochromatin in proliferating cells and in the control of gene expression [215]; (6) the differential regulation of the two main splice variants of the protein (i.e., α and β) in non-cancerous and cancerous cells; (7) the continuous regulation and degradation of Ki-67 by proteasomes in normal and cancerous cells and the extranuclear pathway of protein elimination [203]; (8) changes in expression depending on cell cycle regulation as a reliable indicator of the effect of CDK4/CDK6 inhibitors on cell proliferation [109]; (9) accumulation of the protein during the S, G2, and M phases, and degradation during the G1 and G0 phases; (10) the graded, rather than binary, nature of the protein, with a stable decrease in pKi-67 levels in quiescent cells [210]; (11) the presence of a gradient of Ki-67 expression depending on the phase of the cell cycle, (fast-growing tumors exhibit high levels of this protein in G2 phase cells, while in slow-growing tumors, these levels are notably lower) [216]; (12) the involvement in the regulation of chromosome clustering conditioning the removal of mature ribosomes from the nucleus after mitosis [213]. Although Ki-67 is widely recognized as a proliferation marker, genetic studies indicate that its levels do not correlate directly with this process. Indeed, the downregulation of Ki-67 did not affect the proliferation of HeLa cells [212,214,215], BJ-hTERT cells, and U2OS cells [215].

To evaluate the Ki-67-positive cells (the Ki-67 labeling/proliferating index, LI, PI) in paraffin-embedded sections during histopathology, an antibody called MIB-1 is most commonly used. Sometimes, in the literature, the name pKi-67 is used interchangeably with anti-Ki-67 antibody, or both are used together (Ki-67/MIB-1). Using IHC, it is possible to not only determine the presence of Ki-67 LI but also identify the type of proliferation, which could be a potential prognostic factor [70].

Ki-67 and Clinicopathologic Data in CRC Patients

The study of the tissue expression of Ki-67, as the most common proliferative marker, is widely used to assess tumor grade or stage, predict tumor progression, or identify potential therapeutic targets [106,202,204].

Lower Ki-67 LI with medium intensity has been described in non-neoplastic polyps compared to neoplastic lesions [217]. In colorectal ADs, the Ki-67 expression was lower [218] or comparable to CRC [217]. Moreover, a higher positive rate was observed in AD cases with high atypia and carcinoma in situ [219] and in more severe dysplastic adenomatous lesions [220]. The latter study indicated that the severity of dysplasia is associated with greater cellular proliferation, as opposed to the morphological type of AD (tubular, tubulovillous, and villous).

High levels of Ki-67 expression in pCRC are most often correlated with more severe histopathological changes (stage, grade) [217,218,221–230]. An inverse correlation between Ki-67 expression and the degree of differentiation in non-mucinous AC was observed [231]. A higher Ki-67 LI ($\geq$30%) was present in lymphatic and venous invasion as well as in lymph nodes and CRLMs. The same LI ($\geq$30%) in the primary tumor was associated with a significantly higher incidence of metachronous CRLMs. However, the mean Ki-67 LI was higher in primary tumors compared to CRLMs [221], which was also confirmed at the mRNA level [115]. Moreover, other researchers observed a positive correlation of Ki-67 LI with LN metastasis [88,197,224,228,229,232]. At the same time, Lei et al. showed Ki-67 level $\geq$ 60% to be associated with a high risk of distant metastasis and death, compared with a Ki-67 below this level [230].

Some authors did not show any significant correlation with the clinicopathological data [96,124,126,142,233–235]. In contrast, other authors have shown better clinicopathological variables in CRC patients with higher Ki-67 expression [147,236,237] and an inverse relationship between Ki-67 expression and tumor aggressiveness [115]. Similarly, the percentage of Ki-67-positive cells in poorly differentiated and mucinous AC was significantly lower than in well-differentiated and moderately differentiated AC. In contrast, lower Ki-67 LI in the primary lesion in cases with metachronous liver or lung metastases, compared to synchronous cases, may indicate that metachronous hematogenous metastases occur even in tumors with low proliferative activity [219].

In numerous publications, IHC studies have also evaluated other proliferation markers and their correlation with Ki-67 expression levels. IudR [124] and BrdUrd [126] were positively correlated with Ki-67, while TS expression correlated with Ki-67 in one study of RC [161] but not in others [142,238].

Positive correlations with Ki-67 were observed for cyclin A [141,159,160], cyclin B1 [164], cyclin D1 [160,169], cyclin E [185], cyclin E, and the p21waf1/cip1 cdk inhibitor [179]. Many authors have investigated the extent of cellular proliferation, measured by the expression of Ki-67 and the mutated tumor suppressor gene product p53, as an example of the most common genetic aberration in CRC [125,142,147,218,224,228,232,235,237,239–242]. As for the reciprocal correlations of the two proteins, either a directly proportional correlation [228,235,241], no significant correlation [224,238], or an inverse correlation of Ki-67 and p53 was detected [218].

Ki-67 as a Prognostic Marker in CRC

Cell proliferation is significantly associated with CRC progression and can be used to identify patients with a predicted unfavorable disease outcome after surgery [223,243]. The prognosis of CRC is not solely determined by the proliferative capacity of tumor cells [224]. Many clinicopathological prognostic factors have been documented, related to the advanced pathological TNM stage (pTNM) and the so-called TNM-independent factors (e.g., tumor subtype and histological grade, lymphovascular invasion, tumor-infiltrating lymphocytes, perineural invasion, microvessel density, tumor margin configuration, and poorly differentiated clusters (PDCs) [55,244–246]. One publication provided an algorithm to profile 'bad' and 'good' prognostic biomarkers in CRC that considered the clinical features, histopathology, biochemical markers, and response factors. Of those discussed in this review, typical proliferative markers and, at the same time, unfavorable prognosis factors, included cyclin D, TS, and PCNA [244,245]. Another review reported that more than 100 differentially expressed CRC molecular markers (including proliferative markers), representing more than 1000 biological pathways, have been demonstrated in CRC [55]. It should also be mentioned that MSI-H status and impaired signaling pathways resulting from common gene mutations in CRC (e.g., *WNT, TP53, KRAS, BRAF, PI3K, TGF-β*, phosphatase and tensin homolog protein (*PTEN*)) or amplifications of specific genes (e.g., *IGF-2, IGFBP2, EGFR, VEGF, SMAD*) are usually associated with the overexpression of markers and lead to increased cell proliferation and the inhibition of apoptosis [55,244,245].

Many studies from different regions around the world have also shown the importance of the tissue overexpression of Ki-67 in pCRC and/or CRLM as a poor prognostic predictor of survival for patients with this cancer. Most publications have shown that high Ki-67 expression was associated with inferior OS, but some reports have demonstrated that high Ki-67 expression was correlated with favorable/longer survival [237,247–250], also in CRLM [238]. There was also a study in which the Ki-67 LI analysis results demonstrated various proliferation extents in the central areas of the tumor (cPDCs) (high) and at the tumor periphery (pPDCs) (low) and a range of different correlations with the clinical data [246].

It should be noted that few publications have investigated the prognostic significance of Ki-67 expression in different CRC locations (colon/rectum), resulting in divided opinions. One research group reported no correlation between Ki-67 expression, tumor location, and prognosis [237]. In contrast, Hilska et al. demonstrated a better prognosis for Ki-67 LI values $\geq 5\%$ compared to a lower index, only in the group of patients with rectal cancer [182].

Several authors have indicated Ki-67 as an independent prognostic factor. For some, an increase in Ki-67 is a poor prognostic factor for survival [96,223,228], while others have reported a longer survival in patients with high Ki-67 levels [237,250]. An analysis by Valera et al. showed that tumor Ki-67 PI was an independent prognostic variable, consistently used by the classification and regression tree (CART) algorithm to classify patients with similar clinical features and survival [243]. Studies on Ki-67 expression in CRLM indicate the overexpression of this protein as an independent factor of poor OS prognosis [238,251,252].

The meta-analysis by Luo et al., focused on Ki-67 validation using IHC expression, covering 34 studies based on 6180 primary CRC patients, confirmed that the high expression of Ki-67 is a poor predictor for OS (HR 1.54, 95% CI 1.17–2.02) and DFS (HR 1.43, 95% CI 1.12–1.83) based on an univariate analysis. In multivariate analysis after adjusting for other prognostic factors, an association was shown only for OS (HR 1.50, 95% CI 1.02–2.22) [175]. Another meta-analysis investigated the determination of prognostic biomarkers in CRLM. Ki-67 was included among the 26 independent OS biomarkers in resected CRLM [253].

More than a dozen research publications on Ki-67 as a prognostic factor in CRC have also investigated the prognostic significance of potential apoptosis proteins (e.g., p53, bcl-2, programmed death ligand 1 (PD-L1), survivin) [125,134,142,147,182,197,218,224,228,232, 235,237,238,241,254,255] (Table 3).

There is also a summary of studies on the segmental distribution of some commonly used molecular markers (including proliferative and apoptotic markers) in CRC, which could also potentially affect their prognostic or predictive value [256]. One such marker is Ki-67, a component of the 12-gene Oncotype DX® Colon Cancer Assay, with potential significance for predicting the risk of disease recurrence, DFS, and OS in stages II and III CRC [257]. However, more recent studies indicate that routine use of the Oncotype DX Colon Recurrence Score in stage IIa CC may be unnecessary, especially in patients with normal levels of additional biomarkers [258].

Table 3. Immunohistochemical (IHC) studies on the prognostic relevance of Ki-67 in colorectal cancer (CRC) and CRC with liver metastases (CRLM) (S No. 9, 13, 26, 29, 32).

S No.	Material (No. of Cases) and Methods	Findings	Prognostic Role for Survival	Year of Publication/Country	Ref. No.
1.	pAC (139); IHC, mAb Ki-67, LI; S	↑In mucinous vs. non-mucinous CRC; inverse correlation with grading in non-mucinous AC	No	1990; Italy	[231]
2.	pCRC (125); IHC, LI; S	No correlations with clinicopathological data	No	1994; UK	[124]
3.	CRC (106); IHC, MIB-1, 3 methods of estimation; S	No correlation with clinical outcome	No	1996; Austria	[233]
4.	CRC (70); stages II and III; IHC, MIB-1, LI; S	Relation to disease recurrence, retained in stage II; LI > 45% associated with ↑risk for disease recurrence vs. LI ≤ 45% (MA)	Yes	1997; USA	[125]
5.	CRC (255); Dukes' A–D; IHC, MIB-1, weak (<50%), strong (>50%); S	Level > 50% (62%); <50% (38%); no correlations with clinicopathological variables	No	1997; Sweden	[234]
6.	CRC (56); Dukes' B; survival analysis (47); IHC, anti-Ki-67, morphometry; S	Mean value in luminal border (27.4%), invasive margin (36.8%); ↓LI at the invasive margin correlated with poorer survival (RR 12.1, 95% CI 1.1–1.33) (UA and MA)	Yes	1999; Sweden	[247]
7.	CRC (52); AD (56); IHC, MIB-1, LI; S	↓LI in AD (30.05%) vs. CRC (38.12%); ↑correlated with poor differentiation and Duke's stage	Nd	2000; USA	[218]
8.	CRC (30); IHC, LI; S	No correlation with tumor stage and grade	Nd	2001; France	[127]
9.	CRLM (41); IHC, MIB-1; LI at the hot spot; S	Mean value (38%); LI ≥50% related to shorter survival vs. low scores; ↑score an independent adverse prognostic factor (RR 3.04) (MA)	Yes	2001; Germany	[251]
10.	CRC (25); pTNM; stages I–IV; IHC, MIB-1, LI, morphometry; RT-PCR; S	Median protein LI (61%), median mRNA LI (0.88 amol); better OS for the group with ↓LI and ↓mRNA level vs. median	Yes	2001; Germany	[259]
11.	CRC (100); MSI-H (31), MSI-L (29), MSS (40); IHC, PI; S	↑PI (90.1%) in MSI-H vs. MSI-L (69.5%) and vs. MSS (69.5%); ↑PI showed a trend toward predicting ↑survival only within MSI-H cancers	Probably yes	2001; Australia	[260]
12.	CC (465); Dukes' B2 and C; S alone (151) or S + FU-based CTx (314); IHC, LI	No significant association with clinical outcome	No	2002; USA	[142]
13.	pCRC (74); CRLM (37); IHC, MIB-1, LI; S	LI ≥ 30% more frequently in lymphatic and venous invasion, LN meta, and CRLM; ↑in primary tumors vs. CRLM (24.3 ± 17.9 vs. 5.0 ± 4.2); LI ≥ 30% in pCRC correlated with ↑frequency of metachronous CRLM	Nd	2002; Japan	[221]
14.	CC (706); stages II and III; S alone (275) or S + FU-leucovorin CTx (431); IHC, LI	Tumors with ↑number of (+) cells had improved outcomes vs. tumors with few (+) cells; association with RFS (RR 0.76) and with OS (RR 0.62)	Yes	2003; USA	[147]
15.	CRC (47); IHC, MIB-1, LI; ISH for mRNA with DIG-labelled cRNA probe, LI; S	Median protein LI (59%), mean mRNA LI (42%); ↑protein but ↓mRNA are likely to proliferate more slowly, which possibly explains the pts' improved outcome	No	2003; Germany	[236]
16.	CRC (81); IHC, anti-Ki-67, IRS; S	↑Expression in the low differentiated tumors; inverse correlation to survival	Yes	2003; PL	[222]

Table 3. Cont.

S No.	Material (No. of Cases) and Methods	Findings	Prognostic Role for Survival	Year of Publication/Country	Ref. No.
17.	pCRC (311 including 82 with distant meta); AD and CA in situ (22); IHC, MIB-1; S	↑Rate in AD with severe atypia and CA in situ; ↓rate in poorly differentiated and mucinous AC vs. well- and moderately differentiated tumors	Nd	2003; Japan	[219]
18.	CC (144), RC (90); IHC; MIB-1, semiq estimation; S	↑In LN meta of short-term (505 d) vs. long-term survivors (4150.5 d)	No, but an indicator of survival in Dukes' C	2004; Japan	[240]
19.	RC and rectosigmoid AC (146); IHC, MIB-1, high (>40%) and low (≤40%), hot spot areas (>50%); S	Better OS for ↑values vs. those with ↓values; the presence of hot spot areas associated with better survival (MA); hot spot areas one of the prognostic factor	Yes	2005; Finland	[248]
20.	CRC (106); IHC, MIB-1, PI; S	Mean PI (38.0%); (+) correlation with advanced T status, LN and distant meta, and ↑pTNM stage; an independent prognostic factor for long-term survival; pts with high PI were at greater risk for death (HR 2.1, 95% CI 1.1–4.1) (MA)	Yes	2005; Japan	[223]
21.	CC (53), RC (33); stages I–IV; IHC, MIB-1, group A (<40%) and B (≥40%); S	Mean LI (0.44 ± 0.16); no correlation with sex, age, and clinical stage; ↑level correlated with ↓survival; an independent predictor of survival (MA)	Yes	2005; Brazil	[96]
22.	CRC (pCC + pRC) (363), Dukes' A–D; IHC, LI; S	In RC, pts with a LI ≥ 5% had a better prognosis than those with a lower index	Yes	2005; Finland	[182]
23.	CRC (40); IHC, NCL-Ki67p, PI; S	Mean PI (52.39%); pts who developed either local recurrence or meta had a significantly raised PI; PI ≤ 52.7% with a trend to improved survival	No for OS (MA)	2006; UK	[261]
24.	CRC (38): mucinous (14), non-mucinous (24); stage B1, B2, C1, C; IHC, anti-Ki-67, hot spot, NIH's Image I; S	Median (35%); (+) correlation with age, LN meta, and with Dukes' MAC staging (25% in B1, 60% in C2); ↑with grade	Nd	2007; Romania	[224]
25.	CRC (47): mucinous (5), non-mucinous (42); pT3, G2; IHC, MIB-1, negative <50%; positive >50%; S	(+) Correlation with LN meta	Nd	2009; PL	[197]
26.	CC (40), rectosigmoid or rectal AC (33); CRLM (27); IHC, MIB-1; qRT-PCR; S	pCRC (81.8%) vs. CRLM (36.2%); ↓of the GPS in CRLM and confirmed their ↓proliferative levels by qRT PCR	Nd	2009; New Zealand	[115]
27.	CRC (152), stages I–IV; IHC, rabbit anti-Ki-67, semiq estimation; S	(+) Correlation with the UICC stage and differentiation; (+) pts had the ↓cumulative survival vs. pts with no expression (MA)	Yes	2010; China	[225]
28.	CRC (356); IHC; S	No association with clinicopathological variables	Nd	2010; Korea	[235]
29.	CRLM (188/124 for Ki-67); IHC; S	↑Expression (62%); ↑expression as an independent predictor of poor survival after colon resection (HR 2.6, 95% CI 1.4–4.8)	Yes	2010; USA	[252]
30.	CRC (201); stages I–IV; IHC, anti-Ki-67, semiq estimation, (+) (score ≥ 5); S	(+) Expression (59.7%); (+) correlation with tumor size, grade, invasive depth, LN meta, distant meta, TNM; independent prognostic factor of favorable OS (HR 0.34, 95% CI 0.16–0.72) (MA)	Yes	2011; China	[249]
31.	CRC (31), men with Dukes' B AC; IHC, MIB-1, semiq estimation; S	Median (46.9 ± 19.2%); inverse relationship with OS (r = −0.67)	Yes	2012; Italy	[241]
32.	TMA with CRLM (98); IHC, MIB-1; cut-off value for (+) phenotypes (>50%); S	More (+) pts among the long-term survivors; pts with ↑ expression lived longer (HR 0.82, 95% CI 0.68–0.98) (MA); positive predictor for AS, but not for DFS	Yes	2014; Slovenia	[238]

Table 3. Cont.

S No.	Material (No. of Cases) and Methods	Findings	Prognostic Role for Survival	Year of Publication/Country	Ref. No.
33.	RC (111); IHC, MIB-1, LI; SCRT + S	↑Expression correlated with pTR; in females (+) correlation with pTNM in a long break after SCRT	Nd	2014; PL	[88]
34.	TMA CRC (672), including CRC with LN meta (210); IHC, anti-Ki67, LI; S	Median in pCRC (68.2%), in LN meta (55%); ↑in pCRC vs. CRC LN meta; (+) correlation with tumor penetration and differentiation	No	2015; Portugal	[226]
35.	CRC (110) including Dukes' C; IHC, MIB-1, LI; semiq estimation; S	↑Expression in LN meta vs. pCRC	No	2015; Turkey	[232]
36.	CRC (74) including mucinous AC (5); IHC, LI; S	LI of well (14%), moderate (31%), and poorly differentiated AC (43%); (+) correlation with stage and grade	Nd	2015; India	[227]
37.	CRC (2233), I–IV stage; IHC, MIB-1, low (<50%), high (≥50%); S	Pts in stage III with ↑level had ↑3-yr DFS and OS vs. ↓level pts; improved 3-yr PFS for stage IV pts in the ↑vs. ↓level group	Yes	2016; Germany/pts of Chinese origin	[250]
38.	TMA CRC (1800); IHC, anti-Ki-67, low (0–10%), moderate (>10–25%), high (>25%); S	↑Expression associated with low stage and LN status; an independent prognostic factor of favorable survival	Yes	2016; Germany	[237]
39.	TMA CRC (254), stage II and III; IHC, anti Ki-67, low (<20%) and high (≥20%); S	↑LI associated with ↑TNM stage; ↓LI related to RFS (UA); ↑LI (HR 2.62, 95% CI 1.12–6.14; an independent predictor of unfavorable prognosis (MA)	Yes	2018; China	[228]
40.	RC (46), stage II and III; IHC, MIB-1, Image System (Nikon), LI, cut-off value (30%); CRT + S	No difference between ↓ and ↑expression groups in clinicopathological factors; ↑LI correlated with lower 5-yr DFS vs. group with ↓LI (53% and 88%), as was the 5-yr OS (68% and 100%)	Yes	2018; Japan	[254]
41.	CRC (1090), stage 0-IV; IHC; anti-Ki-67, semiq estimation; cut-off value of 25%; S	(+) Correlation with invasive depth, differentiation, and size, AJCC-8, (+) no. of LN and CTx status; ↑level related to poor prognosis and independently predicts prognosis in the AJCC-8; no differences for DFS and OS in stage IV	Yes	2020; China	[229]
42.	CRC (38), non-neoplastic polyps (2) and AD (20); IHC, anti-Ki-67, LI; S	CRC: ↑LI in higher grade and stage; AD: ↑intensity and high score similar to CRC; non-neoplastic polyps: ↑LI and medium intensity; ↑LI from non-neoplastic to neoplastic cases	Nd	2021; India	[217]
43.	CRC (210), stages I–III; IHC, polyclonal Ab, LI, cut-off value 60%; S	LI ≥60% indicated a high-risk ratio for both distant meta (HR 2.56, 95% CI 1.08–6.06) and death (HR 2.64, 95% CI 1.07–6.54)	Yes	2022; China	[230]
44.	RC (154), RC I–II after RT + S (2–3 d after) (64), RC I–III after S (90); IHC, image analysis application package	↑Level with a survival rate of less than 3 yrs in both pts after RT and S	Yes	2022; Switzerland, Germany, UK	[255]

Legend: ↑/↓—increase (overexpression)/decrease; >/<—higher/lower; (+)—positive; AC—adenocarcinoma; AD(s)—adenoma(s); AJCC—American Joint Committee on Cancer 8th edition; AS—actual survival; C—control; CA—carcinoma; CC—colon cancer; CI—confidence interval; CRT—chemoradiotherapy; CTx—chemotherapy; d—days; DFS—disease-free survival; DIG—digoxygenin; FU—fluorouracil; GPS—multi-gene proliferation signature; HR—hazard ratio; ISH—in situ hybridization; IRS—immunoreactive score; Lbs—laboratories; L(P)I—labeling (proliferation) index; LN—lymph node metastasis; MA—multivariate analysis; mAb—monoclonal antibody; meta—metastasis; MIB-1—antibody against Ki-67 antigen; MSI-H/L—microsatellite instability high/low; MSS—microsatellite stable; nd—not determined; no.—number; OS—overall survival; (p)CRC—(primary) colorectal cancer; PFS—progression-free survival; PL—Poland; pTNM—pathological tumor/node/metastasis; pTR—pathological tumor response; pts—patients; RC—rectal cancer; RFS—relapse-free survival; RR—relative risk; RT—radiotherapy; qRT-PCR—quantitative real-time polymerase chain reaction; RT-PCR—reverse transcriptase-polymerase chain reaction; S—surgery; semiq—semiquantitative; UA—univariate analysis; UICC—International Union Against Cancer; UK—United Kingdom; yr(s)—year(s).

Table 3 shows the potential correlations between Ki-67 expression, clinicopathological data, and survival as prognostic factors in CRC. Moreover, it illustrates the broad geographical coverage of the studies conducted, which include several countries in America, Europe, and Asia. The studies mainly used mAbs (MIB-1) rather than polyclonal antibodies, allowing for better result comparability. However, the publications varied in the semi-quantitative methods used to estimate the results, which may be one reason for the differences between the investigators. Most articles, revealing significant correlations between Ki-67 expression and clinicopathological data, also provided answers regarding the prognosis and survival of patients (OS, DFS).

Traditionally, pathologists examine the expression of IHC markers visually and calculate it semi-quantitatively by considering the intensity and distribution of specific staining. Visual assessment is fraught with problems due to the subjectivity of interpretation. There is a lack of standardized systems for evaluating performance, relying on different cut-off values and inconsistent criteria to define the threshold value of marker/antigen positive expression by IHC. A lower reproducibility of results may also be affected by differences in the preparation conditions, antibodies used, their dilutions, and IHC reaction detection systems [135,136,198,210]. Automated IHC measurements promise to overcome these limitations. Nowadays, spatial visualization methods of digital images are used to quantify IHC data [262].

4.4. Modern Molecular Biology Techniques for the Assessment of Proliferative Markers in CRC

With the rapid development of complex molecular biology techniques (e.g., qRT-PCR, in situ hybridization (ISH), RNA/DNA sequencing, NGS, and DNA methylation detection methods), there is a constant search for new biomarkers of cellular proliferation with potential diagnostic, prognostic, and/or predictive significance in cancers including CRC [115,236,259,263–278].

Quantitative RT-PCR is generally used as the 'gold standard' method to measure RNA expression [115,259,267,276,277]. In situ hybridization is a research tool to detect protein production and provides invaluable information regarding the localization of gene expression in heterogeneous tissues. For example, it was used to detect Ki-67 mRNA in CRC tissues with the digoxigenin-labelled cRNA probe [236].

RNA sequencing is used to study the expression of non-coding RNAs (ncRNAs) [275,276], often complementary to methods for assessing protein expression (e.g., IHC, BrdU staining, Western blotting, qRT-PCR, and ISH). Among the sequencing techniques, NGS is currently the only method that enables the parallel sequencing of thousands of short DNA sequences in a single assay, replacing many less advanced profiling technologies. NGS is used to analyze the genome (whole and partial genome), methylome, transcriptome, or available chromatin using techniques including DNA-Seq, RNA-Seq, or chromatin profiling with methods such as ChIP-Seq. This technology offers a better approach for detecting multiple genetic changes with a minimal amount of DNA. What is particularly important is that it is also possible to sequence RNA transcripts from single cells (scRNA-Seq) [46].

Detection methods for DNA methylation in CRC include methylation-specific polymerase chain reaction (MSR), DNA sequencing (e.g., bisulfide sequencing, pyrosequencing), methylation-specific high resolution melting curve analysis (MS-HRM), and MethyLight assay (reviewed in [278]).

4.4.1. PCNA mRNA Expression

PCNA expression was also studied at the RNA level. Yue et al., using RT-PCR, showed higher PCNA mRNA expression (94.1%) in patients with CRC and venous invasion and LM than in CRC without metastasis (70.6%), confirming the increased production of this marker with CRC progression [263]. However, PCNA was not indicated as a prognostic marker but only as a useful marker for evaluating the LM of cancer cells. In contrast, Cui et al., using qRT-PCR, demonstrated increased PCNA antisense RNA1 (PCNA-AS1) expression in CRC relative to the controls, and detected correlations of this biomarker with the clinical data (tumor invasion and TNM stage). A higher expression of PCNA-AS1 was also confirmed by in vitro studies. These data suggest a role for PCNA-AS1 mainly as a diagnostic rather than a prognostic marker in CRC [264].

4.4.2. Ki-67 mRNA Expression

Possible correlations between the Ki-67 mRNA and clinicopathological data were also analyzed, investigating its prognostic significance in CRC [115,236,259]. A positive correlation was described between protein LI, Ki-67 mRNA, and TNM. The mRNA level was also prognostically important as it correlated with patient survival, similarly to the pKi-67 index [259]. The correlation between pKi-67 LI (median: 59%) and the mRNA level detected using ISH (median: 42%) was slightly more difficult to obtain as a positive correlation was observed in 32/47 resected tumors, with a significant difference detected in 15 cases. In the latter tumors, more than 30% of the cells were pKi-67-positive but did not exhibit the presence of its mRNA. The authors explain this by the likelihood of cell cycle arrest. Interestingly, the latter patients were characterized by a better prognosis. In other words, tumors with high pKi-67 and low mRNA are likely to proliferate more slowly and, hence, be attributed to a better prognosis [236]. On the other hand, comparative studies between pCRC and CRLMs, using qRT-PCR and IHC, showed significantly lower multi-gene proliferation signature (GPS) expression in CRLM and confirmed their lower proliferation rate. Interestingly, proliferative activity was significantly lower for primary cancers with recurrence or those with established metastases than for CRCs that did not metastasize and had no recurrences [115]. Such studies need to be continued, as they may shed new light on tumor proliferation.

4.4.3. Non-Coding RNAs (ncRNAs) Expression

Particular value is attributed to fragments of the human genome that do not encode proteins but play a specific role in many of the biological processes involved in colon carcinogenesis including cell cycle regulation. These are the so-called non-coding RNAs (ncRNAs), among which there are two main classes: small non-coding RNAs with less than 200 nucleotides (nc) (e.g., microRNAs, small interfering RNAs, Piwi-interacting RNAs, small nuclear RNAs, and small circular RNAs) and long non-coding RNAs (lncRNAs) (greater than 200 nc in length [270,273,274].

Studies have consistently demonstrated that the majority of both miRNAs and lncR-NAs are dysregulated in CRC. The role of hundreds of different ncRNAs has been demonstrated in CRC cell proliferation in vivo and in vitro. Non-coding RNAs most often show increased expression in CRC compared to the controls. Depending on what function a given ncRNA has in the tumor (oncogene, tumor suppressor), its overexpression or downregulation enhances proliferative activity and tumor progression [266,268,270,279–281].

Numerous reviews have illustrated the underlying mechanisms of the biological action of miRNAs in CRC and/or reported downstream targets linked to known signaling pathways in colorectal carcinogenesis (mostly responsible for cell proliferation) [276,279,282,283]. For example, microRNAs can activate the KRAS pathway (downregulation of tumor suppressors: miR-96-5b, miR-384, mi-143, Let-7) [279,283] as well as WNT (miR-135, miR-145, miR-17-92) and EGFR signaling (miR-126, miR-143, miR-18a, Let-7, miR-196a, miR-21), and inactivate the TGF-β pathway (miR-200c) [282]. They can result in the downregulation of the TP53 pathway (overexpression of miR-34a, miR-34b, miR-34c, miR-192, miR-194-2, miR-215), epithelial–mesenchymal transition (EMT) (overexpression of miR-181a, miR-17-5p, miR-494; miR-21, miR-22) and SMAD4 (overexpression of miR-20a, miR20a-5p, miR-888). Moreover, the miR-21, miR-31, and miR-200 families are involved in EMT regulation [282,283].

In addition to miRNAs, lncRNAs are also closely involved in enhancing cellular proliferation, acting through the CRC's well-known signaling pathways, as already described in some excellent reviews [268,281,284,285]. These include (i) JAK/STAT (downregulation of cancer susceptibility candidate 2, CASC2), (ii) MAPK (overexpression of H19 imprinted maternally expressed transcript, H19 and a newly discovered lncRNA with a length of 2685 nc, i.e., LINC00858), (iii) EGFR/MAPK (overexpression of solute carrier organic anion transporter family member 4A1-antisense RNA 1, SLCO4A1-AS1), (iv) Ras/MAPK (overexpression of colorectal neoplasia differentially expressed, CRNDE), and (v) AKT (overexpression of nuclear-enriched abundant transcript 1, NEAT1). A further example would be WNT-β-catenin signaling, which is activated by the overexpression of lncRNAs including small nucleolar RNA host gene 1 (SNHG1), HOX transcript antisense RNA (HOTAIR), SLCO4A1-AS1, taurine upregulated gene 1 (TUG1), and the downregulation of growth arrest specific 5 (GAS5). In turn, the TGF-β1 pathway is affected by the downregulation of maternally expressed 3 (MEG3) and the upregulation of LINC00858, whereas TGF-β/Smad is activated by the upregulation of SNHG6. Many lncRNAs are involved in the regulation of the EMT process. These mainly include TUG1, sprouty RTK signaling antagonist 4 intronic transcript 1 (SPRY4-IT1), and promoter of CDKN1A antisense DNA damage activated RNA (PANDAR) [281,284,286,287]. The activation of proliferation through STAT3 or β-catenin-mediated signaling pathways is also mediated by the upregulation of lncRNAs such as BC200, CASC15, colon cancer-associated transcript 2 (CCAT2), focally amplified lncRNA on chromosome 1 (FAL1), SNHG1, and SnaR. The ERK (MAPK)/JNK pathway is also affected by lncRNA DMTF1V4. Moreover, lncRNA SNHG7 acts in the K-RAS/ERK (MAPK)/cyclin D1 pathway (reviewed in [268]), while the MIR22 host gene (MIR22HG) is responsible for blocking the SMAD complex, resulting in the inhibition of EMT signaling [270,288].

Some of the lncRNAs above-mentioned interact with other cell cycle markers. For example, the zinc finger NFXT-type containing 1 antisense RNA 1 (ZFAS1) affects cell proliferation through a mechanism that destabilizes p53 via the CDK1/cyclin B1 complex [289]. Another lncRNA (i.e., ENSG00000254615), inhibits CRC cell proliferation and attenuates CRC resistance to 5-FU by regulating p21 and cyclin D1 expression [290]. Cyclin D1 also belongs to one of the target proteins of lncRNAs such as SNHG1 [291], SNHG7 [292], and XIST [293]. PCNA, on the other hand, is one of the target proteins for the lncRNA FAL1 [294]. These studies suggest a complex network of functional relationships between ncRNAs and classical cell cycle proteins, which may result in their variable expression at different stages of CRC development. In turn, any epigenetic modifications and interactions of lncRNAs with both miRNAs and proteins as well as the action of lncRNAs as precursors or pseudogenes of miRNAs may regulate the expression of multiple genes [272].

The prognostic role of ncRNAs in CRC has also been increasingly demonstrated. A summary of the activity of both subtypes of ncRNAs (miRNAs and lncRNAs) as regulatory and prognostic factors in CRC is provided in other reviews [266,279,280,295].

MicroRNA (miRNAs, miRs)

There has been a rapidly increasing number of original publications and systematic reviews [276,283,296] addressing the prognostic role of miRNAs in CRC. A worse prognosis for survival (worse OS/DFS) is related to both miRNAs that are downregulated and overexpressed in CRC [276,283]. Representative miRNAs detected in tissues and body fluids are often compared in the literature [276]. An analysis of 115 articles identified hundreds of miRNAs with oncogene properties including miR-21, miR-181a, miR-182, miR-183, mi-R210, and miR-224. Overexpression of these miRNAs was associated with CRC progression and shorter patient survival. The most frequently described tumor suppressors among miRNAs included miR-126, miR-199b, and miR-22. Decreased expression of the latter was also associated with poor prognosis and a higher risk of relapse (worse DFS) [283]. A detailed review addresses the mechanisms of methylation of miRNAs as a cause of their silencing and the prognostic value of such altered miRNAs in CRC [296].

In addition, dozens of meta-analyses are available on the prognostic role of single miRNA types (e.g., miR-21 [297], miR-181a/b [298], miR-20a [299], miR-155 [300]) or the entire group of miRNAs tested (e.g., miR-21, miR-215, miR-143-5p, miR-106a, and miR-145) in specific stages of CRC development [301]. Gao et al., in their meta-analysis, showed that the strongest markers of poor prognosis included high levels of miR-141 in blood (HR 2.52, 95% CI 1.68–3.77) and miR-224 in tissue (HR 2.12, 95% CI 1.04–4.34) [302].

Long Non-Coding RNAs (LncRNAs)

Modern molecular techniques and the TCGA dataset allow for the identification of an increasing number of different lncRNA subtypes as new prognostic and predictive factors in CRC [267,272]. Representative lncRNAs detected in CRC tissues and plasma/serum (circulating lncRNAs) have already been compared in the literature [303]. A prognostic role was shown for lncRNAs with tumor suppressor and oncogene properties. For example, the reduced expression of tumor suppressors such as LOC285194 [304] or MIR22HG [288] is associated with poor prognosis. Upregulation of lncRNA-oncogenes in CRC has also been associated with poor prognosis through various mechanisms. These include, among others, plasmacytoma variant translocation 1 (PVT1) [275,305], differentiation antagonizing non-protein coding RNA (DANCR) [306], HOXA distal transcript antisense RNA (HOT-TIP) [307], BRAF-activated non-protein coding RNA (BANCR) [308], SPRY4-IT1 [309], CCAT1/CCAT2 [310], and X inactive specific transcript (XIST) [311].

Although many ncRNAs have been reported as proliferative markers, only a few meta-analyses have provided evidence for the actual role of selected lncRNAs in CRC prognosis [265,312–316]. These include, among others, overexpressed oncogene urothelial cancer-associated 1 (UCA1) for OS (HR 2.25, 95% CI 1.77–2.87) [312], or SNHG6 for OS (HR 1.92, 95% CI 1.48–2.49), and DFS (HR 1.84, 95% CI 1.02–3.34) [313]. As shown in a recent meta-analysis based on 25 publications and more than 2000 patients, the overexpression of various SNHGs (especially SNHG1) is a poor prognostic factor in CRC (HR 1.64, 95% CI 1.40–1.86). The authors also presented all the signaling pathways interacting with this type of lncRNA. Many lncRNAs enhance cancer cell proliferation, acting directly or through different miRNAs [316]. For example, SNHG20 exerts this effect by directly affecting cyclin A1, and its expression is a poor prognostic factor in CRC (HR 2.97, 95% CI 1.51–5.82) [317]. Zhuang et al., in their meta-analysis, showed that the overexpression of lncRNA HNF1A antisense RNA 1 (HNF1A-AS1) could also be a recognized factor for poor prognosis (HR 3.10, 95% CI 1.58–6.11) [318]. A meta-analysis of numerous solid tumors (including CRC) revealed that increased expression of five prime to Xist (FTX) [314] and KCNQ1 opposite strand/antisense transcript 1 (KCNQ1OT1) correlated with shorter OS in CRC [315]. A previous study on metastasis-associated lung adenocarcinoma transcript 1 (MALAT-1/NEAT1) in six different tumors (including CRC) showed that the high expression of MALAT-1 correlated with lymph node and distant metastases (OR 3.52, 95% CI 1.06–11.71) [265]. In contrast, Xie et al. demonstrated a prognostic role for high levels of CRNDE in various cancer types including CRC (poor OS) (HR 2.11, 95% CI 1.63–2.75) [319].

Table 4 summarizes the examples of lncRNAs as prognostic markers in CRC, published in recent years.

Table 4. Prognostic value of selected long non-coding RNAs (lncRNAs) in colorectal cancer (CRC).

Type of lncRNA	Material/Research Model	Expression Level	Findings	Ref. No.
LOC285194	CRC (81); CRC cell lines: CaCO-2, HCT8, LoVo and C (CCC-HIE-2 cells); qRT-PCR	↓	A poor DFS; an independent predictor of DFS (MA)	[303]
PVT1	Pairs of CRC and C (164); CRC cell lines: RKO and HCT116; siRNA transfection; cell proliferation and invasion assays; gene expression array; qRT-PCR; array-CGH and copy no. analysis; gene set enrichment analysis; WB	↑	Promoted cell proliferation; a poor prognosis; an independent risk factor for OS (UA and MA)	[275]
	Pairs of CRC and C (210); qRT-PCR	↑	A shorter DFS and OS; an independent predictor of poor prognosis (MA)	[304]

Table 4. Cont.

Type of lncRNA	Material/Research Model	Expression Level	Findings	Ref. No.
DANCR	CRC (104); qRT-PCR	↑	A shorter OS and DFS; an independent poor prognostic factor for both OS and DFS (MA)	[305]
HOTTIP	CRC (156), C (21); qRT-PCR	↑	An unfavorable as well as an independent poor prognostic factor (MA)	[306]
SNHG20	CRC and C (107)	↑	An independent poor prognostic factor for OS (MA)	[316]
BANCR	CRC (106), C (65); qRT-PCR	↑	A shorter OS; an independent poor prognostic factor (HR 2.24, 95% CI 1.22–4.16)	[307]
SPRY4-IT1	CRC (106); qRT-PCR	↑	A poor OS; an independent prognostic factor (HR 2.34, 95% CI 1.14–4.82)	[308]
CCAT1 and CCAT2	CRC (280) and C (20); qRT-PCR	↑	A poor RFS and OS	[309]
XIST	CRC (196); CRC cell lines: LOVO, HT-29, HCT8, HCT116, SW480, and DLD1 and C (HCoEpics cells); qRT-PCR	↑	Could predict PFS and OS; could act as independent risk factor for poor prognosis	[310]
LINC00858	Pairs of CRC (115); CRC cell lines: T-29, HT-15, SW837 and SW1463; qRT-PCR; siRNA transfection; cell proliferation and apoptosis assays; colony formation assay; dual luciferase reporter assays; RIP; WB	↑	An independent poor prognostic factor	[284]
	Pairs of CRC (50) and 20 female BALB/c nude mouse; qRT-PCR; ISH; MTT assay; BrdU staining; FCM, wound healing, and Transwell assays; luciferase activity assay and RIP; IHC; WB; HE staining	↑	Prognostic factor for OS	[277]
MIR22HG	CRC (79) and C (84); CRC cell lines LoVo and HCT116; bioinformatics screen; qRT-PCR; MTT and Transwell assays; mouse model	↓	A poor OS and DFS; promoted cell survival, proliferation and tumor meta in vitro and in vivo	[287]

Legend: ↑,↓—high (upregulation), low (downregulation); BANCR-BRAF—activated nc RNA; BrdU—bromodeoxyuridine/5-bromo-2′-deoxyuridine; C—control; CCAT1/2—colon cancer-associated transcript 1/2; CGH array—comparative genomic hybridization array; CI—confidence interval; CRC–colorectal cancer; DANCR—anti-differentiation ncRNA; DFS—disease free survival; FCM—flow cytometry; HR—hazard ratio; HNF1A-AS1—HNF1A antisense RNA 1; HE—hematoxylin and eosin; HOTTIP—HOXA transcript at the distal tip; IHC—immunohistochemistry; ISH—in situ hybridization; MA—multivariate analysis; meta—metastasis; MIR22HG—MIR22 host gene; no.—number; OS—overall survival; PFS—poor progression-free survival; PVT1—plasmacytoma variant translocation 1; SNHG20—small nucleolar RNA host gene 20; SPRY4-IT1—sprouty RTK signaling antagonist 4-intronic transcript 1; RIP—RNA immunoprecipitation; qRT-PCR—quantitative real-time polymerase chain reaction; UA—univariate analysis; WB—Western blot analysis; XIST—X-inactive specific transcript.

In a previous review focused on the expression of some ncRNAs (miRNAs and lncRNAs), attention was drawn to the low reproducibility of the results and the poor power of statistical analyses for the reliability of the study. This may be due to both the small amount of material assessed or the over-sampling of ncRNAs, resulting in false positive or negative results [280]. The limitations of ncRNA detection in archival tissue material include high tumor heterogeneity, leading to an increasing preference to detect these molecules in serum/plasma or stool for prognostic purposes [276,303].

It should be noted that protein-coding mRNAs have a short half-life, and their expression changes enormously depending on the physiological/pathological state. Therefore, they are not ideal as prognostic indicators. The correlation between mRNA expression and protein translation is not always guaranteed, especially in heterogeneous tumors (including CRC), prompting the need for more sophisticated molecular techniques to assess the actual expression of biomarkers. In addition, studying complex interactions between different RNA types requires modern technology (e.g., high-throughput CLIP-Seq, degradome-Seq, and RNA–RNA interactome sequencing methods) [46,320].

4.4.4. Prognostic Genetic and Epigenetic Biomarkers

The most relevant genetic and epigenetic alterations have been described as 'potential prognostic markers' [244] or 'potential emerging biomarkers' of clinical utility [321–323]. Initially, numerous panels of genes have been identified for metastatic CRC patients. For example, among the common core of five genes including *BRAF*, *EGFR*, *KRAS*, *NRAS*, and phosphatidylinositol-4,5-biphosphate 3 kinase catalytic subunit alpha (*PIK3CA*), two of them, *EGFR* and *PIK3CA*, have been named as 'emerging biomarkers' [321].

In an era of revolutionary advances in molecular biology techniques and bioinformatical methods, different strategies are being adopted to classify biomarkers in CRC. Considering the mechanisms of carcinogenesis, *KRAS*, *BRAF*, *APC*, and *TP53* genes have a permanent place among genomic biomarkers, whose role can be retrospectively traced to the Vogelstein model [7,45,245,324]. Mutations in protooncogenes (including *KRAS*) confer a strong growth signal to cancer cells and are closely associated with the development of CRC [5,55]. Notably, the *KRAS* mutation is currently the only marker with proven benefit for routine clinical use and selection for anti-EGFR mAbs therapy [324]. However, the presence of *KRAS* mutations does not always correlate with cell proliferation or the survival of patients with CRLMs [251]. In contrast, a meta-analysis by Sorich et al. showed that patients with metastatic CRC without *RAS* mutations (either *KRAS* exon 2 or new *RAS* mutation) treated with anti-EGFR mAbs had longer PFS and OS compared to patients with the presence of these mutations [325]. A recent study performed in a group of 73 CRC patients from South Korea reported no differences in DSF and OS treated with the FOLFOX regimen in groups divided according to the presence of *KRAS* mutations and the expression status of the excision repair cross-complementing 1 (ERCC1) protein. Interestingly, it was shown that the subgroup of patients with wild-type *KRAS* and increased IHC expression of the ERCC1 protein had lower OS compared to the subgroup with decreased ERCC1. No significant difference was found in the group of patients with mutated *KRAS*. In addition, the authors suggest that the presence of wild-type *KRAS* in combination with ERCC1 overexpression may be associated with oxaliplatin resistance. In other words, the *KRAS* status and ERCC1 expression in CRC patients treated with oxaliplatin-based CTx exhibit significant prognostic value [326].

An association has also been found between the loss of *TP53* (17q-*TP53*) and poorer survival rates, but *TP53* is not considered as a useful prognostic marker as the current data are insufficient to validate it [44]. Similarly, mutations in *TGF-β*, rare in CRC, cannot be indicated as significant prognostic factors in this cancer [5]. One meta-analysis showed a weak correlation between short OS and loss of 18q (HR 2.0, 95% CI 1.49–2.69), which encodes two crucial tumor suppressor genes (*SMAD2* and *SMAD4*) of the TGF-β family. Loss of function of these two genes leads, among others, to cell cycle deregulation [327]. In turn, the prognostic value of chromosomal instability in the form of CIN and MSI has been confirmed (also in meta-analyses) [245,327,328]. Erstad et al. listed genes including matrix metalloproteinases (*MMPs*), tumor inhibitor of metalloproteinase-1 (*TIMP-1*), manganese superoxide dismutase (*mnSOD*), *TGF-β*, *Survivin*, and prolactin receptor (*PRLR*) among the prognostic factors of survival. From the classical proliferative markers, they mention the genes for TS and PCNA. The publication also provides an algorithm for the determination of prognostic biomarker profiles in CRC [244]. The following have also been cited as prognostic or predictive markers related to disease recurrence after surgery or resistance to treatment: 'SC signature' circulating tumor (ct)DNA and cell-free (cf)DNA, *RAS*, *PIK3CA* mutations, loss of *PTEN* (shorter PFS), low expression of *EGFR* (increase tumor regression), high density of TILs (better survival), loss of Bcl-2 expression (tumor recurrence), and somatic mutation of *BRAF* (mainly V600E) [323].

Epigenetic alterations in CRC mainly comprise abnormal methylated DNAs, abnormal histone modifications, and changes in the expression levels of abundant ncRNAs [329–331]. The prognostic significance of ncRNAs is described in Section 4.4.3. While the studied epigenetic aberrations in CRC include CIMP [50,323,332], opinions on the prognostic value of this marker differ and are debated by others [323,324].

Several DNA-methylation markers with prognostic value in CRC have also been demonstrated. These include the methylation of genes such as secreted frizzled-related protein (*SFRP*), *p16*, and long interspersed nucleotide element-1 (*LINE-1*). Methylation of *SFRP*, which acts as a tumor suppressor gene, is associated with increased CRC cell proliferation and tumor growth [333]. In turn, the methylation of *LINE-1* is associated with poor prognosis, shorter survival, and advanced stage [334,335]. A meta-analysis on *LINE-1* also suggests that its methylation is significantly related to the survival of CRC patients and may be a prognostic factor [336]. Another gene that undergoes DNA methylation in CRC is the DNA-binding protein Ikaros (*IKZF1*), which regulates the cell cycle. Methylation of the *IKZF1* promoter is associated with the loss of regulation of tumor cell proliferation and differentiation [337].

Recent studies also indicate high sensitivity and specificity in the detection of circulating DNA methylated in branched-chain aminotransferase 1 (*BCAT1*)/*IKZF1* in CRC compared to other cancers (breast, prostate) [338]. Other reviews additionally included methylated biomarkers of prognostic importance such as *p14*, Ras association domain-containing protein 1A (*RASSF1A*) and *APC* (poor prognosis), O-6-methylguanine-DNA methyltransferase (*MGMT*), DNA mismatch repair protein (*hMLH1*) (improved survival), homeodomain-only protein (HOPX-β) (worse prognosis in stage III CRC) and several EMC genes (worse survival), and IGF-2 hypomethylation (poor prognosis, short survival) [245,329]. Moreover, a recent study combined classical histopathology, the IHC method (p53 and Ki-67 expression), and MSP (aberrant methylation of *p16*, E-cadherin, *APC*, RUNX family transcription factor 3 (*RUNX3*), and *hMLH1*) with autofluorescence imaging (AFI) to assess the proliferative capacity of CRC. Abnormal expression of p53 and Ki-67 and the altered methylation of *p16* correlated with a lower AFI intensity [339].

It is important to note that the DNA methylation of genes in CRC also plays a role as predictive markers and/or can be a basis for the development of novel methylation-based therapies. Recent publications point to the important role of selected DNA methylation markers for the screening and early diagnosis of CRC [323,331,340]. One such plasma PCR-based test is the Epi proColon®, which is used to detect methylated *SEPT9* and has been approved by the U.S. Food and Drug Administration (FDA) for CRC screening in the U.S. The test, which is performed in conjunction with a stool test for methylated DNA from CRC cells, is used in patients who reject traditional screening methods [55].

Modern marker testing strategies in CRC potentially allow for the discovery of thousands of new genomic and transcriptomic factors. At least some of these are expected to become sensitive and specific proliferative markers with prognostic significance [55,323,324,340,341].

Considering the mechanisms of colorectal carcinogenesis associated with familial CRC, clinically useful markers such as dMMR, MSI, *KRAS*, *BRAF*, *APC*, *SMAD4*, and *BMPR1A* have already been indicated [47,323]. Markers with crucial roles in the pathogenesis of CRC also include key genes in the cell cycle process [324,328]. Moreover, a range of state-of-the-art molecular technologies used to detect a whole range of diagnostic markers in the human body (blood/plasma, tissue, stool) have also been described [340,342]. There are several recent summaries regarding the available technologies in for the search for the most sensitive, specific, low-cost, and reliable diagnostic, prognostic, and predictive markers in CRC [55,322,323,340,342].

Several publications have summarized the data on the clinical application of NGS technology in CRC [46,321,322,324,342,343]. Additionally, NGS allows for the identification of unknown interactions between genetic variation in CRCs and the relationship of CRCs to the structure of the gut microbiota composition [342].

Regarding the prognostic value in CRC, the activity of many protumoral genes (e.g., *CD74*, *CLCA1*, and *DPEP1*) has been described using this method. Additionally, using this technique revealed intra-tumor cell heterogeneity in ulcerative colitis (UC)-associated CRC [344]. Another study, based on several complementary techniques including scRNA-Seq, revealed that kinesin family member 21B (*KIF21B*) was highly expressed in CRC and was associated with poor survival. *KIF21B* expression was positively correlated with infiltrating CD4+ T cells and neutrophil levels, cell apoptosis, and metastasis. In vitro studies confirmed the role of *KIF21B* in enhancing proliferation, migration, and invasion [345]. In addition, one study based on scRNA-Seq, RNA-Seq, and microarray cohorts established a prognostic model based on the composition of prognosis-related cell subsets in TME including nine specific immune cell lineages [346].

Other publications have described the advantages and technical challenges of using liquid biopsies in the form of circulating tumor cells (CTCs) [347] and ctDNA as a promising alternative to molecular tissue analysis [323,348,349]. ctDNA detection in blood can be used to predict CRC recurrence after surgical resection [323]. In turn, a meta-analysis (2016) showed strong associations between cfDNA, RFS (HR 2.78, 95% CI 2.08–3.72), and OS (HR 3.03, 95% CI 2.51–3.66) in CRC patients. Thus, the appearance of cfDNA in the blood can predict shorter OS and worse RFS regardless of the tumor stage, study size, tumor markers, detection methods, and marker origin [349]. Nonetheless, targeted NGS analysis of cfDNA from TruSight Tumor 170 (TST170) may be useful for the non-invasive detection of gene variants in metastatic CRC patients. TST170 is an NGS panel that covers 170 cancer-related genes including *KRAS* [350]. High compatibility was also detected between cfDNA and tumor DNA in metastatic CRCs using a 10-gene NGS panel. *TP53* was the most frequently mutated gene (63.2%), followed by *APC* (49.5%), *KRAS* (35.8%), and FAT tumor suppressor homolog 4 (*FAT4*) (15.8%). The concordance of mutation patterns in these 10 genes was as high as 91% between the cfDNA and tumor samples. These results also confirmed the high sensitivity (over 88%) and specificity (100%) of the *KRAS* status in cfDNA for predicting mutations of this gene in tumor tissue. Significant prognostic correlations (peritoneal, lung metastasis) between *TP53*, *KRAS*, and *APC* mutations in the tumor were also demonstrated [351].

The use of ctDNA-based genotyping of *KRAS*, *NRAS*, and *BRAF* indicates the utility of predicting patient survival depending on the mutations of these genes. The highest mutation frequency is attributed to *KRAS* (34%). The median OS of patients with *RAS/BRAF* mutations detected in plasma was 26.6 months, and patients with wild-type *RAS/BRAF* did not reach median survival during follow-up. The median RFS for *RAS/BRAF* wild-type and *RAS/BRAF* mutation patients was 12 and 4 months, respectively [352]. Attempts have been made to determine the prognostic role of markers detected by CTC-based techniques in CRC. However, the results are still not convincing enough for recommendation in clinical practice [340,347].

A recent review paper summarized the use of various molecular techniques (e.g., RT-PCR, PCR, and single nucleotide polymorphism (SNP) genotyping assay, NGS, NanoString analysis, Sanger sequencing, MassArray sequencing, quantitative MSP) to investigate changes at the DNA and RNA level that may predict CRC metastasis to the peritoneum. Only *BRAF* mutations were associated with peritoneal metastases in 10/17 studies [353].

The development of modern, especially non-invasive molecular technologies in CRC should improve the specificity of tests (above 90%) primarily for disease screening and therapeutic decisions [55,341,354].

Nowadays, numerous molecular techniques can be chosen, and the decision to use specific markers should balance advantages and limitations that may affect the final results. In the case of NGS-based DNA nucleotide variation testing, the difficulty lies in wide variety of NGS platforms and gene panels and the multi-step nature of the study. In terms of sensitivity, ctDNA NGS techniques cannot compete with digital PCR, prompting the need for PCR result validation. The sensitivity issue is important, particularly in liquid biopsy, as random results (false positive mutations) can be obtained from hematopoietic clones rather than from the tumor itself. The significant number of gene variants of unknown roles obtained in the study is also not accepted by experts due to the lack of clinical utility [321,348]. Another author described the limitations of non-standardized methods, the small cohorts of patients analyzed, and the lack of demonstration of a clear clinical benefit of liquid biopsy studies in CRC [347]. The scientific literature also contains proposals for a systematic review and meta-analysis protocol in detecting *KRAS* mutations in CRC using liquid biopsy samples, with paired tissue samples serving as the control [355].

4.5. Positron Emission Tomography (PET) to Assess Tumor Growth Rate

PET is the most specific and sensitive method of in vivo molecular interaction and pathway imaging, finding an increasing number of applications in oncology [356]. This non-invasive technique for the functional imaging and assessment of CRC growth rate is based on the use of labelled 18-fluoro-3-deoxy-3-fluorothymidine (FLT). The method can reveal the spatial organization of proliferating cells in the tumor and allows for multiple simultaneous in vivo measurements. However, there are some correlations between FLT uptake and tumor proliferative activity [111,112]. FLT was reported to have high sensitivity in detecting extrahepatic disease but poor sensitivity in imaging CRC liver metastases [112]. A better and currently the most commonly used tracer in CRC is 18F-labelled 2-fluoro-2-deoxy-D-glucose (18F-FDG), with its usefulness resulting from increased glucose consumption by malignant cells. Therefore, this tracer's uptake is closely linked to cancer cell proliferation, which depends mainly on glycolysis for energy. Many signal transduction pathways in the malignant transformation of cancer cells are regulated by glycolytic metabolism [357]. Therefore, the combination of PET and 18F-FDG has become an established tool for diagnostic tumor imaging and complete preoperative staging in CRC [112,113,358]. PET–18F-FDG results may have implications for the therapeutic management of patients with CRC [358,359] including metastatic CRC [113]. One review recognized that PET in CRC also allows for the metabolic characterization of lesions suspected of recurrence or the identification of latent metastatic disease [358]. Comparative studies indicate lower FLT versus FDG uptake in patients with CRC. However, no correlation was shown between the two radiotracers used and the proliferative activity assessed by the Ki-67 index [360]. A later meta-analysis only confirmed a moderate correlation between 18F-FDG uptake and Ki-67 expression in CRC [361]. A recent study by Watanabe et al. indicated that tumor proliferation in CRLM is reflected by the standardized uptake value (SUV) from FDG-PET. In addition, the authors showed a high correlation between SUV and Ki-67 expression. SUV was also shown to include factors of glucose metabolism (expression of hypoxia-inducible factor 1 alpha (HIF-1α), pyruvate kinase M2 (PKM2), and glucose transporter 1 (GLUT1)). Thus, this test can be a valuable method to assess the proliferative and metabolic viability of the tumor in advanced CRLM [113].

The remaining limitations of PET comprise its high cost and the lack of necessary equipment in cancer centers, limiting the potential for multidisciplinary PET studies. The most significant limitation for the patient is the need for the administration of radioactive tracers, resulting in potential radiation exposure [356].

Figure 1 summarizes the major categories of prognostic proliferative markers in CRC and the most important signaling pathways that are genetically altered in CRC progression.

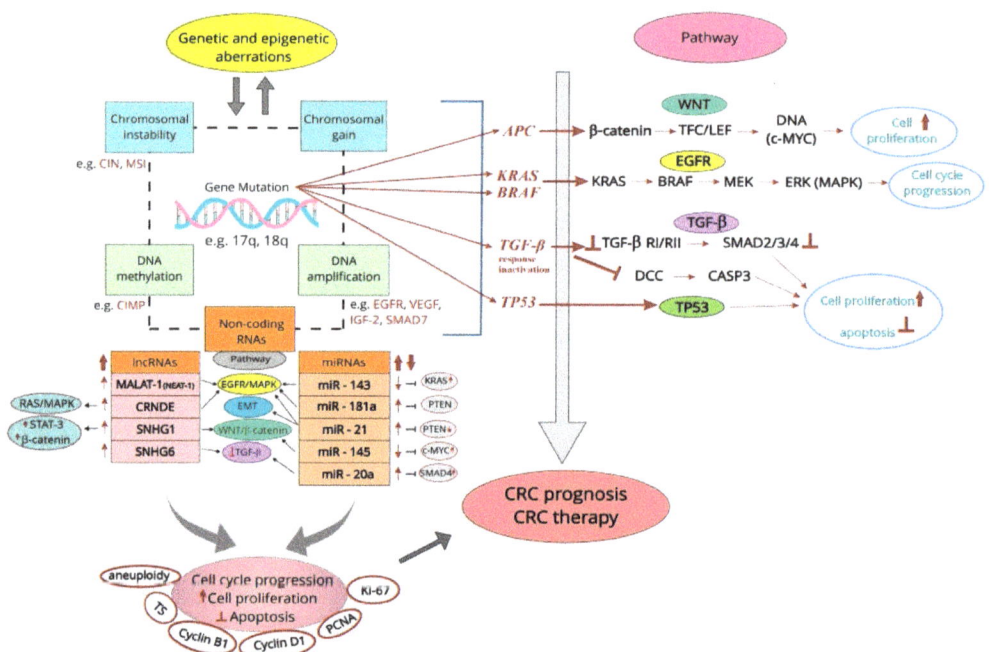

Figure 1. Different categories of proliferative markers with potential prognostic and predictive significance in CRC in association with key signaling pathways that are dysregulated in the 'adenoma–carcinoma sequence.' Dysfunction of the WNT/β-catenin, EGFR/MAPK, TGF-β, and TP53 signaling pathways leads to cell cycle progression, increased proliferation, and the inhibition of cell apoptosis. Classic genetic markers of prognostic significance include the mutated genes (e.g., *APC*, *KRAS/BRAF*, *TGF-β*, and *TP53*). Markers at the chromosome level are CIN and MSI. Epigenetic markers are CIMP and many other candidates including *SERP*, *p14*, *p16*, *LINE-1*, and *RASSF1A* (not shown). Selected genes also undergo amplifications (e.g., *EGFR*, *VEGF*, *SMAD7*, *IGF-2*), enhancing cellular proliferation. Prognostic markers also include ncRNAs. Several representatives were selected based on their proven role in cell cycle progression and enhancement of proliferation, with prognostic value demonstrated in meta-analyses. A prognostic role for aneuploidy and altered expression of conventional IHC proliferating markers in CRC (i.e., TS, cyclin B1, cyclin D1, PCNA, and Ki-67) was shown. Legend: ⇓—regulation; ↑/↓—increase/decrease; ⊥—inhibition; APC—adenomatous polyposis coli; BRAF—protooncogene B-Raf; CASP3—caspase 3; CIMP—CpG island methylator phenotype; CIN—chromosomal instability; c-Myc—protooncogene from Myc family; CRC—colorectal cancer; DCC—deleted in colorectal cancer; EGFR—epidermal growth factor receptor; EMT—epithelial–mesenchymal transition; ERK/MAPK—extracellular signal-regulated kinase or classical MAP kinase; IGF-2—insulin-like growth factor 2; IHC—immunohistochemical; KRAS—Kirsten rat sarcoma virus; LINE-1—long interspersed nucleotide element-1; MEK/MAP2K—mitogen-activated kinase; MSI—microsatellite instability; ncRNAs—non-coding RNAs; PCNA—proliferating cell nuclear antigen; PTEN—phosphatase and tensin homolog deleted on chromosome ten; RAS—rat sarcoma virus, three Ras genes in humans: HRAS, KRAS, and NRAS; RASSF1A–Ras association domain-containing protein 1A; STAT3—signal transducer and activator of transcription 3; TGF-β (RI/RII)—tumor growth factor β (receptor I/II); TS—thymidylate synthase; SERP—secreted frizzled-related protein; SMAD2/3/4/7—mothers against DPP homolog 2/3/4/7; VEGF—vascular endothelial growth factor; WNT—gene wingless + integrated or int-1.

5. Final Remarks and Future Perspectives

The development of IHC and modern molecular biology techniques (qRT-PCR, ISH, RNA/DNA sequencing, NGS, DNA methylation detection methods) has made it possible to determine the prognostic efficacy of many classic IHC markers for the estimation of patient survival, disease-free time, or disease recurrence. The prognostic role of aneuploidy, overexpression of markers such as TS, cyclin B1 (better 5-year survival), cyclin D1 (poor OS and DFS), PCNA (poor OS and CSS), and Ki-67 (poor OS) could be confirmed. Ki-67 antigen was also among 26 independent biomarkers of OS in resected CRLMs. However, studies indicating the overexpression of Ki-67 or other proliferation markers as good predictors of survival remain controversial. It has been suggested that an association between a high Ki-67 index and improved survival is only present in MSI-H status tumors. In turn, RT-PCR studies showed a high positive correlation of Ki-67 mRNA with pKi-67 and confirmed the role of Ki-67 mRNA as a predictor of poor OS. Studies indicate that tumors with high pKi-67 and low mRNA levels are likely to proliferate more slowly and have a better prognosis.

In CRC therapy (especially RT), slowly proliferating cells should also be considered, in addition to rapidly proliferating cells. Such cells provide a reservoir from which cells can be recruited to short-cycle, resulting in accelerated cell repopulation in response to damaging factors (irradiation, hypoxia). However, further research is required to clarify to what extent the pool of slowly proliferating cells includes CSCs that may reside in the G0 phase. So far, an optimal panel of IHC assays with markers of cellular proliferation in CRCs has not been established to predict survival or the effect of adjuvant treatment. While Ki-67 shows some promise as one of the components of the Oncotype Dx Colon Cancer Assay for predicting the risk of recurrence in stages II and III colon cancer, recent studies do not recommend this assay for use in patients with stage II CRC.

Modern molecular biology techniques have confirmed or discovered the role of several genetic and epigenetic markers, mainly as diagnostic and predictive markers in CRC. New technology also allows for the identification of a broad range of candidate prognostic markers. Classic genetic markers of prognostic significance include mutated genes (e.g., *APC, KRAS/BRAF, TGF-β,* and *TP53*), chromosomal markers CIN and MSI, epigenetic markers such as CIMP, and many other candidates including *SERP*, *p14*, *p16*, *LINE-1*, and *RASSF1A*. Further research is required to determine the prognostic role of *KRAS* mutation status in different CRC patient populations worldwide. Similarly, continued research is necessary to determine the contribution of *KRAS* mutations to the mechanisms of drug resistance to oxaliplatin.

The number of long non-coding RNAs (e.g., SNHG1, SNHG6, MALAT-1, CRNDE) and microRNAs (e.g., miR-20a, miR-21, miR-143, miR-145, miR-181a/b) related to proliferation in CRC as confirmed prognostic markers is also increasing. Despite the rather obvious limitations of IHC and new molecular techniques, the standardization of methods for the quantitative assessment of the expression of proliferation markers, or the understanding of endogenous and exogenous (environmental) mechanisms of accelerated cellular proliferation, requires further development. For a more accurate survival prognosis or prediction of therapeutic effects in CRC, it would be ideal to use complementary methods to study cell cycle disruption, apoptosis, and genomic alterations. The expanding development of research techniques is undisputedly contributing to the systematization of knowledge regarding cancer biology. Moreover, the detection of numerous ncRNAs, given their role in cell cycle regulation in CRC, cannot be underestimated. However, the recommendation of a specific ncRNA or a panel of such molecules as clinically useful prognostic markers is still a matter of the future. The previously signaled need to validate large-scale research and conduct multicenter studies on different populations will help to create a base of more reproducible results and identify their potential application in CRC patients.

6. Conclusions

As the reviewed literature reports, the prognostic utility of aneuploidy testing and of some immunocytochemical markers of cellular proliferation in CRC (TS, cyclin B1 and D1, PCNA, and Ki-67) needs to be supplemented by modern molecular biology techniques. The limits of conventional techniques to assess cellular proliferation, the high heterogeneity of tumor tissues, etc., justify the search for a panel of optimally sensitive, specific, and non-invasive CRC biomarkers. A specific expression pattern of ncRNAs (miRNAs and lncRNAs) may prove helpful in effectively identifying patients with a poor prognosis. It is particularly important to confirm known gene mutations/epigenetic alterations and to identify new mutation 'patterns' in different CRC patient populations to determine the prognosis for survival and/or the effects of cytotoxic and biologic regimens. For clinical and personalized medicine purposes, it seems important to construct a commercial test, based on a broad, prospective study, with the independent validation of biomarkers with prognostic/predictive value.

Funding: This research received no external funding.

Conflicts of Interest: The author declares no conflict of interest.

Abbreviations

ABCG2	ATP-binding cassette super-family G member 2
AC	Adenocarcinoma
AD	Adenoma
AKT	Serine/threonine kinase Akt, or protein kinase B (PKB)
ALDH1	Aldehyde dehydrogenase 1
APC	Adenomatous polyposis coli
BMPR1A	Bone morphogenetic protein receptor, type 1A
BRAF	Protooncogene B-Raf; encodes protein called B-Raf
Brd/Id/Urd	Bromo-, iodo-deoxyuridine
CAMs	Cell adhesion molecules
CCND2	G1/S-specific cyclin-D2
CD44	CD44 molecule (Indian blood group), a cell-surface glycoprotein
Cdks	Cyclin-dependent kinases
CEA	Carcinoembryonic antigen
CCS	Colon cancer subtype
CI	Confidence interval
CIMP	CpG island methylator phenotype
CIN	Chromosomal instability
CMS	Consensus molecular subtype
CRC	Colorectal cancer
CRLM(s)	Colorectal cancer liver metastasis(es)
CSCs	Cancer stem cells
CSS	Cancer-specific survival
DCC	Deleted in colorectal cancer
DFS	Disease-free survival
EdU	5-Ethynyl-2'-deoxyuridine
EGFR	Epidermal Growth Factor Receptor (HER1 in humans)
EIF3H	Eukaryotic translation initiation factor 3 subunit H
EMT	Epithelial-mesenchymal transition
ERK	Extracellular signal-regulated kinase or classical MAP kinase (MAPK)
FAP	Familial adenomatous polyposis
FCM	Flow cytometry
FDG	18-Fluoro-2-deoxy-D-glucose
FLT	18-Fluoro-3-deoxy-3-fluorothymidine
GALT	Gut-associated lymphoid tissue
GI	Gastrointestinal
GLUT1	Glucose transporter 1
GREM1	Gremlin 1, DAN family BMP antagonist
HIF-1	Hypoxia-inducible factor 1

HNPCC	Hereditary non-polyposis colorectal cancer
HPs	Hyperplastic polyps
HPFs	High-power fields
HR	Hazard ratio
IGF-2	Insulin growth factor 2
IGFBP2	IGF binding protein 2
IHC	Immunohistochemistry
ISCs	Intestinal stem cells
ISH	In situ hybridization
JAK	Janus kinase
JNK	c-Jun N-terminal kinase
KRAS/K-ras	Kirsten rat sarcoma virus; encodes protein called K-Ras
LGR5	G-protein-coupled receptor 5
LKB1	Serine/threonine-protein kinase STK11
LI	Labeling index
LS	Lynch syndrome
mAb(s)	Monoclonal antibody (antibodies)
MAPK	Mitogen-activated protein kinase
MCC	Colorectal mutant cancer protein
MKI67	Marker of proliferation Ki-67 gene
MLH1, 2, 6	MutL homolog 1, 2, 6
MMR	DNA mismatch repair
MSI-H	High microsatellite instability
MSH2	MutS homolog 2
MSS	Microsatellite stable
MUTYH	*E. coli* MutY homolog
NCAMs	Neural cell adhesion molecules
OS	Overall survival
PCNA	Proliferating cell nuclear antigen
PFS	Progression-free survival
PI	Proliferating index
PI3K	Phosphatidylinositol-3-kinase
PKM2	Pyruvate kinase M2
PMS2	Mismatch repair endonuclease 2
PP1	Protein phosphatase 1
PTEN	Phosphatase and tensin homolog deleted on chromosome ten
RAS	Oncogene "Rat sarcoma virus" from three Ras genes: HRAS, KRAS and NRAS
RC	Rectal cancer
RFS	Relapse/recurrence-free survival
RT	Radiotherapy
RT-PCR/qRT-PCR	Reverse transcriptase-polymerase chain reaction; quantitative real-time PCR
SMAD4	SMAD family member 4, Mothers Against DPP Homolog 4
SOX2	Transcription factor 2, known also as sex determining region Y (SRY)-box 2
SPs	Serrated polyps
SPS	Serrated polyposis syndrome
SSLs	Sessile serrated lesions
STAT3	Signal transducer and activator of transcription 3
TCGA	The cancer genome atlas
TGF-β	Transforming growth factor beta
TMA	Tissue microarray
TME	Tumor microenvironment
TNM	Tumor-node-metastasis
TP53/p53	Tumor gene/protein 53
Tpot	The potential tumor doubling time
Ts	Duration of S phase
TS	Thymidylate synthase
VEGF	Vascular endothelial growth factor
Wnt/WNT	Gene wingless + integrated or int-1

References

1. Ahmed, M. Colon Cancer: A Clinician's Perspective in 2019. *Gastroenterol. Res.* **2020**, *13*, 1–10. [CrossRef] [PubMed]
2. Sung, H.; Ferlay, J.; Siegel, R.L.; Laversanne, M.; Soerjomataram, I.; Jemal, A.; Bray, F. Global Cancer Statistics 2020: GLOBOCAN Estimates of Incidence and Mortality Worldwide for 36 Cancers in 185 Countries. *CA Cancer J. Clin.* **2021**, *71*, 209–249. [CrossRef] [PubMed]
3. Morgan, E.; Arnold, M.; Gini, A.; Lorenzoni, V.; Cabasag, C.J.; Laversanne, M.; Vignat, J.; Ferlay, J.; Murphy, N.; Bray, F. Global burden of colorectal cancer in 2020 and 2040: Incidence and mortality estimates from GLOBOCAN. *Gut* **2023**, *72*, 338–344. [CrossRef] [PubMed]
4. Siegel, R.L.; Miller, K.D.; Wagle, N.S.; Jemal, A. Cancer statistics, 2023. *CA Cancer J. Clin.* **2023**, *73*, 17–48. [CrossRef] [PubMed]
5. Mármol, I.; Sánchez-de-Diego, C.; Pradilla Dieste, A.; Cerrada, E.; Rodriguez Yoldi, M.J. Colorectal Carcinoma: A General Overview and Future Perspectives in Colorectal Cancer. *Int. J. Mol. Sci.* **2017**, *18*, 197. [CrossRef]
6. Xi, Y.; Xu, P. Global colorectal cancer burden in 2020 and projections to 2040. *Transl. Oncol.* **2021**, *14*, 101174. [CrossRef]
7. Vogelstein, B.; Fearon, E.R.; Hamilton, S.R.; Kern, S.E.; Preisinger, A.C.; Leppert, M.; Nakamura, Y.; White, R.; Smits, A.M.; Bos, J.L. Genetic alterations during colorectal-tumor development. *N. Engl. J. Med.* **1988**, *319*, 525–532. [CrossRef]
8. Cho, K.R.; Vogelstein, B. Suppressor gene alterations in the colorectal adenoma-carcinoma sequence. *J. Cell. Biochem. Suppl.* **1992**, *16G*, 137–141. [CrossRef]
9. Dariya, B.; Aliya, S.; Merchant, N.; Alam, A.; Nagaraju, G.P. Colorectal Cancer Biology, Diagnosis, and Therapeutic Approaches. *Crit. Rev. Oncog.* **2020**, *25*, 71–94. [CrossRef]
10. Leedham, S.J.; Schier, S.; Thliveris, A.T.; Halberg, R.B.; Newton, M.A.; Wright, N.A. From gene mutations to tumours—Stem cells in gastrointestinal carcinogenesis. *Cell Prolif.* **2005**, *38*, 387–405. [CrossRef]
11. Ricci-Vitiani, L.; Fabrizi, E.; Palio, E.; De Maria, R. Colon cancer stem cells. *J. Mol. Med.* **2009**, *87*, 1097–1104. [CrossRef] [PubMed]
12. Huang, E.H.; Hynes, M.J.; Zhang, T.; Ginestier, C.; Dontu, G.; Appelman, H.; Fields, J.Z.; Wicha, M.S.; Boman, B.M. Aldehyde dehydrogenase 1 is a marker for normal and malignant human colonic stem cells (SC) and tracks SC overpopulation during colon tumorigenesis. *Cancer Res.* **2009**, *69*, 3382–3389. [CrossRef] [PubMed]
13. Shackleton, M.; Quintana, E.; Fearon, E.R.; Morrison, S.J. Heterogeneity in cancer: Cancer stem cells versus clonal evolution. *Cell* **2009**, *138*, 822–829. [CrossRef]
14. Dieter, S.M.; Ball, C.R.; Hoffmann, C.M.; Nowrouzi, A.; Herbst, F.; Zavidij, O.; Abel, U.; Arens, A.; Weichert, W.; Brand, K.; et al. Distinct types of tumor-initiating cells form human colon cancer tumors and metastases. *Cell Stem Cell* **2011**, *9*, 357–365. [CrossRef] [PubMed]
15. Dieter, S.M.; Glimm, H.; Ball, C.R. Colorectal cancer-initiating cells caught in the act. *EMBO Mol. Med.* **2017**, *9*, 856–858. [CrossRef] [PubMed]
16. Bosman, F.; Yan, P. Molecular pathology of colorectal cancer. *Pol. J. Pathol.* **2014**, *65*, 257–266. [CrossRef]
17. Kinzler, K.W.; Vogelstein, B. Lessons from hereditary colorectal cancer. *Cell* **1996**, *87*, 159–170. [CrossRef]
18. Cheng, L.; Lai, M.D. Aberrant crypt foci as microscopic precursors of colorectal cancer. *World J. Gastroenterol.* **2003**, *9*, 2642–2649. [CrossRef]
19. Kowalczyk, M.; Orłowski, M.; Klepacki, Ł.; Zinkiewicz, K.; Kurpiewski, W.; Kaczerska, D.; Pesta, W.; Zieliński, E.; Siermontowski, P. Rectal aberrant crypt foci (ACF) as a predictor of benign and malignant neoplastic lesions in the large intestine. *BMC Cancer* **2020**, *20*, 133. [CrossRef]
20. Lynch, H.T.; Kimberling, W.; Albano, W.A.; Lynch, J.F.; Biscone, K.; Schuelke, G.S.; Sandberg, A.A.; Lipkin, M.; Deschner, E.E.; Mikol, Y.B.; et al. Hereditary nonpolyposis colorectal cancer (Lynch syndromes I and II). I. Clinical description of resource. *Cancer* **1985**, *56*, 934–938. [CrossRef]
21. Fearon, E.R. Molecular genetics of colorectal cancer. *Annu. Rev. Pathol.* **2011**, *6*, 479–507. [CrossRef] [PubMed]
22. Kim, J.H.; Kang, G.H. Evolving pathologic concepts of serrated lesions of the colorectum. *J. Pathol. Transl. Med.* **2020**, *54*, 276–289. [CrossRef] [PubMed]
23. Jass, J.R. Molecular heterogeneity of colorectal cancer: Implications for cancer control. *Surg. Oncol.* **2007**, *16* (Suppl. S1), S7–S9. [CrossRef]
24. Snover, D.C. Update on the serrated pathway to colorectal carcinoma. *Hum. Pathol.* **2011**, *42*, 1–10. [CrossRef]
25. Patai, A.V.; Molnár, B.; Tulassay, Z.; Sipos, F. Serrated pathway: Alternative route to colorectal cancer. *World J. Gastroenterol.* **2013**, *19*, 607–615. [CrossRef] [PubMed]
26. Thorlacius, H.; Takeuchi, Y.; Kanesaka, T.; Ljungberg, O.; Uedo, N.; Toth, E. Serrated polyps—A concealed but prevalent precursor of colorectal cancer. *Scand. J. Gastroenterol.* **2017**, *52*, 654–661. [CrossRef]
27. Fearon, E.R. Molecular features and mouse models of colorectal cancer. *Trans. Am. Clin. Climatol. Assoc.* **2018**, *129*, 56–62.
28. Lynch, H.T.; de la Chapelle, A. Hereditary colorectal cancer. *N. Engl. J. Med.* **2003**, *348*, 919–932. [CrossRef]
29. Huxley, R.R.; Ansary-Moghaddam, A.; Clifton, P.; Czernichow, S.; Parr, C.L.; Woodward, M. The impact of dietary and lifestyle risk factors on risk of colorectal cancer: A quantitative overview of the epidemiological evidence. *Int. J. Cancer* **2009**, *125*, 171–180. [CrossRef]
30. Mandic, M.; Li, H.; Safizadeh, F.; Niedermaier, T.; Hoffmeister, M.; Brenner, H. Is the association of overweight and obesity with colorectal cancer underestimated? An umbrella review of systematic reviews and meta-analyses. *Eur. J. Epidemiol.* **2023**, *38*, 135–144. [CrossRef]

31. Polyak, K.; Hamilton, S.R.; Vogelstein, B.; Kinzler, K.W. Early alteration of cell-cycle-regulated gene expression in colorectal neoplasia. *Am. J. Pathol.* **1996**, *149*, 381–387. [PubMed]
32. Harada, S.; Morlote, D. Molecular Pathology of Colorectal Cancer. *Adv. Anat. Pathol.* **2020**, *27*, 20–26. [CrossRef]
33. Zhu, S.; Wang, J.; Zellmer, L.; Xu, N.; Liu, M.; Hu, Y.; Ma, H.; Deng, F.; Yang, W.; Liao, D.J. Mutation or not, what directly establishes a neoplastic state, namely cellular immortality and autonomy, still remains unknown and should be prioritized in our research. *J. Cancer* **2022**, *13*, 2810–2843. [CrossRef] [PubMed]
34. Boman, B.M.; Huang, E. Human colon cancer stem cells: A new paradigm in gastrointestinal oncology. *J. Clin. Oncol.* **2008**, *26*, 2828–2838. [CrossRef] [PubMed]
35. Simms, L.; Barraclough, H.; Govindan, R. Biostatistics primer: What a clinician ought to know—Prognostic and predictive factors. *J. Thorac. Oncol.* **2013**, *8*, 808–813. [CrossRef]
36. National Cancer Institute Dictionary of Cancer Terms. Definition of Prognostic Factor. Available online: http://www.cancer.gov/dictionary?CdrID=44245 (accessed on 14 May 2023).
37. Powell, S.M.; Zilz, N.; Beazer-Barclay, Y.; Bryan, T.M.; Hamilton, S.R.; Thibodeau, S.N.; Vogelstein, B.; Kinzler, K.W. APC mutations occur early during colorectal tumorigenesis. *Nature* **1992**, *359*, 235–237. [CrossRef]
38. Cottrell, S.; Bicknell, D.; Kaklamanis, L.; Bodmer, W.F. Molecular analysis of APC mutations in familial adenomatous polyposis and sporadic colon carcinomas. *Lancet* **1992**, *340*, 626–630. [CrossRef]
39. Giles, R.H.; van Es, J.H.; Clevers, H. Caught up in a Wnt storm: Wnt signaling in cancer. *Biochim. Biophys. Acta* **2003**, *1653*, 1–24. [CrossRef]
40. Hedrick, L.; Cho, K.R.; Fearon, E.R.; Wu, T.C.; Kinzler, K.W.; Vogelstein, B. The DCC gene product in cellular differentiation and colorectal tumorigenesis. *Genes Dev.* **1994**, *8*, 1174–1183. [CrossRef]
41. Fearon, E.R.; Pierceall, W.E. The deleted in colorectal cancer (DCC) gene: A candidate tumour suppressor gene encoding a cell surface protein with similarity to neural cell adhesion molecules. *Cancer Surv.* **1995**, *24*, 3–17.
42. Llambi, F.; Causeret, F.; Bloch-Gallego, E.; Mehlen, P. Netrin-1 acts as a survival factor via its receptors UNC5H and DCC. *EMBO J.* **2001**, *20*, 2715–2722. [CrossRef]
43. Nakayama, H.; Ohnuki, H.; Nakahara, M.; Nishida-Fukuda, H.; Sakaue, T.; Fukuda, S.; Higashiyama, S.; Doi, Y.; Mitsuyoshi, M.; Okimoto, T.; et al. Inactivation of axon guidance molecule netrin-1 in human colorectal cancer by an epigenetic mechanism. *Biochem. Biophys. Res. Commun.* **2022**, *611*, 146–150. [CrossRef] [PubMed]
44. Munro, A.J.; Lain, S.; Lane, D.P. P53 abnormalities and outcomes in colorectal cancer: A systematic review. *Br. J. Cancer* **2005**, *92*, 434–444. [CrossRef] [PubMed]
45. Cancer Genome Atlas Network. Comprehensive molecular characterization of human colon and rectal cancer. *Nature* **2012**, *487*, 330–337. [CrossRef] [PubMed]
46. Kothalawala, W.J.; Barták, B.K.; Nagy, Z.B.; Zsigrai, S.; Szigeti, K.A.; Valcz, G.; Takács, I.; Kalmár, A.; Molnár, B. A Detailed Overview About the Single-Cell Analyses of Solid Tumors Focusing on Colorectal Cancer. *Pathol. Oncol. Res.* **2022**, *28*, 1610342. [CrossRef] [PubMed]
47. Cerretelli, G.; Ager, A.; Arends, M.J.; Frayling, I.M. Molecular pathology of Lynch syndrome. *J. Pathol.* **2020**, *250*, 518–531. [CrossRef]
48. Briggs, S.; Tomlinson, I. Germline and somatic polymerase ε and δ mutations define a new class of hypermutated colorectal and endometrial cancers. *J. Pathol.* **2013**, *230*, 148–153. [CrossRef]
49. Nagtegaal, I.D.; Odze, R.D.; Klimstra, D.; Paradis, V.; Rugge, M.; Schirmacher, P.; Washington, K.M.; Carneiro, F.; Cree, I.A. WHO Classification of Tumours Editorial Board. The 2019 WHO classification of tumours of the digestive system. *Histopathology* **2020**, *76*, 182–188. [CrossRef]
50. Teodoridis, J.M.; Hardie, C.; Brown, R. CpG island methylator phenotype (CIMP) in cancer: Causes and implications. *Cancer Lett.* **2008**, *268*, 177–186. [CrossRef]
51. Arnau-Collell, C.; Soares de Lima, Y.; Díaz-Gay, M.; Muñoz, J.; Carballal, S.; Bonjoch, L.; Moreira, L.; Lozano, J.J.; Ocaña, T.; Cuatrecasas, M.; et al. Colorectal cancer genetic variants are also associated with serrated polyposis syndrome susceptibility. *J. Med. Genet.* **2020**, *57*, 677–682. [CrossRef]
52. Hang, D.; Joshi, A.D.; He, X.; Chan, A.T.; Jovani, M.; Gala, M.K.; Ogino, S.; Kraft, P.; Turman, C.; Peters, U.; et al. Colorectal cancer susceptibility variants and risk of conventional adenomas and serrated polyps: Results from three cohort studies. *Int. J. Epidemiol.* **2020**, *49*, 259–269. [CrossRef] [PubMed]
53. Rubio, C.A.; Puppa, G.; de Petris, G.; Kis, L.; Schmidt, P.T. The third pathway of colorectal carcinogenesis. *J. Clin. Pathol.* **2018**, *71*, 7–11. [CrossRef]
54. Sadanandam, A.; Wang, X.; de Sousa E Melo, F.; Gray, J.W.; Vermeulen, L.; Hanahan, D.; Medema, J.P. Reconciliation of classification systems defining molecular subtypes of colorectal cancer: Interrelationships and clinical implications. *Cell Cycle* **2014**, *13*, 353–357. [CrossRef] [PubMed]
55. Kamel, F.; Eltarhoni, K.; Nisar, P.; Soloviev, M. Colorectal Cancer Diagnosis: The Obstacles We Face in Determining a Non-Invasive Test and Current Advances in Biomarker Detection. *Cancers* **2022**, *14*, 1889. [CrossRef] [PubMed]
56. Suryadinata, R.; Sadowski, M.; Sarcevic, B. Control of cell cycle progression by phosphorylation of cyclin-dependent kinase (CDK) substrates. *Biosci. Rep.* **2010**, *30*, 243–255. [CrossRef]
57. Malumbres, M. Cyclin-dependent kinases. *Genome Biol.* **2014**, *15*, 122. [CrossRef] [PubMed]

58. Martínez-Alonso, D.; Malumbres, M. Mammalian cell cycle cyclins. *Semin. Cell Dev. Biol.* **2020**, *107*, 28–35. [CrossRef]
59. Dang, F.; Nie, L.; Wei, W. Ubiquitin signaling in cell cycle control and tumorigenesis. *Cell Death Differ.* **2021**, *28*, 427–438. [CrossRef]
60. Malumbres, M.; Barbacid, M. To cycle or not to cycle: A critical decision in cancer. *Nat. Rev. Cancer* **2001**, *1*, 222–231. [CrossRef]
61. Doonan, J.H.; Kitsios, G. Functional evolution of cyclin-dependent kinases. *Mol. Biotechnol.* **2009**, *42*, 14–29. [CrossRef]
62. Loyer, P.; Trembley, J.H. Roles of CDK/Cyclin complexes in transcription and pre-mRNA splicing: Cyclins L and CDK11 at the cross-roads of cell cycle and regulation of gene expression. *Semin. Cell Dev. Biol.* **2020**, *107*, 36–45. [CrossRef] [PubMed]
63. Kontomanolis, E.N.; Koutras, A.; Syllaios, A.; Schizas, D.; Mastoraki, A.; Garmpis, N.; Diakosavvas, M.; Angelou, K.; Tsatsaris, G.; Pagkalos, A.; et al. Role of Oncogenes and Tumor-suppressor Genes in Carcinogenesis: A Review. *Anticancer Res.* **2020**, *40*, 6009–6015. [CrossRef] [PubMed]
64. Patergnani, S.; Danese, A.; Bouhamida, E.; Aguiari, G.; Previati, M.; Pinton, P.; Giorgi, C. Various Aspects of Calcium Signaling in the Regulation of Apoptosis, Autophagy, Cell Proliferation, and Cancer. *Int. J. Mol. Sci.* **2020**, *21*, 8323. [CrossRef] [PubMed]
65. Sonnenschein, C.; Soto, A.M.; Rangarajan, A.; Kulkarni, P. Competing views on cancer. *J. Biosci.* **2014**, *39*, 281–302. [CrossRef]
66. Hanahan, D. Hallmarks of Cancer: New Dimensions. *Cancer Discov.* **2022**, *12*, 31–46. [CrossRef] [PubMed]
67. Pardee, A.B. A restriction point for control of normal animal cell proliferation. *Proc. Natl. Acad. Sci. USA* **1974**, *71*, 1286–1290. [CrossRef]
68. Wilson, G.D. Proliferation models in tumours. *Int. J. Radiat. Biol.* **2003**, *79*, 525–530. [CrossRef]
69. Baisch, H.; Otto, U.; Hatje, U.; Fack, H. Heterogeneous cell kinetics in tumors analyzed with a simulation model for bromodeoxyuridine single and multiple labeling. *Cytometry* **1995**, *21*, 52–61. [CrossRef]
70. Shackney, S.E.; Shankey, T.V. Cell cycle models for molecular biology and molecular oncology: Exploring new dimensions. *Cytometry* **1999**, *35*, 97–116. [CrossRef]
71. Blanpain, C.; Horsley, V.; Fuchs, E. Epithelial stem cells: Turning over new leaves. *Cell* **2007**, *128*, 445–458. [CrossRef]
72. Sender, R.; Milo, R. The distribution of cellular turnover in the human body. *Nat. Med.* **2021**, *7*, 45–48. [CrossRef] [PubMed]
73. Hammarlund, E.U.; Amend, S.R.; Pienta, K.J. The issues with tissues: The wide range of cell fate separation enables the evolution of multicellularity and cancer. *Med. Oncol.* **2020**, *37*, 62. [CrossRef] [PubMed]
74. Tomasetti, C.; Vogelstein, B. Cancer etiology. Variation in cancer risk among tissues can be explained by the number of stem cell divisions. *Science* **2015**, *347*, 78–81. [CrossRef] [PubMed]
75. Huels, D.J.; Sansom, O.J. Stem vs non-stem cell origin of colorectal cancer. *Br. J. Cancer* **2015**, *113*, 1–5. [CrossRef]
76. Shih, I.M.; Wang, T.L.; Traverso, G.; Romans, K.; Hamilton, S.R.; Ben-Sasson, S.; Kinzler, K.W.; Vogelstein, B. Top-down morphogenesis of colorectal tumors. *Proc. Natl. Acad. Sci. USA* **2001**, *98*, 2640–2645. [CrossRef]
77. Preston, S.L.; Wong, W.M.; Chan, A.O.; Poulsom, R.; Jeffery, R.; Goodlad, R.A.; Mandir, N.; Elia, G.; Novelli, M.; Bodmer, W.F.; et al. Bottom-up histogenesis of colorectal adenomas: Origin in the monocryptal adenoma and initial expansion by crypt fission. *Cancer Res.* **2003**, *63*, 3819–3825.
78. Cortina, C.; Turon, G.; Stork, D.; Hernando-Momblona, X.; Sevillano, M.; Aguilera, M.; Tosi, S.; Merlos-Suárez, A.; Stephan-Otto Attolini, C.; Sancho, E.; et al. A genome editing approach to study cancer stem cells in human tumors. *EMBO Mol. Med.* **2017**, *9*, 869–879. [CrossRef]
79. De Sousa e Melo, F.; Kurtova, A.V.; Harnoss, J.M.; Kljavin, N.; Hoeck, J.D.; Hung, J.; Anderson, J.E.; Storm, E.E.; Modrusan, Z.; Koeppen, H.; et al. A distinct role for Lgr5$^+$ stem cells in primary and metastatic colon cancer. *Nature* **2017**, *543*, 676–680. [CrossRef]
80. Shimokawa, M.; Ohta, Y.; Nishikori, S.; Matano, M.; Takano, A.; Fujii, M.; Date, S.; Sugimoto, S.; Kanai, T.; Sato, T. Visualization and targeting of LGR5$^+$ human colon cancer stem cells. *Nature* **2017**, *545*, 187–192. [CrossRef]
81. Szaryńska, M.; Olejniczak, A.; Kobiela, J.; Spychalski, P.; Kmieć, Z. Therapeutic strategies against cancer stem cells in human colorectal cancer. *Oncol. Lett.* **2017**, *14*, 7653–7668. [CrossRef]
82. Alowaidi, F.; Hashimi, S.M.; Alqurashi, N.; Alhulais, R.; Ivanovski, S.; Bellette, B.; Meedenyia, A.; Lam, A.; Wood, S. Assessing stemness and proliferation properties of the newly established colon cancer 'stem' cell line, CSC480 and novel approaches to identify dormant cancer cells. *Oncol. Rep.* **2018**, *39*, 2881–2891. [CrossRef] [PubMed]
83. Thirlwell, C.; Will, O.C.; Domingo, E.; Graham, T.A.; McDonald, S.A.; Oukrif, D.; Jeffrey, R.; Gorman, M.; Rodriguez-Justo, M.; Chin-Aleong, J.; et al. Clonality assessment and clonal ordering of individual neoplastic crypts shows polyclonality of colorectal adenomas. *Gastroenterology* **2010**, *138*, 1441–1454. [CrossRef] [PubMed]
84. Thliveris, A.T.; Clipson, L.; White, A.; Waggoner, J.; Plesh, L.; Skinner, B.L.; Zahm, C.D.; Sullivan, R.; Dove, W.F.; Newton, M.A.; et al. Clonal structure of carcinogen-induced intestinal tumors in mice. *Cancer Prev. Res.* **2011**, *4*, 916–923. [CrossRef] [PubMed]
85. Roy, P.; Paganelli, G.M.; Faivre, J.; Biasco, G.; Scheppach, W.; Saldanha, M.H.; Beckly, D.E. Pattern of epithelial cell proliferation in colorectal mucosa of patients with large bowel adenoma or cancer: An ECP case-control study. European cancer prevention. *Eur. J. Cancer Prev.* **1999**, *8*, 401–407. [CrossRef]
86. Tubiana, M. The kinetics of tumour cell proliferation and radiotherapy. *Br. J. Radiol.* **1971**, *44*, 325–347. [CrossRef]
87. Colak, S.; Medema, J.P. Cancer stem cells—Important players in tumor therapy resistance. *FEBS J.* **2014**, *281*, 4779–4791. [CrossRef]
88. Gasinska, A.; Adamczyk, A.; Niemiec, J.; Biesaga, B.; Darasz, Z.; Skolyszewski, J. Gender-related differences in pathological and clinical tumor response based on immunohistochemical proteins expression in rectal cancer patients treated with short course of preoperative radiotherapy. *J. Gastrointest. Surg.* **2014**, *18*, 1306–1318. [CrossRef]

89. Trott, K.R.; Kummermehr, J. What is known about tumour proliferation rates to choose between accelerated fractionation or hyperfractionation? *Radiother. Oncol.* **1985**, *3*, 1–9. [CrossRef]
90. Wilson, G.D. Cell kinetics. *Clin. Oncol. R. Coll. Radiol.* **2007**, *19*, 370–384. [CrossRef]
91. Jin, F.; Luo, H.; Zhou, J.; Wu, Y.; Sun, H.; Liu, H.; Zheng, X.; Wang, Y. Dose-time fractionation schedules of preoperative radiotherapy and timing to surgery for rectal cancer. *Ther. Adv. Med. Oncol.* **2020**, *12*, 1758835920907537. [CrossRef]
92. Das, P.K.; Islam, F.; Lam, A.K. The Roles of Cancer Stem Cells and Therapy Resistance in Colorectal Carcinoma. *Cells* **2020**, *9*, 1392. [CrossRef] [PubMed]
93. Hen, O.; Barkan, D. Dormant disseminated tumor cells and cancer stem/progenitor-like cells: Similarities and opportunities. *Semin. Cancer Biol.* **2020**, *60*, 157–165. [CrossRef] [PubMed]
94. Colak, S.; Zimberlin, C.D.; Fessler, E.; Hogdal, L.; Prasetyanti, P.R.; Grandela, C.M.; Letai, A.; Medema, J.P. Decreased mitochondrial priming determines chemoresistance of colon cancer stem cells. *Cell Death Differ.* **2014**, *21*, 1170–1177. [CrossRef] [PubMed]
95. Takahashi, H.; Ishii, H.; Nishida, N.; Takemasa, I.; Mizushima, T.; Ikeda, M.; Yokobori, T.; Mimori, K.; Yamamoto, H.; Sekimoto, M.; et al. Significance of Lgr5(+ve) cancer stem cells in the colon and rectum. *Ann. Surg. Oncol.* **2011**, *18*, 1166–1174. [CrossRef]
96. Oshima, C.T.; Iriya, K.; Forones, N.M. Ki-67 as a prognostic marker in colorectal cancer but not in gastric cancer. *Neoplasma* **2005**, *52*, 420–424.
97. Ahadi, M.; Sokolova, A.; Brown, I.; Chou, A.; Gill, A.J. The 2019 World Health Organization Classification of appendiceal, colorectal and anal canal tumours: An update and critical assessment. *Pathology* **2021**, *53*, 454–461. [CrossRef]
98. Cree, I.A.; Tan, P.H.; Travis, W.D.; Wesseling, P.; Yagi, Y.; White, V.A.; Lokuhetty, D.; Scolyer, R.A. Counting mitoses: SI(ze) matters! *Mod. Pathol.* **2021**, *34*, 1651–1657. [CrossRef]
99. Potten, C.S.; Kellett, M.; Roberts, S.A.; Rew, D.A.; Wilson, G.D. Measurement of in vivo proliferation in human colorectal mucosa using bromodeoxyuridine. *Gut* **1992**, *33*, 71–78. [CrossRef]
100. Palmqvist, R.; Oberg, A.; Bergström, C.; Rutegård, J.N.; Zackrisson, B.; Stenling, R. Systematic heterogeneity and prognostic significance of cell proliferation in colorectal cancer. *Br. J. Cancer* **1998**, *77*, 917–925. [CrossRef]
101. Salud, A.; Porcel, J.M.; Raikundalia, B.; Camplejohn, R.S.; Taub, N.A. Prognostic significance of DNA ploidy, S-phase fraction, and P-glycoprotein expression in colorectal cancer. *J. Surg. Oncol.* **1999**, *72*, 167–174. [CrossRef]
102. Rew, D.A.; Wilson, G.D. Cell production rates in human tissues and tumours and their significance. Part 1: An introduction to the techniques of measurement and their limitations. *Eur. J. Surg. Oncol.* **2000**, *26*, 227–238. [CrossRef] [PubMed]
103. Biasco, G.; Paganelli, G.M.; Santucci, R.; Brandi, G.; Barbara, L. Methodological problems in the use of rectal cell proliferation as a biomarker of colorectal cancer risk. *J. Cell. Biochem. Suppl.* **1994**, *19*, 55–60. [PubMed]
104. Paganelli, G.M.; Lalli, E.; Facchini, A.; Biasco, G.; Santucci, R.; Brandi, G.; Barbara, L. Flow cytometry and in vitro tritiated thymidine labeling in normal rectal mucosa of patients at high risk of colorectal cancer. *Am. J. Gastroenterol.* **1994**, *89*, 220–224. [PubMed]
105. Gerdes, J.; Lemke, H.; Baisch, H.; Wacker, H.H.; Schwab, U.; Stein, H. Cell cycle analysis of a cell proliferation-associated human nuclear antigen defined by the monoclonal antibody Ki-67. *J. Immunol.* **1984**, *133*, 1710–1715. [CrossRef] [PubMed]
106. Scholzen, T.; Gerdes, J. The Ki-67 protein: From the known and the unknown. *J. Cell. Physiol.* **2000**, *182*, 311–322. [CrossRef]
107. Hall, P.A.; Levison, D.A. Review: Assessment of cell proliferation in histological material. *J. Clin. Pathol.* **1990**, *43*, 184–192. [CrossRef]
108. Sawtell, R.M.; Rew, D.A.; Stradling, R.N.; Wilson, G.D. Pan cycle expression of proliferating cell nuclear antigen in human colorectal cancer and its proliferative correlations. *Cytometry* **1995**, *22*, 190–199. [CrossRef]
109. Sobecki, M.; Mrouj, K.; Colinge, J.; Gerbe, F.; Jay, P.; Krasinska, L.; Dulic, V.; Fisher, D. Cell-Cycle Regulation Accounts for Variability in Ki-67 Expression Levels. *Cancer Res.* **2017**, *77*, 2722–2734. [CrossRef]
110. Wang, Y.L.; Zhang, H.W.; Mo, Y.Q.; Zhong, H.; Liu, W.M.; Lei, Y.; Lin, F. Application of dual-layer spectral detector computed tomography to evaluate the expression of Ki-67 in colorectal cancer. *J. Chin. Med. Assoc.* **2022**, *85*, 610–616. [CrossRef]
111. Francis, D.L.; Freeman, A.; Visvikis, D.; Costa, D.C.; Luthra, S.K.; Novelli, M.; Taylor, I.; Ell, P.J. In vivo imaging of cellular proliferation in colorectal cancer using positron emission tomography. *Gut* **2003**, *52*, 1602–1606. [CrossRef]
112. Francis, D.L.; Visvikis, D.; Costa, D.C.; Arulampalam, T.H.; Townsend, C.; Luthra, S.K.; Taylor, I.; Ell, P.J. Potential impact of [18F]3′-deoxy-3′-fluorothymidine versus [18F]fluoro-2-deoxy-D-glucose in positron emission tomography for colorectal cancer. *Eur. J. Nucl. Med. Mol. Imaging* **2003**, *30*, 988–994. [CrossRef] [PubMed]
113. Watanabe, A.; Harimoto, N.; Yokobori, T.; Araki, K.; Kubo, N.; Igarashi, T.; Tsukagoshi, M.; Ishii, N.; Yamanaka, T.; Handa, T.; et al. FDG-PET reflects tumor viability on SUV in colorectal cancer liver metastasis. *Int. J. Clin. Oncol.* **2020**, *25*, 322–329. [CrossRef] [PubMed]
114. Biasco, G.; Paganelli, G.M.; Miglioli, M.; Barbara, L. Cell proliferation biomarkers in the gastrointestinal tract. *J. Cell. Biochem. Suppl.* **1992**, *16G*, 73–78. [CrossRef] [PubMed]
115. Anjomshoaa, A.; Nasri, S.; Humar, B.; McCall, J.L.; Chatterjee, A.; Yoon, H.S.; McNoe, L.; Black, M.A.; Reeve, A.E. Slow proliferation as a biological feature of colorectal cancer metastasis. *Br. J. Cancer* **2009**, *101*, 822–828. [CrossRef]
116. Tomita, T. DNA ploidy and proliferating cell nuclear antigen in colonic adenomas and adenocarcinomas. *Dig. Dis. Sci.* **1995**, *40*, 996–1004. [CrossRef]
117. Barletta, A.; Marzullo, F.; Pellecchia, A.; Montemurro, S.; Labriola, A.; Lomonaco, R.; Grammatica, L.; Paradiso, A. DNA flow cytometry, p53 levels and proliferative cell nuclear antigen in human colon dysplastic, precancerous and cancerous tissues. *Anticancer Res.* **1998**, *18*, 1677–1682.

118. Yigit, N.; Gunal, A.; Kucukodaci, Z.; Karslioglu, Y.; Onguru, O.; Ozcan, A. Are we counting mitoses correctly? *Ann. Diagn. Pathol.* **2013**, *17*, 536–539. [CrossRef]
119. Kim, D.; Pantanowitz, L.; Schüffler, P.; Yarlagadda, D.V.K.; Ardon, O.; Reuter, V.E.; Hameed, M.; Klimstra, D.S.; Hanna, M.G. (Re) Defining the High-Power Field for Digital Pathology. *J. Pathol. Inform.* **2020**, *11*, 33. [CrossRef]
120. Orr, B.; Godek, K.M.; Compton, D. Aneuploidy. *Curr. Biol.* **2015**, *25*, R538–R542. [CrossRef]
121. Brás, R.; Sunkel, C.E.; Resende, L.P. Tissue stem cells: The new actors in the aneuploidy field. *Cell Cycle* **2019**, *18*, 1813–1823. [CrossRef]
122. Ben-David, U.; Amon, A. Context is everything: Aneuploidy in cancer. *Nat. Rev. Genet.* **2020**, *21*, 44–62. [CrossRef] [PubMed]
123. Lazaris, A.C.; Davaris, P.; Nakopoulou, L.; Theodoropoulos, G.E.; Koullias, G.; Golematis, B.C. Correlation between immunohistochemical expression of proliferating cell nuclear antigen and flow cytometry parameters in colorectal neoplasia. *Dis. Colon Rectum* **1994**, *37*, 1083–1089. [CrossRef] [PubMed]
124. Wilson, M.S.; Anderson, E.; Bell, J.C.; Pearson, J.M.; Haboubi, N.Y.; James, R.D.; Schofield, P.F. An evaluation of five different methods for estimating proliferation in human colorectal adenocarcinomas. *Surg. Oncol.* **1994**, *3*, 263–273. [CrossRef] [PubMed]
125. Chen, Y.T.; Henk, M.J.; Carney, K.J.; Wong, W.D.; Rothenberger, D.A.; Zheng, T.; Feygin, M.; Madoff, R.D. Prognostic significance of tumor markers in colorectal cancer patients: DNA index, S-phase fraction, p53 expression, and Ki-67 index. *J. Gastrointest. Surg.* **1997**, *1*, 266–272, discussion 273. [CrossRef]
126. Le Pessot, F.; Michel, P.; Paresy, M.; Lemoine, F.; Hellot, M.F.; Paillot, B.; Scotte, M.; Peillon, C.; Hemet, J. Cell proliferation in colorectal adenocarcinomas: Comparison between Ki-67 immunostaining and bromodeoxyuridine uptake detected by immunohistochemistry and flow cytometry. *Pathol. Res. Pract.* **2001**, *197*, 411–418. [CrossRef]
127. Laubert, T.; Freitag-Wolf, S.; Linnebacher, M.; König, A.; Vollmar, B.; Habermann, J.K. North German Tumorbank of Colorectal Cancer (ColoNet) consortium. Stage-specific frequency and prognostic significance of aneuploidy in patients with sporadic colorectal cancer—A meta-analysis and current overview. *Int. J. Color. Dis.* **2015**, *30*, 1015–1028. [CrossRef]
128. Lin, J.K.; Chang, S.C.; Yang, S.H.; Jiang, J.K.; Chen, W.C.; Lin, T.C. Prognostic value of DNA ploidy patterns of colorectal adenocarcinoma. *Hepatogastroenterology* **2003**, *50*, 1927–1932.
129. Araujo, S.E.; Bernardo, W.M.; Habr-Gama, A.; Kiss, D.R.; Cecconello, I. DNA ploidy status and prognosis in colorectal cancer: A meta-analysis of published data. *Dis. Colon Rectum* **2007**, *50*, 1800–1810. [CrossRef]
130. Crissman, J.D.; Zarbo, R.J.; Ma, C.K.; Visscher, D.W. Histopathologic parameters and DNA analysis in colorectal adenocarcinomas. *Pathol. Annu.* **1989**, *24*, 103–147.
131. Michel, P.; Paresy, M.; Lepessot, F.; Hellot, M.F.; Paillot, B.; Scotte, M.; Peillon, C.; Ducrotté, P.; Hemet, J. Pre-operative kinetic parameter determination of colorectal adenocarcinomas. Prognostic significance. *Eur. J. Gastroenterol. Hepatol.* **2000**, *12*, 275–280. [CrossRef]
132. Zarbo, R.J.; Nakhleh, R.E.; Brown, R.D.; Kubus, J.J.; Ma, C.K.; Mackowiak, P. Prognostic significance of DNA ploidy and proliferation in 309 colorectal carcinomas as determined by two-color multiparametric DNA flow cytometry. *Cancer* **1997**, *79*, 2073–2086. [CrossRef]
133. Rew, D.A.; Wilson, G.D.; Taylor, I.; Weaver, P.C. Proliferation characteristics of human colorectal carcinomas measured in vivo. *Br. J. Surg.* **1991**, *78*, 60–66. [CrossRef] [PubMed]
134. Gasinska, A.; Skolyszewski, J.; Popiela, T.; Richter, P.; Darasz, Z.; Nowak, K.; Niemiec, J.; Biesaga, B.; Adamczyk, A.; Bucki, K.; et al. Bromodeoxyuridine labeling index as an indicator of early tumor response to preoperative radiotherapy in patients with rectal cancer. *J. Gastrointest. Surg.* **2007**, *11*, 520–528. [CrossRef] [PubMed]
135. Magaki, S.; Hojat, S.A.; Wei, B.; So, A.; Yong, W.H. An Introduction to the Performance of Immunohistochemistry. *Methods Mol. Biol.* **2019**, *1897*, 289–298. [CrossRef]
136. Mauriello, S.; Treglia, M.; Pallocci, M.; Bonfiglio, R.; Giacobbi, E.; Passalacqua, P.; Cammarano, A.; D'Ovidio, C.; Marsella, L.T.; Scimeca, M. Antigenicity Preservation Is Related to Tissue Characteristics and the Post-Mortem Interval: Immunohistochemical Study and Literature Review. *Healthcare* **2022**, *10*, 1495. [CrossRef]
137. Koo, M.; Squires, J.M.; Ying, D.; Huang, J. Making a Tissue Microarray. *Methods Mol. Biol.* **2019**, *1897*, 313–323. [CrossRef]
138. Johnston, P.G.; Liang, C.M.; Henry, S.; Chabner, B.A.; Allegra, C.J. Production and characterization of monoclonal antibodies that localize human thymidylate synthase in the cytoplasm of human cells and tissue. *Cancer Res.* **1991**, *51*, 6668–6676.
139. Showalter, S.L.; Showalter, T.N.; Witkiewicz, A.; Havens, R.; Kennedy, E.P.; Hucl, T.; Kern, S.E.; Yeo, C.J.; Brody, J.R. Evaluating the drug-target relationship between thymidylate synthase expression and tumor response to 5-fluorouracil. Is it time to move forward? *Cancer Biol. Ther.* **2008**, *7*, 986–994. [CrossRef]
140. Rahman, L.; Voeller, D.; Rahman, M.; Lipkowitz, S.; Allegra, C.; Barrett, J.C.; Kaye, F.J.; Zajac-Kaye, M. Thymidylate synthase as an oncogene: A novel role for an essential DNA synthesis enzyme. *Cancer Cell* **2004**, *5*, 341–351. [CrossRef]
141. Edler, D.; Glimelius, B.; Hallström, M.; Jakobsen, A.; Johnston, P.G.; Magnusson, I.; Ragnhammar, P.; Blomgren, H. Thymidylate synthase expression in colorectal cancer: A prognostic and predictive marker of benefit from adjuvant fluorouracil-based chemotherapy. *J. Clin. Oncol.* **2002**, *20*, 1721–1728. [CrossRef]
142. Allegra, C.J.; Parr, A.L.; Wold, L.E.; Mahoney, M.R.; Sargent, D.J.; Johnston, P.; Klein, P.; Behan, K.; O'Connell, M.J.; Levitt, R.; et al. Investigation of the prognostic and predictive value of thymidylate synthase, p53, and Ki-67 in patients with locally advanced colon cancer. *J. Clin. Oncol.* **2002**, *20*, 1735–1743. [CrossRef]

143. Badary, D.M.; Elkabsh, M.M.; Mady, H.H.; Gabr, A.; Kroosh, S.S. Prognostic and Predictive Role of Excision Repair Cross-complementation Group 1 and Thymidylate Synthase in Colorectal Carcinoma Patients Received FOLFOX Chemotherapy: An Immunohistochemical Study. *Appl. Immunohistochem. Mol. Morphol.* **2020**, *28*, 741–747. [CrossRef] [PubMed]
144. Kumar, A.; Singh, A.K.; Singh, H.; Thareja, S.; Kumar, P. Regulation of thymidylate synthase: An approach to overcome 5-FU resistance in colorectal cancer. *Med. Oncol.* **2022**, *40*, 3. [CrossRef] [PubMed]
145. Johnston, P.G.; Fisher, E.R.; Rockette, H.E.; Fisher, B.; Wolmark, N.; Drake, J.C.; Chabner, B.A.; Allegra, C.J. The role of thymidylate synthase expression in prognosis and outcome of adjuvant chemotherapy in patients with rectal cancer. *J. Clin. Oncol.* **1994**, *12*, 2640–2647. [CrossRef] [PubMed]
146. Van Triest, B.; Pinedo, H.M.; Blaauwgeers, J.L.; van Diest, P.J.; Schoenmakers, P.S.; Voorn, D.A.; Smid, K.; Hoekman, K.; Hoitsma, H.F.; Peters, G.J. Prognostic role of thymidylate synthase, thymidine phosphorylase/platelet-derived endothelial cell growth factor, and proliferation markers in colorectal cancer. *Clin. Cancer Res.* **2000**, *6*, 1063–1072. [PubMed]
147. Allegra, C.J.; Paik, S.; Colangelo, L.H.; Parr, A.L.; Kirsch, I.; Kim, G.; Klein, P.; Johnston, P.G.; Wolmark, N.; Wieand, H.S. Prognostic value of thymidylate synthase, Ki-67, and p53 in patients with Dukes' B and C colon cancer: A National Cancer Institute-National Surgical Adjuvant Breast and Bowel Project collaborative study. *J. Clin. Oncol.* **2003**, *21*, 241–250. [CrossRef]
148. Ciaparrone, M.; Quirino, M.; Schinzari, G.; Zannoni, G.; Corsi, D.C.; Vecchio, F.M.; Cassano, A.; La Torre, G.; Barone, C. Predictive role of thymidylate synthase, dihydropyrimidine dehydrogenase and thymidine phosphorylase expression in colorectal cancer patients receiving adjuvant 5-fluorouracil. *Oncology* **2006**, *70*, 366–377. [CrossRef]
149. Kim, S.H.; Kwon, H.C.; Oh, S.Y.; Lee, D.M.; Lee, S.; Lee, J.H.; Roh, M.S.; Kim, D.C.; Park, K.; Choi, H.J.; et al. Prognostic value of ERCC1, thymidylate synthase, and glutathione S-transferase pi for 5-FU/oxaliplatin chemotherapy in advanced colorectal cancer. *Am. J. Clin. Oncol.* **2009**, *32*, 38–43. [CrossRef]
150. Tsourouflis, G.; Theocharis, S.E.; Sampani, A.; Giagini, A.; Kostakis, A.; Kouraklis, G. Prognostic and predictive value of thymidylate synthase expression in colon cancer. *Dig. Dis. Sci.* **2008**, *53*, 1289–1296. [CrossRef]
151. Popat, S.; Matakidou, A.; Houlston, R.S. Thymidylate synthase expression and prognosis in colorectal cancer: A systematic review and meta-analysis. *J. Clin. Oncol.* **2004**, *22*, 529–536. [CrossRef]
152. Aschele, C.; Debernardis, D.; Tunesi, G.; Maley, F.; Sobrero, A. Thymidylate synthase protein expression in primary colorectal cancer compared with the corresponding distant metastases and relationship with the clinical response to 5-fluorouracil. *Clin. Cancer Res.* **2000**, *6*, 4797–4802. [PubMed]
153. Niedzwiecki, D.; Hasson, R.M.; Lenz, H.J.; Ye, C.; Redston, M.; Ogino, S.; Fuchs, C.S.; Compton, C.C.; Mayer, R.J.; Goldberg, R.M.; et al. A Study of Thymidylate Synthase Expression as a Biomarker for Resectable Colon Cancer: Alliance (Cancer and Leukemia Group B) 9581 and 89803. *Oncologist* **2017**, *22*, 107–114. [CrossRef] [PubMed]
154. Ma, Z.; Wu, Y.; Jin, J.; Yan, J.; Kuang, S.; Zhou, M.; Zhang, Y.; Guo, A.Y. Phylogenetic analysis reveals the evolution and diversification of cyclins in eukaryotes. *Mol. Phylogenet. Evol.* **2013**, *66*, 1002–1010. [CrossRef] [PubMed]
155. Bondi, J.; Husdal, A.; Bukholm, G.; Nesland, J.M.; Bakka, A.; Bukholm, I.R. Expression and gene amplification of primary (A, B1, D1, D3, and E) and secondary (C and H) cyclins in colon adenocarcinomas and correlation with patient outcome. *J. Clin. Pathol.* **2005**, *58*, 509–514. [CrossRef]
156. Yam, C.H.; Fung, T.K.; Poon, R.Y. Cyclin A in cell cycle control and cancer. *Cell. Mol. Life Sci.* **2002**, *59*, 1317–1326. [CrossRef]
157. Köhler, K.; Sanchez-Pulido, L.; Höfer, V.; Marko, A.; Ponting, C.P.; Snijders, A.P.; Feederle, R.; Schepers, A.; Boos, D. The Cdk8/19-cyclin C transcription regulator functions in genome replication through metazoan Sld7. *PLoS Biol.* **2019**, *17*, e2006767. [CrossRef]
158. Koff, A.; Cross, F.; Fisher, A.; Schumacher, J.; Leguellec, K.; Philippe, M.; Roberts, J.M. Human cyclin E, a new cyclin that interacts with two members of the CDC2 gene family. *Cell* **1991**, *66*, 1217–1228. [CrossRef]
159. Handa, K.; Yamakawa, M.; Takeda, H.; Kimura, S.; Takahashi, T. Expression of cell cycle markers in colorectal carcinoma: Superiority of cyclin A as an indicator of poor prognosis. *Int. J. Cancer* **1999**, *84*, 225–233. [CrossRef]
160. Bahnassy, A.A.; Zekri, A.R.; El-Houssini, S.; El-Shehaby, A.M.; Mahmoud, M.R.; Abdallah, S.; El-Serafi, M. Cyclin A and cyclin D1 as significant prognostic markers in colorectal cancer patients. *BMC Gastroenterol.* **2004**, *4*, 22. [CrossRef]
161. Edler, D.; Hallström, M.; Ragnhammar, P.; Blomgren, H. Thymidylate synthase expression in rectal cancer and proliferation, assessed by cyclin A and Ki-67 expression. *Anticancer Res.* **2002**, *22*, 3113–3116.
162. Nozoe, T.; Inutsuka, S.; Honda, M.; Ezaki, T.; Korenaga, D. Clinicopathologic significance of cyclin A expression in colorectal carcinoma. *J. Exp. Clin. Cancer Res.* **2004**, *23*, 127–133.
163. Zhao, D.B.; Chandler, I.; Chen, Z.M.; Pan, H.C.; Popat, S.; Shao, Y.F.; Houlston, R.S. Mismatch repair, minichromosome maintenance complex component 2, cyclin A, and transforming growth factor β receptor type II as prognostic factors for colorectal cancer: Results of a 10-year prospective study using tissue microarray analysis. *Chin. Med. J.* **2011**, *124*, 483–490. [PubMed]
164. Li, J.Q.; Kubo, A.; Wu, F.; Usuki, H.; Fujita, J.; Bandoh, S.; Masaki, T.; Saoo, K.; Takeuchi, H.; Kobayashi, S.; et al. Cyclin B1, unlike cyclin G1, increases significantly during colorectal carcinogenesis and during later metastasis to lymph nodes. *Int. J. Oncol.* **2003**, *22*, 1101–1110. [CrossRef] [PubMed]
165. Grabsch, H.; Lickvers, K.; Hansen, O.; Takeno, S.; Willers, R.; Stock, W.; Gabbert, H.E.; Mueller, W. Prognostic value of cyclin B1 protein expression in colorectal cancer. *Am. J. Clin. Pathol.* **2004**, *122*, 511–516. [CrossRef] [PubMed]

166. Fang, Y.; Liang, X.; Jiang, W.; Li, J.; Xu, J.; Cai, X. Cyclin b1 suppresses colorectal cancer invasion and metastasis by regulating e-cadherin. *PLoS ONE* **2015**, *10*, e0126875. [CrossRef]
167. Ye, C.; Wang, J.; Wu, P.; Li, X.; Chai, Y. Prognostic role of cyclin B1 in solid tumors: A meta-analysis. *Oncotarget* **2017**, *8*, 2224–2232. [CrossRef]
168. Firestein, R.; Shima, K.; Nosho, K.; Irahara, N.; Baba, Y.; Bojarski, E.; Giovannucci, E.L.; Hahn, W.C.; Fuchs, C.S.; Ogino, S. CDK8 expression in 470 colorectal cancers in relation to beta-catenin activation, other molecular alterations and patient survival. *Int. J. Cancer* **2010**, *126*, 2863–2873. [CrossRef]
169. Palaiologos, P.; Chrysikos, D.; Theocharis, S.; Kouraklis, G. The Prognostic Value of G1 Cyclins, p21 and Rb Protein in Patients with Colon Cancer. *Anticancer Res.* **2019**, *39*, 6291–6297. [CrossRef]
170. Li, Y.; Wei, J.; Xu, C.; Zhao, Z.; You, T. Prognostic significance of cyclin D1 expression in colorectal cancer: A meta-analysis of observational studies. *PLoS ONE* **2014**, *9*, e94508. [CrossRef]
171. Jun, S.Y.; Kim, J.; Yoon, N.; Maeng, L.S.; Byun, J.H. Prognostic Potential of Cyclin D1 Expression in Colorectal Cancer. *J. Clin. Med.* **2023**, *12*, 572. [CrossRef]
172. Maeda, K.; Chung, Y.; Kang, S.; Ogawa, M.; Onoda, N.; Nishiguchi, Y.; Ikehara, T.; Nakata, B.; Okuno, M.; Sowa, M. Cyclin D1 overexpression and prognosis in colorectal adenocarcinoma. *Oncology* **1998**, *55*, 145–151. [CrossRef]
173. Sarkar, R.; Hunter, I.A.; Rajaganeshan, R.; Perry, S.L.; Guillou, P.; Jayne, D.G. Expression of cyclin D2 is an independent predictor of the development of hepatic metastasis in colorectal cancer. *Color. Dis.* **2010**, *12*, 316–323. [CrossRef] [PubMed]
174. Mao, Y.; Li, Z.; Lou, C.; Zhang, Y. Expression of phosphorylated Stat5 predicts expression of cyclin D1 and correlates with poor prognosis of colonic adenocarcinoma. *Int. J. Color. Dis.* **2011**, *26*, 29–35. [CrossRef] [PubMed]
175. Luo, W.X.; Chen, Y.; Li, Y.T.; Tang, J.; Ding, J.; Du, Y.; Wu, Q.; Liu, J.Y. Selected proliferation markers correlated with dynamics of growth in colorectal cancer. *Eur. J. Cancer Prev.* **2019**, *28*, 181–187. [CrossRef]
176. Babic, A.; Miladinovic, N.; Milin Lazovic, J.; Milenkovic, S. Decreased ERβ expression and high cyclin D1 expression may predict early CRC recurrence in high-risk Duk's B and Duke's C stage. *J. BUON* **2021**, *26*, 536–543. [PubMed]
177. Palmqvist, R.; Stenling, R.; Oberg, A.; Landberg, G. Expression of cyclin D1 and retinoblastoma protein in colorectal cancer. *Eur. J. Cancer* **1998**, *34*, 1575–1581. [CrossRef] [PubMed]
178. Schwandner, O.; Bruch, H.P.; Broll, R. p21, p27, cyclin D1, and p53 in rectal cancer: Immunohistology with prognostic significance? *Int. J. Color. Dis.* **2002**, *17*, 11–19. [CrossRef]
179. Ioachim, E. Expression patterns of cyclins D1, E and cyclin-dependent kinase inhibitors p21waf1/cip1, p27kip1 in colorectal carcinoma: Correlation with other cell cycle regulators (pRb, p53 and Ki-67 and PCNA) and clinicopathological features. *Int. J. Clin. Pract.* **2008**, *62*, 1736–1743. [CrossRef]
180. Al-Maghrabi, J.; Mufti, S.; Gomaa, W.; Buhmeida, A.; Al-Qahtani, M.; Al-Ahwal, M. Immunoexpression of cyclin D1 in colorectal carcinomas is not correlated with survival outcome. *J. Microsc. Ultrastruct.* **2015**, *3*, 62–67. [CrossRef]
181. Ogino, S.; Nosho, K.; Irahara, N.; Kure, S.; Shima, K.; Baba, Y.; Toyoda, S.; Chen, L.; Giovannucci, E.L.; Meyerhardt, J.A.; et al. A cohort study of cyclin D1 expression and prognosis in 602 colon cancer cases. *Clin. Cancer Res.* **2009**, *15*, 4431–4438. [CrossRef]
182. Hilska, M.; Collan, Y.U.; O Laine, V.J.; Kössi, J.; Hirsimäki, P.; Laato, M.; Roberts, P.J. The significance of tumor markers for proliferation and apoptosis in predicting survival in colorectal cancer. *Dis. Colon Rectum* **2005**, *48*, 2197–2208. [CrossRef] [PubMed]
183. Holland, T.A.; Elder, J.; McCloud, J.M.; Hall, C.; Deakin, M.; Fryer, A.A.; Elder, J.B.; Hoban, P.R. Subcellular localisation of cyclin D1 protein in colorectal tumours is associated with p21(WAF1/CIP1) expression and correlates with patient survival. *Int. J. Cancer* **2001**, *95*, 302–306. [CrossRef] [PubMed]
184. Yan, H.; Jiang, F.; Yang, J. Association of β-Catenin, APC, SMAD3/4, Tp53, and Cyclin D1 Genes in Colorectal Cancer: A Systematic Review and Meta-Analysis. *Genet. Res.* **2022**, *2022*, 5338956. [CrossRef] [PubMed]
185. Li, W.; Zhang, G.; Wang, H.L.; Wang, L. Analysis of expression of cyclin E, p27kip1 and Ki67 protein in colorectal cancer tissues and its value for diagnosis, treatment and prognosis of disease. *Eur. Rev. Med. Pharmacol. Sci.* **2016**, *20*, 4874–4879. [PubMed]
186. Melincovici, C.S.; Mihu, C.M.; Mărginean, M.; Boşca, A.B.; Coneac, A.; Moldovan, I.; Crişan, M. The prognostic significance of p53, Bax, Bcl-2 and cyclin E protein overexpression in colon cancer—An immunohistochemical study using the tissue microarray technique. *Rom. J. Morphol. Embryol.* **2016**, *7*, 81–89.
187. Boehm, E.M.; Gildenberg, M.S.; Washington, M.T. The Many Roles of PCNA in Eukaryotic DNA Replication. *Enzymes* **2016**, *39*, 231–254. [CrossRef]
188. Lavezzi, A.M.; Ottaviani, G.; De Ruberto, F.; Fichera, G.; Matturri, L. Prognostic significance of different biomarkers (DNA content, PCNA, karyotype) in colorectal adenomas. *Anticancer Res.* **2002**, *22*, 2077–2081.
189. Al-Sheneber, I.F.; Shibata, H.R.; Sampalis, J.; Jothy, S. Prognostic significance of proliferating cell nuclear antigen expression in colorectal cancer. *Cancer* **1993**, *71*, 1954–1959. [CrossRef]
190. Choi, H.J.; Jung, I.K.; Kim, S.S.; Hong, S.H. Proliferating cell nuclear antigen expression and its relationship to malignancy potential in invasive colorectal carcinomas. *Dis. Colon Rectum* **1997**, *40*, 51–59. [CrossRef]
191. Neoptolemos, J.P.; Oates, G.D.; Newbold, K.M.; Robson, A.M.; McConkey, C.; Powell, J. Cyclin/proliferation cell nuclear antigen immunohistochemistry does not improve the prognostic power of Dukes' or Jass' classifications for colorectal cancer. *Br. J. Surg.* **1995**, *82*, 184–187. [CrossRef]

192. Mayer, A.; Takimoto, M.; Fritz, E.; Schellander, G.; Kofler, K.; Ludwig, H. The prognostic significance of proliferating cell nuclear antigen, epidermal growth factor receptor, and mdr gene expression in colorectal cancer. *Cancer* **1993**, *71*, 2454–2460. [CrossRef] [PubMed]
193. Teixeira, C.R.; Tanaka, S.; Haruma, K.; Yoshihara, M.; Sumii, K.; Kajiyama, G. Proliferating cell nuclear antigen expression at the invasive tumor margin predicts malignant potential of colorectal carcinomas. *Cancer* **1994**, *73*, 575–579. [CrossRef] [PubMed]
194. Nakamura, T.; Tabuchi, Y.; Nakae, S.; Ohno, M.; Saitoh, Y. Serum carcinoembryonic antigen levels and proliferating cell nuclear antigen labeling index for patients with colorectal carcinoma. Correlation with tumor progression and survival. *Cancer* **1996**, *77*, 1741–1746. [CrossRef]
195. Sandler, R.S.; Baron, J.A.; Tosteson, T.D.; Mandel, J.S.; Haile, R.W. Rectal mucosal proliferation and risk of colorectal adenomas: Results from a randomized controlled trial. *Cancer Epidemiol. Biomark. Prev.* **2000**, *9*, 653–656.
196. Kunihiro, M.; Tanaka, S.; Haruma, K.; Yoshihara, M.; Sumii, K.; Kajiyama, G.; Shimamoto, F. Combined expression of HLA-DR antigen and proliferating cell nuclear antigen correlate with colorectal cancer prognosis. *Oncology* **1998**, *55*, 326–333. [CrossRef]
197. Guzińska-Ustymowicz, K.; Pryczynicz, A.; Kemona, A.; Czyzewska, J. Correlation between proliferation markers: PCNA, Ki-67, MCM-2 and antiapoptotic protein Bcl-2 in colorectal cancer. *Anticancer Res.* **2009**, *29*, 3049–3052.
198. Zhou, H.; Huang, T.; Xiong, Y.; Peng, L.; Wang, R.; Zhang, G.J. The prognostic value of proliferating cell nuclear antigen expression in colorectal cancer: A meta-analysis. *Medicine* **2018**, *97*, e13574. [CrossRef]
199. Gerdes, J.; Schwab, U.; Lemke, H.; Stein, H. Production of a mouse monoclonal antibody reactive with a human nuclear antigen associated with cell proliferation. *Int. J. Cancer* **1983**, *31*, 13–20. [CrossRef]
200. Schlüter, C.; Duchrow, M.; Wohlenberg, C.; Becker, M.H.; Key, G.; Flad, H.D.; Gerdes, J. The cell proliferation-associated antigen of antibody Ki-67: A very large, ubiquitous nuclear protein with numerous repeated elements, representing a new kind of cell cycle-maintaining proteins. *J. Cell Biol.* **1993**, *123*, 513–522. [CrossRef]
201. Gerdes, J.; Li, L.; Schlueter, C.; Duchrow, M.; Wohlenberg, C.; Gerlach, C.; Stahmer, I.; Kloth, S.; Brandt, E.; Flad, H.D. Immunobiochemical and molecular biologic characterization of the cell proliferation-associated nuclear antigen that is defined by monoclonal antibody Ki-67. *Am. J. Pathol.* **1991**, *138*, 867–873.
202. Brown, D.C.; Gatter, K.C. Monoclonal antibody Ki-67: Its use in histopathology. *Histopathology* **1990**, *17*, 489–503. [CrossRef]
203. Chierico, L.; Rizzello, L.; Guan, L.; Joseph, A.S.; Lewis, A.; Battaglia, G. The role of the two splice variants and extranuclear pathway on Ki-67 regulation in non-cancer and cancer cells. *PLoS ONE* **2017**, *12*, e0171815. [CrossRef]
204. Menon, S.S.; Guruvayoorappan, C.; Sakthivel, K.M.; Rasmi, R.R. Ki-67 protein as a tumour proliferation marker. *Clin. Chim. Acta* **2019**, *491*, 39–45. [CrossRef]
205. Remnant, L.; Kochanova, N.Y.; Reid, C.; Cisneros-Soberanis, F.; Earnshaw, W.C. The intrinsically disordered story of Ki-67. *Open Biol.* **2021**, *11*, 210120. [CrossRef]
206. Andrés-Sánchez, N.; Fisher, D.; Krasinska, L. Physiological functions and roles in cancer of the proliferation marker Ki-67. *J. Cell Sci.* **2022**, *135*, jcs258932. [CrossRef]
207. Luo, Z.W.; Zhu, M.G.; Zhang, Z.Q.; Ye, F.J.; Huang, W.H.; Luo, X.Z. Increased expression of Ki-67 is a poor prognostic marker for colorectal cancer patients: A meta analysis. *BMC Cancer* **2019**, *19*, 123. [CrossRef]
208. Cheutin, T.; O'Donohue, M.F.; Beorchia, A.; Klein, C.; Kaplan, H.; Ploton, D. Three-dimensional organization of pKi-67: A comparative fluorescence and electron tomography study using FluoroNanogold. *J. Histochem. Cytochem.* **2003**, *51*, 1411–1423. [CrossRef]
209. Bullwinkel, J.; Baron-Lühr, B.; Lüdemann, A.; Wohlenberg, C.; Gerdes, J.; Scholzen, T. Ki-67 protein is associated with ribosomal RNA transcription in quiescent and proliferating cells. *J. Cell. Physiol.* **2006**, *206*, 624–635. [CrossRef]
210. Miller, I.; Min, M.; Yang, C.; Tian, C.; Gookin, S.; Carter, D.; Spencer, S.L. Ki67 is a Graded Rather than a Binary Marker of Proliferation versus Quiescence. *Cell Rep.* **2018**, *24*, 1105–1112.e5. [CrossRef]
211. Stamatiou, K.; Vagnarelli, P. Chromosome clustering in mitosis by the nuclear protein Ki-67. *Biochem. Soc. Trans.* **2021**, *49*, 2767–2776. [CrossRef]
212. Cuylen, S.; Blaukopf, C.; Politi, A.Z.; Müller-Reichert, T.; Neumann, B.; Poser, I.; Ellenberg, J.; Hyman, A.A.; Gerlich, D.W. Ki-67 acts as a biological surfactant to disperse mitotic chromosomes. *Nature* **2016**, *535*, 308–312. [CrossRef] [PubMed]
213. Cuylen-Haering, S.; Petrovic, M.; Hernandez-Armendariz, A.; Schneider, M.W.G.; Samwer, M.; Blaukopf, C.; Holt, L.J.; Gerlich, D.W. Chromosome clustering by Ki-67 excludes cytoplasm during nuclear assembly. *Nature* **2020**, *587*, 285–290. [CrossRef]
214. Booth, D.G.; Takagi, M.; Sanchez-Pulido, L.; Petfalski, E.; Vargiu, G.; Samejima, K.; Imamoto, N.; Ponting, C.P.; Tollervey, D.; Earnshaw, W.C.; et al. Ki-67 is a PP1-interacting protein that organises the mitotic chromosome periphery. *Elife* **2014**, *27*, e01641. [CrossRef] [PubMed]
215. Sobecki, M.; Mrouj, K.; Camasses, A.; Parisis, N.; Nicolas, E.; Llères, D.; Gerbe, F.; Prieto, S.; Krasinska, L.; David, A.; et al. The cell proliferation antigen Ki-67 organises heterochromatin. *Elife* **2016**, *5*, e13722. [CrossRef] [PubMed]
216. Sales Gil, R.; Vagnarelli, P. Ki-67: More Hidden behind a 'Classic Proliferation Marker'. *Trends Biochem. Sci.* **2018**, *43*, 747–748. [CrossRef] [PubMed]
217. Nayak, J.; Mohanty, P.; Lenka, A.; Sahoo, N.; Agrawala, S.; Panigrahi, S.K. Histopathological and Immunohistochemical Evaluation of CDX2 and Ki67 in Colorectal Lesions with their Expression Pattern in Different Histologic Variants, Grade, and Stage of Colorectal Carcinomas. *J. Microsc. Ultrastruct.* **2021**, *9*, 183–189. [CrossRef]

218. Saleh, H.A.; Jackson, H.; Banerjee, M. Immunohistochemical expression of bcl-2 and p53 oncoproteins: Correlation with Ki67 proliferation index and prognostic histopathologic parameters in colorectal neoplasia. *Appl. Immunohistochem. Mol. Morphol.* **2000**, *8*, 175–812. [CrossRef]
219. Ishida, H.; Sadahiro, S.; Suzuki, T.; Ishikawa, K.; Kamijo, A.; Tajima, T.; Makuuchi, H.; Murayama, C. Proliferative, infiltrative, and metastatic activities in colorectal tumors assessed by MIB-1 antibody. *Oncol. Rep.* **2003**, *10*, 1741–1745. [CrossRef]
220. Woodland, J.G. CDX-2 and MIB-1 expression in the colorectum: Correlation with morphological features of adenomatous lesions. *Br. J. Biomed. Sci.* **2006**, *63*, 68–73. [CrossRef]
221. Kitabatake, T.; Kojima, K.; Fukasawa, M.; Beppu, T.; Futagawa, S. Correlation of thymidine phosphorylase staining and the Ki-67 labeling index to clinicopathologic factors and hepatic metastasis in patients with colorectal cancer. *Surg. Today* **2002**, *32*, 322–328. [CrossRef]
222. Dziegiel, P.; Forgacz, J.; Suder, E.; Surowiak, P.; Kornafel, J.; Zabel, M. Prognostic significance of metallothionein expression in correlation with Ki-67 expression in adenocarcinomas of large intestine. *Histol. Histopathol.* **2003**, *18*, 401–407. [CrossRef] [PubMed]
223. Valera, V.; Yokoyama, N.; Walter, B.; Okamoto, H.; Suda, T.; Hatakeyama, K. Clinical significance of Ki-67 proliferation index in disease progression and prognosis of patients with resected colorectal carcinoma. *Br. J. Surg.* **2005**, *92*, 1002–1007. [CrossRef] [PubMed]
224. Gurzu, S.; Jung, J.; Mezei, T.; Pávai, Z. The correlation between the immunostains for p53 and Ki67 with bcl-2 expression and classical prognostic factors in colorectal carcinomas. *Rom. J. Morphol. Embryol.* **2007**, *48*, 95–99.
225. Ma, Y.L.; Peng, J.Y.; Zhang, P.; Liu, W.J.; Huang, L.; Qin, H.L. Immunohistochemical analysis revealed CD34 and Ki67 protein expression as significant prognostic factors in colorectal cancer. *Med. Oncol.* **2010**, *27*, 304–309. [CrossRef] [PubMed]
226. Martins, S.F.; Amorim, R.; Mota, S.C.; Costa, L.; Pardal, F.; Rodrigues, M.; Longatto-Filho, A. Ki-67 Expression in CRC Lymph Node Metastasis Does Not Predict Survival. *Biomed Res. Int.* **2015**, *2015*, 131685. [CrossRef] [PubMed]
227. Sen, A.; Mitra, S.; Das, R.N.; Dasgupta, S.; Saha, K.; Chatterjee, U.; Mukherjee, K.; Datta, C.; Chattopadhyay, B.K. Expression of CDX-2 and Ki-67 in different grades of colorectal adenocarcinomas. *Indian J. Pathol. Microbiol.* **2015**, *58*, 158–162. [CrossRef] [PubMed]
228. Wang, L.; Liu, Z.; Fisher, K.W.; Ren, F.; Lv, J.; Davidson, D.D.; Baldridge, L.A.; Du, X.; Cheng, L. Prognostic value of programmed death ligand 1, p53, and Ki-67 in patients with advanced-stage colorectal cancer. *Hum. Pathol.* **2018**, *71*, 20–29. [CrossRef]
229. Tong, G.; Zhang, G.; Liu, J.; Zheng, Z.; Chen, Y.; Niu, P.; Xu, X. Cutoff of 25% for Ki67 expression is a good classification tool for prognosis in colorectal cancer in the AJCC-8 stratification. *Oncol. Rep.* **2020**, *43*, 1187–1198. [CrossRef]
230. Lei, H.T.; Yan, S.; He, Y.H.; Xu, N.; Zhao, M.; Yu, C.J.; Li, H.L.; Kuang, S.; Cui, Z.H.; Fang, J. Ki67 testing in the clinical management of patients with non-metastatic colorectal cancer: Detecting the optimal cut-off value based on the Restricted Cubic Spline model. *Oncol. Lett.* **2022**, *24*, 420. [CrossRef]
231. Lanza, G., Jr.; Cavazzini, L.; Borghi, L.; Ferretti, S.; Buccoliero, F.; Rubbini, M. Immunohistochemical assessment of growth fractions in colorectal adenocarcinomas with monoclonal antibody Ki-67. Relation to clinical and pathological variables. *Pathol. Res. Pract.* **1990**, *186*, 608–618. [CrossRef]
232. Meteoglu, I.; Erdogdu, I.H.; Tuncyurek, P.; Coskun, A.; Culhaci, N.; Erkus, M.; Barutca, S. Nuclear Factor Kappa B, Matrix Metalloproteinase-1, p53, and Ki-67 Expressions in the Primary Tumors and the Lymph Node Metastases of Colorectal Cancer Cases. *Gastroenterol. Res. Pract.* **2015**, *2015*, 945392. [CrossRef] [PubMed]
233. Ofner, D.; Grothaus, A.; Riedmann, B.; Larcher, P.; Maier, H.; Bankfalvi, A.; Schmid, K.W. MIB1 in colorectal carcinomas: Its evaluation by three different methods reveals lack of prognostic significance. *Anal. Cell. Pathol.* **1996**, *12*, 61–70. [PubMed]
234. Jansson, A.; Sun, X.F. Ki-67 expression in relation to clinicopathological variables and prognosis in colorectal adenocarcinomas. *APMIS* **1997**, *105*, 730–734. [CrossRef] [PubMed]
235. Huh, J.W.; Lee, J.H.; Kim, H.R. Expression of p16, p53, and Ki-67 in colorectal adenocarcinoma: A study of 356 surgically resected cases. *Hepatogastroenterology* **2010**, *57*, 734–740.
236. Duchrow, M.; Ziemann, T.; Windhövel, U.; Bruch, H.P.; Broll, R. Colorectal carcinomas with high MIB-1 labelling indices but low pKi67 mRNA levels correlate with better prognostic outcome. *Histopathology* **2003**, *42*, 566–574. [CrossRef]
237. Melling, N.; Kowitz, C.M.; Simon, R.; Bokemeyer, C.; Terracciano, L.; Sauter, G.; Izbicki, J.R.; Marx, A.H. High Ki67 expression is an independent good prognostic marker in colorectal cancer. *J. Clin. Pathol.* **2016**, *69*, 209–214. [CrossRef]
238. Ivanecz, A.; Kavalar, R.; Palfy, M.; Pivec, V.; Sremec, M.; Horvat, M.; Potrč, S. Can we improve the clinical risk score? The prognostic value of p53, Ki-67 and thymidylate synthase in patients undergoing radical resection of colorectal liver metastases. *HPB* **2014**, *16*, 235–242. [CrossRef]
239. Fernebro, E.; Bendahl, P.O.; Dictor, M.; Persson, A.; Fernö, M.; Nilbert, M. Immunohistochemical patterns in rectal cancer: Application of tissue microarray with prognostic correlations. *Int. J. Cancer* **2004**, *111*, 921–928. [CrossRef]
240. Ishida, H.; Miwa, H.; Tatsuta, M.; Masutani, S.; Imamura, H.; Shimizu, J.; Ezumi, K.; Kato, H.; Kawasaki, T.; Furukawa, H.; et al. Ki-67 and CEA expression as prognostic markers in Dukes' C colorectal cancer. *Cancer Lett.* **2004**, *207*, 109–115. [CrossRef]
241. Lumachi, F.; Orlando, R.; Marino, F.; Chiara, G.B.; Basso, S.M. Expression of p53 and Ki-67 as prognostic factors for survival of men with colorectal cancer. *Anticancer Res.* **2012**, *32*, 3965–3967.
242. Hur, H.; Tulina, I.; Cho, M.S.; Min, B.S.; Koom, W.S.; Lim, J.S.; Ahn, J.B.; Kim, N.K. Biomarker-Based Scoring System for Prediction of Tumor Response After Preoperative Chemoradiotherapy in Rectal Cancer by Reverse Transcriptase Polymerase Chain Reaction Analysis. *Dis. Colon Rectum* **2016**, *59*, 1174–1182. [CrossRef]

243. Valera, V.A.; Walter, B.A.; Yokoyama, N.; Koyama, Y.; Iiai, T.; Okamoto, H.; Hatakeyama, K. Prognostic groups in colorectal carcinoma patients based on tumor cell proliferation and classification and regression tree (CART) survival analysis. *Ann. Surg. Oncol.* **2007**, *14*, 34–40. [CrossRef] [PubMed]
244. Erstad, D.J.; Tumusiime, G.; Cusack, J.C., Jr. Prognostic and Predictive Biomarkers in Colorectal Cancer: Implications for the Clinical Surgeon. *Ann. Surg. Oncol.* **2015**, *22*, 3433–3450. [CrossRef] [PubMed]
245. Das, V.; Kalita, J.; Pal, M. Predictive and prognostic biomarkers in colorectal cancer: A systematic review of recent advances and challenges. *Biomed. Pharmacother.* **2017**, *87*, 8–19. [CrossRef] [PubMed]
246. Caramaschi, S.; Mangogna, A.; Salviato, T.; Ammendola, S.; Barresi, V.; Manco, G.; Canu, P.G.; Zanelli, G.; Bonetti, L.R. Cytoproliferative activity in colorectal poorly differentiated clusters: Biological significance in tumor setting. *Ann. Diagn. Pathol.* **2021**, *53*, 151772. [CrossRef]
247. Palmqvist, R.; Sellberg, P.; Oberg, A.; Tavelin, B.; Rutegård, J.N.; Stenling, R. Low tumour cell proliferation at the invasive margin is associated with a poor prognosis in Dukes' stage B colorectal cancers. *Br. J. Cancer* **1999**, *79*, 577–581. [CrossRef]
248. Salminen, E.; Palmu, S.; Vahlberg, T.; Roberts, P.J.; Söderström, K.O. Increased proliferation activity measured by immunoreactive Ki67 is associated with survival improvement in rectal/recto sigmoid cancer. *World J. Gastroenterol.* **2005**, *11*, 3245–3249. [CrossRef]
249. Xi, H.Q.; Zhao, P. Clinicopathological significance and prognostic value of EphA3 and CD133 expression in colorectal carcinoma. *J. Clin. Pathol.* **2011**, *64*, 498–503. [CrossRef]
250. Li, P.; Xiao, Z.T.; Braciak, T.A.; Ou, Q.J.; Chen, G.; Oduncu, F.S. Association between Ki67 Index and Clinicopathological Features in Colorectal Cancer. *Oncol. Res. Treat.* **2016**, *39*, 696–702. [CrossRef]
251. Petrowsky, H.; Sturm, I.; Graubitz, O.; Kooby, D.A.; Staib-Sebler, E.; Gog, C.; Köhne, C.H.; Hillebrand, T.; Daniel, P.T.; Fong, Y.; et al. Relevance of Ki-67 antigen expression and K-ras mutation in colorectal liver metastases. *Eur. J. Surg. Oncol.* **2001**, *27*, 80–87. [CrossRef]
252. Nash, G.M.; Gimbel, M.; Shia, J.; Nathanson, D.R.; Ndubuisi, M.I.; Zeng, Z.S.; Kemeny, N.; Paty, P.B. KRAS mutation correlates with accelerated metastatic progression in patients with colorectal liver metastases. *Ann. Surg. Oncol.* **2010**, *17*, 572–578. [CrossRef] [PubMed]
253. Torén, W.; Ansari, D.; Andersson, R. Immunohistochemical investigation of prognostic biomarkers in resected colorectal liver metastases: A systematic review and meta-analysis. *Cancer Cell Int.* **2018**, *18*, 217. [CrossRef] [PubMed]
254. Yoshikawa, K.; Shimada, M.; Higashijima, J.; Nakao, T.; Nishi, M.; Takasu, C.; Kashihara, H.; Eto, S.; Bando, Y. Ki-67 and Survivin as Predictive Factors for Rectal Cancer Treated with Preoperative Chemoradiotherapy. *Anticancer Res.* **2018**, *38*, 1735–1739. [CrossRef] [PubMed]
255. Taha, A.; Taha-Mehlitz, S.; Petzold, S.; Achinovich, S.L.; Zinovkin, D.; Enodien, B.; Pranjol, M.Z.I.; Nadyrov, E.A. Prognostic Value of Immunohistochemical Markers for Locally Advanced Rectal Cancer. *Molecules* **2022**, *27*, 596. [CrossRef]
256. Papagiorgis, P.C. Segmental distribution of some common molecular markers for colorectal cancer (CRC): Influencing factors and potential implications. *Tumour Biol.* **2016**, *37*, 5727–5734. [CrossRef]
257. Reimers, M.S.; Zeestraten, E.C.; Kuppen, P.J.; Liefers, G.J.; van de Velde, C.J. Biomarkers in precision therapy in colorectal cancer. *Gastroenterol. Rep.* **2013**, *1*, 166–183. [CrossRef]
258. Allar, B.G.; Messaris, E.; Poylin, V.Y.; Schlechter, B.L.; Cataldo, T.E. Oncotype DX testing does not affect clinical practice in stage IIa colon cancer. *Med. Oncol.* **2022**, *39*, 59. [CrossRef]
259. Duchrow, M.; Häsemeyer, S.; Broll, R.; Bruch, H.P.; Windhövel, U. Assessment of proliferative activity in colorectal carcinomas by quantitative reverse transcriptase-polymerase chain reaction (RT-PCR). *Cancer Investig.* **2001**, *19*, 588–596. [CrossRef]
260. Michael-Robinson, J.M.; Reid, L.E.; Purdie, D.M.; Biemer-Hüttmann, A.E.; Walsh, M.D.; Pandeya, N.; Simms, L.A.; Young, J.P.; Leggett, B.A.; Jass, J.R.; et al. Proliferation, apoptosis, and survival in high-level microsatellite instability sporadic colorectal cancer. *Clin. Cancer Res.* **2001**, *7*, 2347–2356.
261. Evans, C.; Morrison, I.; Heriot, A.G.; Bartlett, J.B.; Finlayson, C.; Dalgleish, A.G.; Kumar, D. The correlation between colorectal cancer rates of proliferation and apoptosis and systemic cytokine levels; plus their influence upon survival. *Br. J. Cancer* **2006**, *94*, 1412–1419. [CrossRef]
262. Kaczmarek, E.; Banasiewicz, T.; Seraszek-Jaros, A.; Krokowicz, P.; Grochowalski, M.; Majewski, P.; Zurawski, J.; Paszkowski, J.; Drews, M. Digital image analysis of inflammation markers in colorectal mucosa by using a spatial visualization method. *Pathol. Res. Pract.* **2014**, *210*, 147–154. [CrossRef] [PubMed]
263. Yue, S.Q.; Yang, Y.L.; Dou, K.F.; Li, K.Z. Expression of PCNA and CD44mRNA in colorectal cancer with venous invasion and its relationship to liver metastasis. *World J. Gastroenterol.* **2003**, *9*, 2863–2865. [CrossRef] [PubMed]
264. Cai, F.; Li, J.; Pan, X.; Zhang, C.; Wei, D.; Gao, C. Increased Expression of PCNA-AS1 in Colorectal Cancer and its Clinical Association. *Clin. Lab.* **2017**, *63*, 1809–1814. [CrossRef] [PubMed]
265. Zhu, L.; Liu, J.; Ma, S.; Zhang, S. Long Noncoding RNA MALAT-1 Can Predict Metastasis and a Poor Prognosis: A Meta-Analysis. *Pathol. Oncol. Res.* **2015**, *21*, 1259–1264. [CrossRef]
266. Perakis, S.O.; Thomas, J.E.; Pichler, M. Non-coding RNAs Enabling Prognostic Stratification and Prediction of Therapeutic Response in Colorectal Cancer Patients. *Adv. Exp. Med. Biol.* **2016**, *937*, 183–204. [CrossRef] [PubMed]
267. Yamada, A.; Yu, P.; Lin, W.; Okugawa, Y.; Boland, C.R.; Goel, A. A RNA-Sequencing approach for the identification of novel long non-coding RNA biomarkers in colorectal cancer. *Sci. Rep.* **2018**, *8*, 575. [CrossRef]
268. Chen, B.; Zhang, R.N.; Fan, X.; Wang, J.; Xu, C.; An, B.; Wang, Q.; Wang, J.; Leung, E.L.; Sui, X.; et al. Clinical diagnostic value of long non-coding RNAs in Colorectal Cancer: A systematic review and meta-analysis. *J. Cancer* **2020**, *11*, 5518–5526. [CrossRef]

269. Chen, S.; Shen, X. Long noncoding RNAs: Functions and mechanisms in colon cancer. *Mol. Cancer* **2020**, *19*, 167. [CrossRef]
270. Zhang, L.; Li, C.; Su, X. Emerging impact of the long noncoding RNA MIR22HG on proliferation and apoptosis in multiple human cancers. *J. Exp. Clin. Cancer Res.* **2020**, *39*, 271. [CrossRef]
271. Zhang, J.; Li, K.; Zheng, H.; Zhu, Y. Research progress review on long non-coding RNA in colorectal cancer. *Neoplasma* **2021**, *68*, 240–252. [CrossRef]
272. Lulli, M.; Napoli, C.; Landini, I.; Mini, E.; Lapucci, A. Role of Non-Coding RNAs in Colorectal Cancer: Focus on Long Non-Coding RNAs. *Int. J. Mol. Sci.* **2022**, *23*, 13431. [CrossRef] [PubMed]
273. St Laurent, G.; Wahlestedt, C.; Kapranov, P. The Landscape of long noncoding RNA classification. *Trends Genet.* **2015**, *31*, 239–251. [CrossRef] [PubMed]
274. Hombach, S.; Kretz, M. Non-coding RNAs: Classification, Biology and Functioning. *Adv. Exp. Med. Biol.* **2016**, *937*, 3–17. [CrossRef] [PubMed]
275. Takahashi, Y.; Sawada, G.; Kurashige, J.; Uchi, R.; Matsumura, T.; Ueo, H.; Takano, Y.; Eguchi, H.; Sudo, T.; Sugimachi, K.; et al. Amplification of PVT-1 is involved in poor prognosis via apoptosis inhibition in colorectal cancers. *Br. J. Cancer* **2014**, *110*, 164–171. [CrossRef] [PubMed]
276. To, K.K.; Tong, C.W.; Wu, M.; Cho, W.C. MicroRNAs in the prognosis and therapy of colorectal cancer: From bench to bedside. *World J. Gastroenterol.* **2018**, *24*, 2949–2973. [CrossRef] [PubMed]
277. Zhan, W.; Liao, X.; Chen, Z.; Li, L.; Tian, T.; Yu, L.; Li, R. LINC00858 promotes colorectal cancer by sponging miR-4766-5p to regulate PAK2. *Cell Biol. Toxicol.* **2020**, *36*, 333–347. [CrossRef]
278. Zhan, Y.X.; Luo, G.H. DNA methylation detection methods used in colorectal cancer. *World J. Clin. Cases* **2019**, *7*, 2916–2929. [CrossRef]
279. Ragusa, M.; Barbagallo, C.; Statello, L.; Condorelli, A.G.; Battaglia, R.; Tamburello, L.; Barbagallo, D.; Di Pietro, C.; Purrello, M. Non-coding landscapes of colorectal cancer. *World J. Gastroenterol.* **2015**, *21*, 11709–11739. [CrossRef]
280. Wang, J.; Song, Y.X.; Ma, B.; Wang, J.J.; Sun, J.X.; Chen, X.W.; Zhao, J.H.; Yang, Y.C.; Wang, Z.N. Regulatory Roles of Non-Coding RNAs in Colorectal Cancer. *Int. J. Mol. Sci.* **2015**, *16*, 19886–19919. [CrossRef]
281. He, J.; Wu, M. Comprehensive landscape and future perspectives of long noncoding RNAs (lncRNAs) in colorectal cancer (CRC): Based on a bibliometric analysis. *Noncoding RNA Res.* **2022**, *8*, 33–52. [CrossRef]
282. Fadaka, A.O.; Pretorius, A.; Klein, A. Biomarkers for Stratification in Colorectal Cancer: MicroRNAs. *Cancer Control* **2019**, *26*, 1073274819862784. [CrossRef] [PubMed]
283. Dos Santos, I.L.; Penna, K.G.B.D.; Dos Santos Carneiro, M.A.; Libera, L.S.D.; Ramos, J.E.P.; Saddi, V.A. Tissue micro-RNAs associated with colorectal cancer prognosis: A systematic review. *Mol. Biol. Rep.* **2021**, *48*, 1853–1867. [CrossRef] [PubMed]
284. Zhang, Q.; Zhong, C.; Duan, S. The tumorigenic function of LINC00858 in cancer. *Biomed. Pharmacother.* **2021**, *143*, 112235. [CrossRef] [PubMed]
285. Sha, Q.K.; Chen, L.; Xi, J.Z.; Song, H. Long non-coding RNA LINC00858 promotes cells proliferation, migration and invasion by acting as a ceRNA of miR-22-3p in colorectal cancer. *Artif. Cells Nanomed. Biotechnol.* **2019**, *47*, 1057–1066. [CrossRef] [PubMed]
286. Li, X.; Wang, F.; Sun, Y.; Fan, Q.; Cui, G. Expression of long non-coding RNA PANDAR and its prognostic value in colorectal cancer patients. *Int. J. Biol. Markers* **2017**, *32*, e218–e223. [CrossRef]
287. Rivandi, M.; Pasdar, A.; Hamzezadeh, L.; Tajbakhsh, A.; Seifi, S.; Moetamani-Ahmadi, M.; Ferns, G.A.; Avan, A. The prognostic and therapeutic values of long noncoding RNA PANDAR in colorectal cancer. *J. Cell. Physiol.* **2019**, *234*, 1230–1236. [CrossRef]
288. Xu, J.; Shao, T.; Song, M.; Xie, Y.; Zhou, J.; Yin, J.; Ding, N.; Zou, H.; Li, Y.; Zhang, J. MIR22HG acts as a tumor suppressor via TGFβ/SMAD signaling and facilitates immunotherapy in colorectal cancer. *Mol. Cancer* **2020**, *19*, 51. [CrossRef]
289. Thorenoor, N.; Faltejskova-Vychytilova, P.; Hombach, S.; Mlcochova, J.; Kretz, M.; Svoboda, M.; Slaby, O. Long non-coding RNA ZFAS1 interacts with CDK1 and is involved in p53-dependent cell cycle control and apoptosis in colorectal cancer. *Oncotarget* **2016**, *7*, 622–637. [CrossRef]
290. Fu, Y.; Huang, R.; Li, J.; Xie, X.; Deng, Y. LncRNA ENSG00000254615 Modulates Proliferation and 5-FU Resistance by Regulating p21 and Cyclin D1 in Colorectal Cancer. *Cancer Investig.* **2021**, *39*, 696–710. [CrossRef]
291. Yang, H.; Wang, S.; Kang, Y.J.; Wang, C.; Xu, Y.; Zhang, Y.; Jiang, Z. Long non-coding RNA SNHG1 predicts a poor prognosis and promotes colon cancer tumorigenesis. *Oncol. Rep.* **2018**, *40*, 261–271. [CrossRef]
292. Liu, K.L.; Wu, J.; Li, W.K.; Li, N.S.; Li, Q.; Lao, Y.Q. LncRNA SNHG7 is an Oncogenic Biomarker Interacting with MicroRNA-193b in Colon Carcinogenesis. *Clin. Lab.* **2019**, *65*, 2199–2204. [CrossRef] [PubMed]
293. Sun, N.; Zhang, G.; Liu, Y. Long non-coding RNA XIST sponges miR-34a to promotes colon cancer progression via Wnt/β-catenin signaling pathway. *Gene* **2018**, *665*, 141–148. [CrossRef] [PubMed]
294. Wu, K.; Zhang, N.; Ma, J.; Huang, J.; Chen, J.; Wang, L.; Zhang, J. Long noncoding RNA FAL1 promotes proliferation and inhibits apoptosis of human colon cancer cells. *IUBMB Life* **2018**, *70*, 1093–1100. [CrossRef] [PubMed]
295. Andrabi, M.Q.; Kesavan, Y.; Ramalingam, S. Non-Coding RNA as Biomarkers for Survival in Colorectal Cancer Patients. *Curr. Aging Sci.* **2023**. [CrossRef]
296. Baharudin, R.; Rus Bakarurraini, N.Q.; Ismail, I.; Lee, L.H.; Ab Mutalib, N.S. MicroRNA Methylome Signature and Their Functional Roles in Colorectal Cancer Diagnosis, Prognosis, and Chemoresistance. *Int. J. Mol. Sci.* **2022**, *23*, 7281. [CrossRef]
297. Peng, Q.; Zhang, X.; Min, M.; Zou, L.; Shen, P.; Zhu, Y. The clinical role of microRNA-21 as a promising biomarker in the diagnosis and prognosis of colorectal cancer: A systematic review and meta-analysis. *Oncotarget* **2017**, *8*, 44893–44909. [CrossRef]

298. Gu, X.; Jin, R.; Mao, X.; Wang, J.; Yuan, J.; Zhao, G. Prognostic value of miRNA-181a/b in colorectal cancer: A meta-analysis. *Biomark. Med.* **2018**, *12*, 299–308. [CrossRef]
299. Moody, L.; Dvoretskiy, S.; An, R.; Mantha, S.; Pan, Y.X. The Efficacy of miR-20a as a Diagnostic and Prognostic Biomarker for Colorectal Cancer: A Systematic Review and Meta-Analysis. *Cancers* **2019**, *11*, 1111. [CrossRef]
300. Wu, Y.; Hong, Q.; Lu, F.; Zhang, Z.; Li, J.; Nie, Z.; He, B. The Diagnostic and Prognostic Value of miR-155 in Cancers: An Updated Meta-analysis. *Mol. Diagn. Ther.* **2023**, *27*, 283–301. [CrossRef]
301. Sabarimurugan, S.; Madhav, M.R.; Kumarasamy, C.; Gupta, A.; Baxi, S.; Krishnan, S.; Jayaraj, R. Prognostic Value of MicroRNAs in Stage II Colorectal Cancer Patients: A Systematic Review and Meta-Analysis. *Mol. Diagn. Ther.* **2020**, *24*, 15–30. [CrossRef]
302. Gao, S.; Zhao, Z.Y.; Wu, R.; Zhang, Y.; Zhang, Z.Y. Prognostic value of microRNAs in colorectal cancer: A meta-analysis. *Cancer Manag. Res.* **2018**, *10*, 907–929. [CrossRef] [PubMed]
303. Galamb, O.; Barták, B.K.; Kalmár, A.; Nagy, Z.B.; Szigeti, K.A.; Tulassay, Z.; Igaz, P.; Molnár, B. Diagnostic and prognostic potential of tissue and circulating long non-coding RNAs in colorectal tumors. *World J. Gastroenterol.* **2019**, *25*, 5026–5048. [CrossRef] [PubMed]
304. Qi, P.; Xu, M.D.; Ni, S.J.; Huang, D.; Wei, P.; Tan, C.; Zhou, X.Y.; Du, X. Low expression of LOC285194 is associated with poor prognosis in colorectal cancer. *J. Transl. Med.* **2013**, *11*, 122. [CrossRef] [PubMed]
305. Fan, H.; Zhu, J.H.; Yao, X.Q. Long non-coding RNA PVT1 as a novel potential biomarker for predicting the prognosis of colorectal cancer. *Int. J. Biol. Markers* **2018**, *33*, 415–422. [CrossRef]
306. Liu, Y.; Zhang, M.; Liang, L.; Li, J.; Chen, Y.X. Over-expression of lncRNA DANCR is associated with advanced tumor progression and poor prognosis in patients with colorectal cancer. *Int. J. Clin. Exp. Pathol.* **2015**, *8*, 11480–11484.
307. Ren, Y.K.; Xiao, Y.; Wan, X.B.; Zhao, Y.Z.; Li, J.; Li, Y.; Han, G.S.; Chen, X.B.; Zou, Q.Y.; Wang, G.C.; et al. Association of long non-coding RNA HOTTIP with progression and prognosis in colorectal cancer. *Int. J. Clin. Exp. Pathol.* **2015**, *8*, 11458–11463.
308. Shen, X.; Bai, Y.; Luo, B.; Zhou, X. Upregulation of lncRNA BANCR associated with the lymph node metastasis and poor prognosis in colorectal cancer. *Biol. Res.* **2017**, *50*, 32. [CrossRef]
309. Tan, W.; Song, Z.Z.; Xu, Q.; Qu, X.; Li, Z.; Wang, Y.; Yu, Q.; Wang, S. Up-Regulated Expression of SPRY4-IT1 Predicts Poor Prognosis in Colorectal Cancer. *Med. Sci. Monit.* **2017**, *23*, 309–314. [CrossRef]
310. Ozawa, T.; Matsuyama, T.; Toiyama, Y.; Takahashi, N.; Ishikawa, T.; Uetake, H.; Yamada, Y.; Kusunoki, M.; Calin, G.; Goel, A. CCAT1 and CCAT2 long noncoding RNAs, located within the 8q.24.21 'gene desert', serve as important prognostic biomarkers in colorectal cancer. *Ann. Oncol.* **2017**, *28*, 1882–1888. [CrossRef]
311. Zhang, X.T.; Pan, S.X.; Wang, A.H.; Kong, Q.Y.; Jiang, K.T.; Yu, Z.B. Long Non-Coding RNA (lncRNA) X-Inactive Specific Transcript (XIST) Plays a Critical Role in Predicting Clinical Prognosis and Progression of Colorectal Cancer. *Med. Sci. Monit.* **2019**, *25*, 6429–6435. [CrossRef]
312. Liu, X.; Liu, X.; Qiao, T.; Chen, W. Prognostic and clinicopathological significance of long non-coding RNA UCA1 in colorectal cancer: Results from a meta-analysis. *Medicine* **2019**, *98*, e18031. [CrossRef] [PubMed]
313. Yao, X.; Lan, Z.; Lai, Q.; Li, A.; Liu, S.; Wang, X. LncRNA SNHG6 plays an oncogenic role in colorectal cancer and can be used as a prognostic biomarker for solid tumors. *J. Cell. Physiol.* **2020**, *235*, 7620–7634. [CrossRef] [PubMed]
314. Chen, W.; Li, Y.; Guo, L.; Zhang, C.; Tang, S. Long non-coding RNA FTX predicts a poor prognosis of human cancers: A meta-analysis. *Biosci. Rep.* **2021**, *41*, BSR20203995. [CrossRef] [PubMed]
315. Lin, Z.B.; Long, P.; Zhao, Z.; Zhang, Y.R.; Chu, X.D.; Zhao, X.X.; Ding, H.; Huan, S.W.; Pan, Y.L.; Pan, J.H. Long Noncoding RNA KCNQ1OT1 is a Prognostic Biomarker and mediates CD8$^+$ T cell exhaustion by regulating CD155 Expression in Colorectal Cancer. *Int. J. Biol. Sci.* **2021**, *17*, 1757–1768. [CrossRef] [PubMed]
316. Luo, P.; Du, J.; Li, Y.; Ma, J.; Shi, W. Association between small nucleolar RNA host gene expression and survival outcome of colorectal cancer patients: A meta-analysis based on PRISMA and bioinformatics analysis. *Front. Oncol.* **2023**, *13*, 1094131. [CrossRef]
317. Li, C.; Zhou, L.; He, J.; Fang, X.Q.; Zhu, S.W.; Xiong, M.M. Increased long noncoding RNA SNHG20 predicts poor prognosis in colorectal cancer. *BMC Cancer* **2016**, *16*, 655. [CrossRef]
318. Zhuang, C.; Zheng, L.; Wang, P. Prognostic role of long non-coding RNA HNF1A-AS1 in Chinese cancer patients: A meta-analysis. *Onco Targets Ther.* **2018**, *11*, 5325–5332. [CrossRef]
319. Xie, H.; Ma, B.; Gao, Q.; Zhan, H.; Liu, Y.; Chen, Z.; Ye, S.; Li, J.; Yao, L.; Huang, W. Long non-coding RNA CRNDE in cancer prognosis: Review and meta-analysis. *Clin. Chim. Acta* **2018**, *485*, 262–271. [CrossRef]
320. Li, X.; Liang, Q.X.; Lin, J.R.; Peng, J.; Yang, J.H.; Yi, C.; Yu, Y.; Zhang, Q.C.; Zhou, K.R. Epitranscriptomic technologies and analyses. *Sci. China Life Sci.* **2020**, *63*, 501–515. [CrossRef]
321. Fontanges, Q.; De Mendonca, R.; Salmon, I.; Le Mercier, M.; D'Haene, N. Clinical Application of Targeted Next Generation Sequencing for Colorectal Cancers. *Int. J. Mol. Sci.* **2016**, *17*, 2117. [CrossRef]
322. Lee, M.K.C.; Loree, J.M. Current and emerging biomarkers in metastatic colorectal cancer. *Curr. Oncol.* **2019**, *26* (Suppl. S1), S7–S15. [CrossRef] [PubMed]
323. Koulis, C.; Yap, R.; Engel, R.; Jardé, T.; Wilkins, S.; Solon, G.; Shapiro, J.D.; Abud, H.; McMurrick, P. Personalized Medicine-Current and Emerging Predictive and Prognostic Biomarkers in Colorectal Cancer. *Cancers* **2020**, *12*, 812. [CrossRef] [PubMed]
324. Luo, X.J.; Zhao, Q.; Liu, J.; Zheng, J.B.; Qiu, M.Z.; Ju, H.Q.; Xu, R.H. Novel Genetic and Epigenetic Biomarkers of Prognostic and Predictive Significance in Stage II/III Colorectal Cancer. *Mol. Ther.* **2021**, *29*, 587–596. [CrossRef] [PubMed]

325. Sorich, M.J.; Wiese, M.D.; Rowland, A.; Kichenadasse, G.; McKinnon, R.A.; Karapetis, C.S. Extended RAS mutations and anti-EGFR monoclonal antibody survival benefit in metastatic colorectal cancer: A meta-analysis of randomized, controlled trials. *Ann. Oncol.* **2015**, *26*, 13–21. [CrossRef]
326. Park, S.M.; Choi, S.B.; Lee, Y.S.; Lee, I.K. Predictive value of KRAS mutation and excision repair cross-complementing 1 (ERCC1) protein overexpression in patients with colorectal cancer administered FOLFOX regimen. *Asian J. Surg.* **2021**, *44*, 715–722. [CrossRef]
327. Popat, S.; Houlston, R.S. A systematic review and meta-analysis of the relationship between chromosome 18q genotype, DCC status and colorectal cancer prognosis. *Eur. J. Cancer* **2005**, *41*, 2060–2070. [CrossRef]
328. Whitfield, M.L.; George, L.K.; Grant, G.D.; Perou, C.M. Common markers of proliferation. *Nat. Rev. Cancer* **2006**, *6*, 99–106. [CrossRef]
329. Coppedè, F.; Lopomo, A.; Spisni, R.; Migliore, L. Genetic and epigenetic biomarkers for diagnosis, prognosis and treatment of colorectal cancer. *World J. Gastroenterol.* **2014**, *20*, 943–956. [CrossRef]
330. Zhang, H.; Dong, S.; Feng, J. Epigenetic profiling and mRNA expression reveal candidate genes as biomarkers for colorectal cancer. *J. Cell. Biochem.* **2019**, *120*, 10767–10776. [CrossRef]
331. Kong, C.; Fu, T. Value of methylation markers in colorectal cancer (Review). *Oncol. Rep.* **2021**, *46*, 177. [CrossRef]
332. Lee, S.; Cho, N.Y.; Choi, M.; Yoo, E.J.; Kim, J.H.; Kang, G.H. Clinicopathological features of CpG island methylator phenotype-positive colorectal cancer and its adverse prognosis in relation to KRAS/BRAF mutation. *Pathol. Int.* **2008**, *58*, 104–113. [CrossRef] [PubMed]
333. Boughanem, H.; Cabrera-Mulero, A.; Hernández-Alonso, P.; Clemente-Postigo, M.; Casanueva, F.F.; Tinahones, F.J.; Morcillo, S.; Crujeiras, A.B.; Macias-Gonzalez, M. Association between variation of circulating 25-OH vitamin D and methylation of secreted frizzled-related protein 2 in colorectal cancer. *Clin. Epigenet.* **2020**, *12*, 83. [CrossRef] [PubMed]
334. Barchitta, M.; Quattrocchi, A.; Maugeri, A.; Vinciguerra, M.; Agodi, A. LINE-1 hypomethylation in blood and tissue samples as an epigenetic marker for cancer risk: A systematic review and meta-analysis. *PLoS ONE* **2014**, *9*, e109478. [CrossRef] [PubMed]
335. Boughanem, H.; Martin-Nuñez, G.M.; Torres, E.; Arranz-Salas, I.; Alcaide, J.; Morcillo, S.; Tinahones, F.J.; Crujeiras, A.B.; Macias-Gonzalez, M. Impact of Tumor *LINE-1* Methylation Level and Neoadjuvant Treatment and Its Association with Colorectal Cancer Survival. *J. Pers. Med.* **2020**, *10*, 219. [CrossRef] [PubMed]
336. Ye, D.; Jiang, D.; Li, Y.; Jin, M.; Chen, K. The role of LINE-1 methylation in predicting survival among colorectal cancer patients: A meta-analysis. *Int. J. Clin. Oncol.* **2017**, *22*, 749–757. [CrossRef] [PubMed]
337. Javierre, B.M.; Rodriguez-Ubreva, J.; Al-Shahrour, F.; Corominas, M.; Graña, O.; Ciudad, L.; Agirre, X.; Pisano, D.G.; Valencia, A.; Roman-Gomez, J.; et al. Long-range epigenetic silencing associates with deregulation of Ikaros targets in colorectal cancer cells. *Mol. Cancer Res.* **2011**, *9*, 1139–1151. [CrossRef]
338. Winter, J.M.; Sheehan-Hennessy, L.; Yao, B.; Pedersen, S.K.; Wassie, M.M.; Eaton, M.; Chong, M.; Young, G.P.; Symonds, E.L. Detection of hypermethylated BCAT1 and IKZF1 DNA in blood and tissues of colorectal, breast and prostate cancer patients. *Cancer Biomark.* **2022**, *34*, 493–503. [CrossRef]
339. Moriichi, K.; Fujiya, M.; Kobayashi, Y.; Murakami, Y.; Iwama, T.; Kunogi, T.; Sasaki, T.; Ijiri, M.; Takahashi, K.; Tanaka, K.; et al. Autofluorescence Imaging Reflects the Nuclear Enlargement of Tumor Cells as well as the Cell Proliferation Ability and Aberrant Status of the *p53*, Ki-67, and *p16* Genes in Colon Neoplasms. *Molecules* **2019**, *24*, 1106. [CrossRef]
340. Zygulska, A.L.; Pierzchalski, P. Novel Diagnostic Biomarkers in Colorectal Cancer. *Int. J. Mol. Sci.* **2022**, *23*, 852. [CrossRef]
341. Cerrito, M.G.; Grassilli, E. Identifying Novel Actionable Targets in Colon Cancer. *Biomedicines* **2021**, *9*, 579. [CrossRef]
342. Abbes, S.; Baldi, S.; Sellami, H.; Amedei, A.; Keskes, L. Molecular methods for colorectal cancer screening: Progress with next-generation sequencing evolution. *World J. Gastrointest. Oncol.* **2023**, *15*, 425–442. [CrossRef] [PubMed]
343. Del Vecchio, F.; Mastroiaco, V.; Di Marco, A.; Compagnoni, C.; Capece, D.; Zazzeroni, F.; Capalbo, C.; Alesse, E.; Tessitore, A. Next-generation sequencing: Recent applications to the analysis of colorectal cancer. *J. Transl. Med.* **2017**, *15*, 246. [CrossRef]
344. Wang, Q.; Wang, Z.; Zhang, Z.; Zhang, W.; Zhang, M.; Shen, Z.; Ye, Y.; Jiang, K.; Wang, S. Landscape of cell heterogeneity and evolutionary trajectory in ulcerative colitis-associated colon cancer revealed by single-cell RNA sequencing. *Chin. J. Cancer Res.* **2021**, *33*, 271–288. [CrossRef]
345. Xu, S.; Li, Y.; Huang, H.; Miao, X.; Gu, Y. Identification of KIF21B as a Biomarker for Colorectal Cancer and Associated with Poor Prognosis. *J. Oncol.* **2022**, *2022*, 7905787. [CrossRef] [PubMed]
346. Liu, Y.; Liu, X.; Xu, Q.; Gao, X.; Linghu, E. A Prognostic Model of Colon Cancer Based on the Microenvironment Component Score via Single Cell Sequencing. *In Vivo* **2022**, *36*, 753–763. [CrossRef] [PubMed]
347. Normanno, N.; Cervantes, A.; Ciardiello, F.; De Luca, A.; Pinto, C. The liquid biopsy in the management of colorectal cancer patients: Current applications and future scenarios. *Cancer Treat. Rev.* **2018**, *70*, 1–8. [CrossRef] [PubMed]
348. Kastrisiou, M.; Zarkavelis, G.; Pentheroudakis, G.; Magklara, A. Clinical Application of Next-Generation Sequencing as A Liquid Biopsy Technique in Advanced Colorectal Cancer: A Trick or A Treat? *Cancers* **2019**, *11*, 1573. [CrossRef]
349. Basnet, S.; Zhang, Z.Y.; Liao, W.Q.; Li, S.H.; Li, P.S.; Ge, H.Y. The Prognostic Value of Circulating Cell-Free DNA in Colorectal Cancer: A Meta-Analysis. *J. Cancer* **2016**, *7*, 1105–1113. [CrossRef]
350. Rodríguez-Casanova, A.; Bao-Caamano, A.; Lago-Lestón, R.M.; Brozos-Vázquez, E.; Costa-Fraga, N.; Ferreirós-Vidal, I.; Abdulkader, I.; Vidal-Insua, Y.; Rivera, F.V.; Candamio Folgar, S.; et al. Evaluation of a Targeted Next-Generation Sequencing Panel for the Non-Invasive Detection of Variants in Circulating DNA of Colorectal Cancer. *J. Clin. Med.* **2021**, *10*, 4487. [CrossRef]

351. Lan, Y.T.; Chang, S.C.; Lin, P.C.; Lin, C.H.; Liang, W.Y.; Chen, W.S.; Jiang, J.K.; Yang, S.H.; Lin, J.K. High concordance of mutation patterns in 10 common mutated genes between tumor tissue and cell-free DNA in metastatic colorectal cancer. *Am. J. Cancer Res.* **2021**, *11*, 2228–2237.
352. Güttlein, L.; Luca, M.R.; Esteso, F.; Fresno, C.; Mariani, J.; Otero Pizarro, M.; Brest, E.; Starapoli, S.; Kreimberg, K.; Teves, P.; et al. Liquid biopsy for *KRAS*, *NRAS* and *BRAF* mutation testing in advanced colorectal cancer patients: The Argentinean experience. *Future Oncol.* **2022**, *18*, 3277–3287. [CrossRef] [PubMed]
353. Heuvelings, D.J.I.; Wintjens, A.G.W.E.; Luyten, J.; Wilmink, G.E.W.A.; Moonen, L.; Speel, E.M.; de Hingh, I.H.J.T.; Bouvy, N.D.; Peeters, A. DNA and RNA Alterations Associated with Colorectal Peritoneal Metastases: A Systematic Review. *Cancers* **2023**, *15*, 549. [CrossRef] [PubMed]
354. Koveitypour, Z.; Panahi, F.; Vakilian, M.; Peymani, M.; Seyed Forootan, F.; Nasr Esfahani, M.H.; Ghaedi, K. Signaling pathways involved in colorectal cancer progression. *Cell Biosci.* **2019**, *9*, 97. [CrossRef] [PubMed]
355. Ye, P.; Cai, P.; Xie, J.; Wei, Y. The diagnostic accuracy of digital PCR, ARMS and NGS for detecting KRAS mutation in cell-free DNA of patients with colorectal cancer: A protocol for systematic review and meta-analysis. *Medicine* **2020**, *99*, e20708. [CrossRef] [PubMed]
356. Jones, T.; Townsend, D. History and future technical innovation in positron emission tomography. *J. Med. Imaging* **2017**, *4*, 011013. [CrossRef]
357. Lunt, S.Y.; Vander Heiden, M.G. Aerobic glycolysis: Meeting the metabolic requirements of cell proliferation. *Annu. Rev. Cell Dev. Biol.* **2011**, *27*, 441–464. [CrossRef]
358. Pelosi, E.; Deandreis, D. The role of 18F-fluoro-deoxy-glucose positron emission tomography (FDG-PET) in the management of patients with colorectal cancer. *Eur. J. Surg. Oncol.* **2007**, *33*, 1–6. [CrossRef]
359. Flamen, P.; Stroobants, S.; Van Cutsem, E.; Dupont, P.; Bormans, G.; De Vadder, N.; Penninckx, F.; Van Hoe, L.; Mortelmans, L. Additional value of whole-body positron emission tomography with fluorine-18-2-fluoro-2-deoxy-D-glucose in recurrent colorectal cancer. *J. Clin. Oncol.* **1999**, *17*, 894–901. [CrossRef]
360. Yamamoto, Y.; Kameyama, R.; Izuishi, K.; Takebayashi, R.; Hagiike, M.; Asakura, M.; Haba, R.; Nishiyama, Y. Detection of colorectal cancer using ^{18}F-FLT PET: Comparison with ^{18}F-FDG PET. *Nucl. Med. Commun.* **2009**, *30*, 841–845. [CrossRef]
361. Deng, S.M.; Zhang, W.; Zhang, B.; Chen, Y.Y.; Li, J.H.; Wu, Y.W. Correlation between the Uptake of 18F-Fluorodeoxyglucose (18F-FDG) and the Expression of Proliferation-Associated Antigen Ki-67 in Cancer Patients: A Meta-Analysis. *PLoS ONE* **2015**, *10*, e0129028. [CrossRef]

Disclaimer/Publisher's Note: The statements, opinions and data contained in all publications are solely those of the individual author(s) and contributor(s) and not of MDPI and/or the editor(s). MDPI and/or the editor(s) disclaim responsibility for any injury to people or property resulting from any ideas, methods, instructions or products referred to in the content.

MDPI
St. Alban-Anlage 66
4052 Basel
Switzerland
www.mdpi.com

Cancers Editorial Office
E-mail: cancers@mdpi.com
www.mdpi.com/journal/cancers

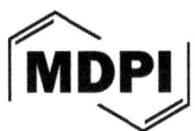

Disclaimer/Publisher's Note: The statements, opinions and data contained in all publications are solely those of the individual author(s) and contributor(s) and not of MDPI and/or the editor(s). MDPI and/or the editor(s) disclaim responsibility for any injury to people or property resulting from any ideas, methods, instructions or products referred to in the content.

www.ingramcontent.com/pod-product-compliance
Lightning Source LLC
LaVergne TN
LVHW070730100526
838202LV00013B/1203